Fatal Contact

Aboriginal and Torres Strait Islander people should be aware that this book contains the names of deceased persons.

Fatal Contact

How Epidemics Nearly Wiped Out Australia's First Peoples

Peter Dowling

MONASH
UNIVERSITY
PUBLISHING

Fatal Contact: How Epidemics Nearly Wiped Out Australia's First Peoples

Monash University Publishing
Matheson Library Annexe
40 Exhibition Walk
Monash University
Clayton, Victoria 3800, Australia
publishing.monash.edu/

Monash University Publishing brings to the world publications which advance the best traditions of humane and enlightened thought.

Monash University Publishing titles pass through a rigorous process of independent peer review.

ISBN: 9781922464460 (paperback)
ISBN: 9781922464477 (pdf)
ISBN: 9781922464484 (epub)

Edited by Kerry Davies AE
Internal design by Les Thomas
Cover design by Les Thomas
Typeset by Jo Mullins

A catalogue record for this book is available from the National Library of Australia.

CONTENTS

LIST OF TABLES

For those First Nation People who suffered from the epidemics.
Most of them nameless to history and in many cases unknown to history.
Left out and missing from the human story of Australia.

ACKNOWLEDGEMENTS

Putting this tome on the shelves of bookshops has been a long process lasting over two decades. I have not done this alone. During its course I have had the help, advice and comment of many people along the way and to them I owe a deep and lasting gratitude. It is with their unquestioned help, willingness and support that this book has been produced.

First and foremost is my wife, Dianne, who at all stages supported, carried and guided me through this whole process from beginning to end.

I am especially grateful to Dr Robert Attenborough, my primary PhD supervisor at the Australian National University, who, with a red pen in hand, reviewed each chapter of my thesis making it a much better document and which now has formed the basis of this book.

Professor Isabel McBryde, my second PhD supervisor, guided me to the historic collections in the state libraries and archives and showed me how to interpret them and then persuaded me to put everything together and publish as a book. It has taken some time but that is down to me.

Professor Judith Littleton was a fellow post-graduate student in biological anthropology at ANU, a supporter and constructive critic of my work, who has become a long-term friend.

The late Professor Colin Groves was my MA supervisor at ANU who was the first to comment and guide me in writing on this subject.

My former colleagues and friends from the ANU: Dr Goran Şevo, who has also graciously read sections of the draft manuscript for this book and commented where I strayed on medical interpretations; Dr Jan Klaver, Dr Kate Stockhausen, Dr Helen Cooke and Dr Keiko Tamura, who at various stages assisted me in field research and listened to me in the early days of my research into this project.

During my time at ANU I had the great honour and privilege to mentor and tutor students studying archaeology and biological anthropology through the Tjabal Indigenous Higher Education Centre. They came from different parts of Australia and their ages varied from the younger to the senior. But they were all eager to learn. While I may have influenced them in some way, I know that I learned a lot from the experience. I thank them for assisting and influencing me.

I also thank Dr Elizabeth Williams who thoughtfully discussed this project, providing help over coffees at the National Library of Australia, and Dr Fenja Theden-Ringl for kindly reading and commenting on the introduction.

A special thanks to Georgia Harrison-Dowling, my much-valued research assistant, particularly in the latter stages of this book, for giving her time during her third year at Monash University to help her grandfather continue research in the midst of a developing COVID-19 pandemic and subsequent lockdown.

My family in Melbourne, Michael, Deborah, Georgia, Charlie, Jamie, and Mia for showing interest, encouragement and support in this project and for giving me the opportunities to tune out a bit and get back to the realities of family life.

I also gratefully thank my extended family in South Australia, Tasmania, and the Australian Capital Territory for willingly helping me in field and archival research and for their unconditional support over the years I have been engaged in this project. Also David and Jessie in Dubai for their encouragement.

To Derrick (Noddy) and Leann Brassington for many years of friendship, dinners and coffee.

During the research and writing of this book the National Library of Australia gave me a quiet place in the Petherick Reading Room among the books and manuscripts, many of which have been used in this story. My appreciation goes to the staff for their endless, professional help. A special thanks must go to one, Sarah Schindeler at the NLA, who first encouraged and invited me to join the Petherick Readers group. And so, a grateful thanks must also go to my fellow Petherick readers for the coffee breaks and lively discussions we all enjoyed while plodding on with our various research topics.

The Canberra and District Historical Society and the National Trust ACT gave me access to their libraries and collections. I spent many quiet and industrious hours in their offices all the while trying not to get distracted by the wealth of historic material they held.

I am especially indebted to the team and reviewers at Monash University Publishing who received a very scratchy draft manuscript from me but saw in it something of Australia's history that needed to be told and agreed to publish. I hope I have done them some justice in their decision. Thank you to Les Thomas for his evocative cover, and to Madeleine Davis for her thorough index. Finally, I am particularly grateful to a very formidable and professional editing duo, Kerry Davies AE who polished the prose, and Joanne Mullins who put it all together. I was writing in Canberra, and they were in Brisbane and Melbourne respectively, but we got the job done; and it was done during the strange and worrying time of an unpredictable pandemic.

Thank you all.

Peter Dowling
Canberra 2021

FOREWORD

We write in the midst of a shocking pandemic – one of us from New Zealand, a nation coping rather well at present, and the other from the UK, a nation clearly not coping – to commend Peter Dowling's book on a world of infectious disease that must have been far more terrifying to experience: that of Indigenous Australians in the long aftermath of British invasion.

Despite the contrasts between current global circumstances and those that this book will draw to your attention, it is a good time to reflect on infection. All the more so if we ever thought infectious disease was a problem conquered, at least in the developed world. Now, more than at any time in living memory, we have been sensitised to the impact of infectious disease on everyday lives, national economies and global politics. Interestingly, as the current pandemic progresses, attention has drifted from the world's broader causes (environmental change, human treatment of animals, social and economic inequality, global networks of trade and information) to focus on a single virus – as if the virus itself were the enemy. This is also how the collapse of indigenous populations was viewed: as if it were the 'germs, not these imperialists themselves, for all their brutality and callousness, that were chiefly responsible for sweeping aside the indigenes'.[1]

In 1983, Noel Butlin's very influential book, *Our Original Aggression*, made a (then controversial) case that early colonial impacts in south-eastern Australia had led to massive depopulation.[2] This stimulated debate around the introduction of smallpox (who, when, where and how), focused on that single causative agent and time. Butlin and subsequent writers argued that specific diseases like smallpox had devastating impacts on Aboriginal populations – in some parts of Australia, even before the physical arrival of European colonialists.

Four years later, in 1987, Peter Dowling began researching the contentious area of Aboriginal infectious disease and population decline. This new book is the fruit of his devoted and tenacious researches ever since, which both of us have followed with great interest from their very beginnings. Peter has trawled through historical records – official correspondence, parliamentary inquiries, newspapers, journals and diaries – through which he demonstrates the slow grind of disease, and how even minor conditions could become fatal in the context of massive disruption. Since his PhD thesis on this topic in 1997, Peter has expanded his geographic scope, and he has further deepened his involvement in both archaeological and historical perspectives on his topic.

He has also extended his chronological scope, with a public involvement, to more recent history, particularly around World War One. As a result, while there is a solid perspective from biological anthropology at the heart of the book, ensuring that the nature of disease is read in a comparative and analytical context, it has also developed in historical richness.

Peter shows that it was the cumulative impact of infectious diseases in concert with economic, environmental and social devastation that ravaged communities. In many places people were driven from their traditional lands and cooped up alongside others who had not been close neighbours. Nor – and this point is crucial – was this a moment of collapse, but rather a long drawn-out cascade. Population numbers – crude measure of wellbeing as they are – continued to decline, reaching a nadir probably only in the 1930s. Nonetheless, Aboriginal culture and people persisted, demonstrating resilience despite great social suffering. This is achingly spelled out in Peter's account of Truganini's life and death, where the detail behind the numbers is made horrifyingly vivid.

The disruption that followed European contact is unimaginable. But to emphasise a single aspect of depopulation, whether disease or violence, in the years immediately following 1788 is to oversimplify the complexity and duration of the social and epidemiological processes, and to render the agency and resilience of Aboriginal people and culture invisible. In this book, social suffering is writ through both the numbers and the details. In an era when we often tally the latest infection country by country, that more local and more human perspective is an important one to remember.

Judith Littleton
Department of Anthropology
University of Auckland

Robert Attenborough
Department of Archaeology
University of Cambridge
&
School of Archaeology & Anthropology
Australian National University

INTRODUCTION

A Brief Flight over History

A few years ago, I was on a flight from Sydney to Singapore, crossing the centre of the Australian continent. I was lucky enough to have a window seat and even luckier to be flying on a clear, sunny and cloudless day. At ten kilometres above the ground, the view of the landscape was fascinating. First into view was the Murray–Darling Basin region, with its scattering of settlements slowly giving way to the arid Strzelecki Desert, where the state borders of South Australia, New South Wales and Queensland meet. As we travelled on a north-westerly course, we passed over the long parallel systems of windblown sand dunes snaking across the lands of the Lake Eyre and Simpson Basins. The massive Uluru (Ayres Rock) and Kata Tjuta (Mount Olga) features came into view and, when the captain announced that we would fly over them, there was a scramble for the few vacant window seats. With Uluru and Kata Tjuta behind us, most went back to their seats.

But what fascinated me for the next few hours as we travelled towards the northern coastline were the clear outlines of the ancient lake, river and creek systems that flowed many hundreds of kilometres across the basins from the higher ranges to the east and west. Intermittent Pleistocene lake beds could be seen juxtaposed between the more recent long backbones of sandy dunes. Between the ancient lakes were the connecting creeks and riverbeds. Some wide, others long and narrow. The most impressive I could see was the Lake Amadeus system, but I had to quickly cross the aisle and grab another spare window seat to glimpse it in the far distance. Most of the lakes and river systems I knew held little water, or were near to dry, at the time because the country was in a period of drought. The annual monsoons had moved north of the equator and were no longer supplying the rainwater that would once again flow through the system next season. It was a compelling sight to see an ancient landscape unrolling through the small window, while other passengers were glued to their video screens watching the latest in-flight movies. Apart from a quick viewing of Uluru, they were missing the natural geomorphological history of this vast part of Australia.

Looking over this landscape from far above I could not help but wonder about the people who had walked the surface of the ancient land, about how they lived, managed and interacted with the land and the plants and animals, and how they related to their fellow humans across the vastness of the continent. As a biological anthropologist and an archaeologist, I had a fair idea but was nevertheless left in awe with my nose pressed up against the small window of the giant jet. Then into view came the enigmatic Gibson Desert and last of all the Great Sandy Desert and the tropic zones. We crossed the northern coastline of Australia and the view was taken up by a seemingly grey, velvety sea.

My thoughts returned to thinking about the fate of these people of the inland, and of the whole of the continent, when far-off Europe (my ultimate destination on that trip) reached out, crossed the enormous expanse of sea and clashed so profoundly with these people almost 250 years ago. What follows is part of that story, the biological consequences of contact between two vastly different cultures. In particular, I focus on the major epidemics of introduced infectious diseases that the Europeans brought with them.

* * *

The first humans to set foot on Australian soil happened at least 65,000 years ago, as far as our current archaeological and genetic knowledge tells us.[1] They came from, or via, the Asian continent, as it was in the deep past, and entered what was then the northern coastline of Australia. Even though the Australian continent (Sahul) included what is now New Guinea, at least the final part of the journey from Asia was by island hopping to the mainland in watercraft. Over the following centuries these adventurous people spread around the coastline and into to the inland areas, north to south and east to west, finally occupying the entire continent.

At first they would have relied on the natural resources available in this new untrodden land, but soon their ingenuity and management of the plants and animals transformed the ecosystems. They used fire to create new open spaces in the forested areas, creating more favourable habitats suited to them and their food sources. They soon learned how to propagate the natural grasses, cultivating, managing and harvesting them when the heads were ripe with seed, then grinding the seeds to make a flour and storing the rest for leaner times. They controlled water resources by diverting streams and built stone dams and structures along shorelines and riverine systems to control the movement of fish, crustaceans, shellfish and eels. Across the landscapes they created a mosaic of open grasslands and bordering woodlands. They quickly learned how to occupy and flourish in the arid interior deserts, the tropical regions of the north and colder climates of the far south, even living above the glacier valleys of Tasmania. Some built solid stone and timber structures, creating village settlements capable of housing hundreds in times of plenty. Others chose to move regularly across their country. Wherever they went they carved or painted their history and lore onto the rock surfaces or the trunks of trees for future generations to understand and learn.

They came to manage and appreciate the country they occupied, incorporating the landscape features into their cultures and languages by creating songs and stories that were regularly reinforced by ritual celebrations handed down from generation to generation. They recognised the climate variations of the land and knew how to endure the periods of drought when the land cried out for rain and the resources were few. In the arid desert regions they dug wells to capture and store the artesian streams that lay deep below the surface. They saw the sea levels rise and create new shorelines, bays and islands. They saw old habitats disappear under water and new ones created by the encroaching seas. In the inland areas they saw rivers diverted by the tectonic shaping of the land and lake systems that once enabled large populations to live and thrive dry up completely. They saw the large megafauna species that once dominated the land slowly die out, never to return. They experienced the fire, smoke and violence of volcanos. They witnessed the planet's climate change from the coldness of the Pleistocene to the warmer times of the Holocene. They stared up into the night skies and created a cosmology of their own that explained the creation of their being and the land in which they lived.

Throughout the vast expanse of Australia the people did not live in isolation from each other. They developed trading and cultural-exchange ties and routes that criss-crossed the continent and many languages along the way. Pathways through the lands provided the physical access to neighbouring groups and 'songlines' – stories telling of the origin of landforms and the routes to travel – provided mental maps to find their way over long distances. Their meetings with other groups were elegantly planned affairs, often with hundreds congregating to exchange their experiences, share in seasonally abundant food resources, exchange trading goods, reinforce cultural and social ties (networking as it is referred to today) and to acquire wives and husbands (a vital practice to enable a steady gene flow across the land). And they incorporated all in their story of what is today known as the Dreaming.

But in one respect they were isolated, with little connection to the outer world. There was some contact with New Guinea via the islands off the north coast and with fishing fleets that came mainly from Macassar (Ujung Pandang) visiting much of Australia's north coast for perhaps a thousand years until

1906, when the newly formed Australian Government banned them. As the populations of Europe, Asia and Africa developed and fluctuated, experiencing periods of peace, war, famine and disease over thousands of years, the people of Australia were on their own, so to speak, particularly in the last 10,000 years when sea levels cut into the Sahul continent, creating the islands of New Guinea and extending the sea distances to Asia. While this isolation created a human culture unique to Australia, it also facilitated a biological time bomb that was to explode across the continent, bringing untold suffering, death by the thousands and cultural collapse. It began in January 1788, when Europeans from the other side of the world came to stay.

That time bomb was a part of their own biology and part that of the Old World. Because of their isolation from the world populations, Australia's Indigenous peoples (like those of the Americas and the islands of Oceania) had developed an immune system that adequately protected them from the range of naturally occurring pathogens they encountered in their daily lives. Their immune systems were attuned to the habitats they occupied and were able to produce the right proteins (antibodies) to attack the invading pathogens, whether a virus or bacterium, and in most cases counter their effect.

The human immune system is a wonderous thing, able to deal with thousands of potentially dangerous invaders that a person encounters day by day and still maintain a healthy body. But, to enable it to recognise what is dangerous to the health of the individual (and conversely what is beneficial or harmless), a part of the immune system must first 'learn', then 'remember', the nature of the invader before it can produce the right antibodies to nullify the effect of a pathogen. In most cases this is achieved only by first encountering the invader, successfully defending against it and then retaining the ability to fight the invader when encountered again. This ability of the immune system is why we in the modern world receive vaccinations against a range of diseases that work by preparing our immune systems to protect us into the future. The active ingredient of vaccinations can be variously a live but weakened (attenuated) pathogen, one that is killed and inactive, a biosynthetic version of the pathogen itself or a toxin or chemical that is made by a virus or bacterium when it invades the human body. The immune systems of Australia's Aboriginal people, while working well for thousands of years, had never experienced the pathogens that were brought from Europe or the diseases they caused. As a result, they were often slow in recognising an unknown invader and unable to mount a speedy defence before the invading pathogens were able to replicate in amounts that caused serious illness and death. They were a virgin-soil population. The immune systems of the human invaders from the Old World were well experienced with the local and endemic pathogens they carried, causing in most cases mild illness but at the same time transferring the pathogens to the non-immune Aboriginal people they encountered. It was in most respects a one-way exchange, and a deadly exchange at that.

Infectious diseases, alien to the many thousands of years of human history in Australia, were introduced following the 1788 British colonisation of the continent. The diseases were introduced in different places across the continent and at different times. Some, like smallpox, measles and influenza, spread like destructive wildfires at great speed through the populations, causing a great deal of sickness and mortality. Others, like syphilis and tuberculosis, were more insidious, creeping slowly, surely but constantly, often causing long and chronic illnesses and eventual death. Whichever way these diseases infiltrated the Aboriginal populations, they caused the destruction of long-standing cultural and social structures, which in many cases have never recovered. Languages, cultural ceremonies, social interactions, trade and reciprocity obligations, marriage customs and intergroup contacts were either destroyed or forever changed, along with the massive death toll of individuals and clans. If these separate diseases, their courses and destruction are viewed as components of a larger single epidemic or pandemic lasting for over 150 years of continual destruction, then perhaps a picture of the magnitude of the event can begin to emerge. Perhaps.

When the European colonists arrived on the shores of Botany Bay and Sydney Harbour in 1788, they brought with them a whole host of viruses and bacteria, many of which were pathogens and many foreign to Australian biota. With subsequent continual arrivals from Europe over the ensuing decades, more were brought into the country as the colonial borders spread out along the coastline and into the inland. It was inevitable that, with the European population increasing and the colonial boundaries expanding, more and more Europeans came into close contact with Aboriginal people. Along with this close contact came the diseases, in many cases spreading not only with the colonists but far ahead of the colonial boundaries. Sickness and death came from a long distance for many Aboriginal people. While many foreign pathogens were introduced into Australia during the colonial period (as there are even today) several stand out in terms of the destruction they caused. It is these diseases – smallpox, measles, the sexually transmitted diseases of syphilis and gonorrhoea, tuberculosis, influenza and other respiratory diseases – that are of concern here.

When these diseases are considered today, they are often thought of as either sweeping through large population centres such as cities, towns and even rural villages, where people live closely together, or as diseases that are always present (endemic) in large populations, flaring up every now and then to cause more sickness and death than usual. Medical science has a term for such diseases – 'crowd diseases'. It is a generic term applied to any disease-causing pathogen that requires large immune-susceptible host populations to infect, where they then reproduce, infect more susceptible hosts and spread. If a pathogen, such as the smallpox virus, has only one host it can infect, it requires a constantly large population of that host in which to continue reproducing. Without that large population the disease will ultimately burn out and the pathogens will have to find more susceptibles. Other human diseases have alternative hosts they can invade if the human population has become too low or has reached a degree of immunity to the invading pathogen.

The influenza virus has the great advantage of being able to reside in wild waterfowl, domestic ducks and pigs, to reproduce (and in some cases genetically change) before attacking the human populations again. Large populations of immunologically susceptible human hosts or alternative animal hosts are what keeps these pathogens, and in consequence the diseases they cause, alive and biologically sustainable. A question now arises: were there such population centres in Aboriginal Australia large enough to suffer severely from a crowd disease? The short answer to that is yes. There were large population centres in Australia prior to European arrival and, what is more, they were often sedentary and always interconnected and susceptible. Just the right environment for a 'new' pathogen to enter and cause destruction.

So how did these Aboriginal people exist in such numbers in what even many of today's Australians would consider as groups of hunters and gatherers moving constantly around the landscapes in small numbers, chasing food resources, eking out a precarious existence? This is a concept that I have heard many times. Common enough, but misguided. Paul Memmott, who studied Aboriginal structures and architectural styles in his book *Gunyah Goondie + Wurley*, and Bruce Pascoe, author of a small but influential book, *Dark Emu, Black Seeds*,[2] claim that this is entirely the wrong concept modern Australia has of Aboriginal people. Both have reviewed many of the journals and diaries made by the early explorers, along with later ethnographic research, and found that they contain numerous firsthand accounts of large population groups, up to a thousand in some places, living in villages with substantial numbers of organised constructions. Along the Darling River, for example, one of Australia's best known explorers, Charles Sturt, encountered a village (or perhaps a township) of 70 domed constructions capable of holding up to 15 people. He described them being

> … made of strong boughs, fitted in a circle in the ground, so as to meet in a common centre; on these there was … a thick seam of grass and leaves and over this a compact coating of clay. They were from eight to ten feet in diameter, and about four and a half feet high, the opening into them not being larger than to allow a man to creep in. These huts also faced north-west, and each one had a smaller one attached.[3]

Aboriginal people hunted and collected their food sources but also utilised native grasses. Clearing away trees and bushes, they created large areas of land to become grasslands that, when in season, were able to be harvested and the grain stored for later times. In many other areas in the temperate, tropical and arid regions, they tilled the surface of the land and propagated large areas of natural root crops that were dug up when ripe, and eaten or stored. The explorer George Grey saw such crops firsthand while exploring the area between Gantheaume Bay and the Hutt River estuary in Western Australia. Following well-used Aboriginal pathways in the late 1830s, he recorded in his diary:

> And as we wound along the native path my wonder augment; the path increased in breadth and in its beaten appearance, whilst along the side of it we found frequent wells, some of which were ten and twelve feet deep; and were altogether executed in a superior manner. We now crossed the dry bed of a stream, and from that emerged upon a tract of light fertile soil quite overrun with warran plants [*Dioscorea hastifolia* or native yam], the root of which is a favourite article of food with the natives. This was the first time we had yet seen this plant on our journey, and now for three and a half consecutive miles we traversed a fertile piece of land, literally perforated with the holes the natives had made to dig this root; indeed, we could with difficulty walk it on that account, whilst this tract extended east and west as far as we could see.
>
> It was now evident that we had entered the most thickly-populated district of Australia that I had yet observed, and moreover one which must have been inhabited for a long series of years, for more had been done to secure a provision from the ground by hard manual labour than I could have believed it in the power of uncivilised man to accomplish. After crossing a low limestone range, we came down upon another equally fertile warran ground, bounded eastward by a high range of rocky limestone hills, luxuriantly grassed and westward by a low range of similar formation. The native path, about two miles further on,

> crossed this latter range, and we found ourselves in a grassy valley, about four miles wide, bounded seawards by sandy downs. Along its centre lay a chain of reedy freshwater swamps, and native paths ran in from all quarters, to one main line of communication leading southward.[4]

Grey was to find more evidence of large Aboriginal villages, yam fields, grass fields and well-trodden pathways as he made his way south to the Perth settlement.

Pascoe claims that Aboriginal people throughout most of the country practised agriculture, as well as hunting and gathering, and lived permanently or semi-permanently in village-like lifestyles. He is most likely close to the point when he claims they were perhaps the earliest agriculturalists in the world. But that is another story. The focus here is that large population centres existed in pre-European Australia, along with regular movements and associations with large population numbers. It was a social and physical scenario readily suited to the transfer of infectious pathogens and the spread of introduced diseases originating from the other side of the world.

* * *

I began being involved in this subject of introduced infectious diseases among Aboriginal populations in the 1980s. During my undergraduate years studying biological anthropology at the Australian National University, Canberra, I began reading as many books and papers on the Aboriginal history of this country I could get my hands on. I soon found that many historians writing on the subject would tend to acknowledge that 'introduced diseases' caused much sickness and mortality and were part of the huge population decline following colonisation, but did not elaborate much further. Some would give a paragraph or two, sometimes even a page or two, often mentioning the 1789 smallpox epidemic at Sydney and then leave it at that. There was a whole lot missing in our knowledge of the biological consequences surrounding the meeting of these two cultures. I then became intrigued. Which diseases were responsible for the population decline, when and where did they occur, how severe where they, how long did they last and which diseases were more devastating? What were the diseases that inflicted Aboriginal populations before the arrival of Europeans?

I began with an MA thesis investigating the biological consequences of European and Aboriginal contact along the Murray River in South Australia.

My interest then developed into a PhD project covering south-eastern Australia from 1788 to 1901. Finishing the thesis, I then put it all aside in my professional life but never forgot what I had uncovered and how much was yet to be dealt with. Now I have come to grapple with it all again, covering most of the continent and extending into the 20th century, and even some reflection on the 21st. In doing so I have come to the realisation that Australians (including me) have not yet reached a full understanding of the magnitude of despair and destruction the diseases have caused the Aboriginal people of Australia. Perhaps we never will, but I can at least hope that by writing about the events I can bring some degree of understanding to Australians, and the rest of the world, today. But I tend to think that the real understanding and depth of cultural feeling will always lie with the Aboriginal people themselves.

The following chapters examine each of what I consider the main epidemics causing excessive morbidity and mortality, and their pathways through Aboriginal populations. The focus of each chapter is the disease, its path and its effects on the Aboriginal people. But to focus on the close and personal detail I at first wished is not possible in this book as the events and mortality the diseases caused are just too immense. I have therefore limited the discussions to particular places, times and events, while considering that together these will develop into an image of what happened in Australia after 1788. And what happened is the greatest human tragedy that Australia has ever experienced. I hope it will never happen again.

* * *

Several factors influence the quality and reliability of historic health data concerning Aboriginal people in Australia's colonial period. Here I have focused on sources written by trained medical personnel. Their observations on symptoms and the course of the epidemics overall may be considered more reliable than descriptions from witnesses without medical backgrounds. Nevertheless, when the latter sources are compliant with those of trained medical observations, they can be considered reliable, but should be used with caution. However, observations by trained medical practitioners must also be used with a degree of caution as their medical observations were limited, being based on patient symptoms without necropsy or laboratory confirmation. An exception in this case is the series of post-mortem reports done by medical practitioners on Aboriginal inmates at Flinders Island (considered in later chapters). Euro-Australian medical beliefs and training in the 19th century, together with personal ethnocentric biases, can also colour and misinterpret an epidemic situation.

As most of the medical practitioners who observed Aboriginal people during epidemics were concerned with the provision of medical aid, particularly during acute phases of the epidemics, systematic enumeration of morbidity and mortality cases were rarely taken. Most of the reports consist of subjective assessment of the major visible aspects of the epidemic, sometimes supplemented with cursory statistics concerning mortality. Statements such as 'a great deal of sickness', 'hundreds died' or 'over half the population has been lost' are often all we have in terms of enumeration. It was not until the mid–late 19th century, when institutionalisation became the main colonial government policy and records of births, deaths and marriages were kept on the Aboriginal stations and missionary settlements, that enumerated cases and causes of death can begin to be seen.

Despite these limitations, the collective subjective impressions of medical observers do show substantial agreement on the causative disease and the severity, timing and geographical locations of the major epidemics. Taken together, and used with awareness and caution by the historian, the existing sources can be used with a sense of reliability to gather an insight into the epidemiological, environmental and socio-cultural aspects of the epidemics. But there is always the overriding fact that these accounts are the very nature of the historical sources available and to dismiss them out of hand for being sources from a former medical philosophy and understanding would be to lose a valuable window into the past and its influence on present times.

A Note on Traditional Cultures

This discussion ranges in time and space across the continent of Australia. In pre-colonial times this vast area was occupied by more the 250 different socio-linguistic groups that had developed cultural differences jointly and independently over a period of more than 65,000 years. When names of groups (or 'tribes') were recorded by Europeans they were often inaccurate, through a misunderstanding of the traditional relationships to land and a lack of knowledge of the traditional social structures and language differences.

In 1996 the Australian Institute of Aboriginal and Torres Strait Islander Studies (AIATSIS) produced a map of the linguistic groups and their areas throughout the continent, with the warning that the boundaries of the groups were not definitive and may not be agreed to by some traditional custodians, and the map was not claimed to be exact. But, with these restraints in mind, the map does offer valuable guidance to the historian who is concerned with the continental view as a whole.

Following the arrival of Europeans, many of the linguistic groups suffered severe population decline through the exotic disease epidemics and displacement from traditional lands, with people forced to abandon their country. The traditional (pre-1788) boundaries dissipated. Bearing this in mind, throughout this book I have referred to the traditional occupants either with such general terminology as 'First Nations peoples', 'Indigenous people/s', 'Aboriginal people/s', 'Aboriginal groups' and 'Torres Strait Islanders'. However, in cases where there can be some certainty of traditional linguistic boundaries and culture intact, I use the traditional names recognised by the AIATSIS map, with some minor variations in spelling.

It is also important to note that traditional beliefs are still held by many Aboriginal people today, particularly in remote communities, but also in more urban settings. Where this book refers to past beliefs and practices, I acknowledge that these may still be held and performed in communities today. Use of the past tense is not meant to imply that the belief or practice is not also current for some.

Protection of Aboriginal People?

When the British landed on the east coast of Australia in 1788, the Indigenous people were considered to be subjects of the Crown and therefore under the protection of British law. Such a decision was made without any consultation with Indigenous people, who had no concept of British law, and consequently the British lawmakers had little or no concept of Indigenous culture, society and land custodianship. Nevertheless, the legal processes of a faraway land were brought to bear on people who had lived in this land for many millennia.

Aboriginal protection laws were established by the colonial governments ostensibly to shield Aboriginal people from the negative influences of Europeans. But they were more of a legal mechanism to control their lives and deny the groups the very civil rights afforded to the non-Indigenous population. Although the content of the laws differed from colony to colony, and from time to time, the essence of the acts allowed the governments to restrict and control freedom of movement of Aboriginal people across country they had held for thousands of years, controlling their associations within their family and extended social networks. The acts extended further into control of property ownership, marriage, wages and earnings, and prohibited Aboriginal people from drinking or carrying guns.[5]

Although each colony differed to some extent in their administrations of the acts, each formed management boards that acted independently of each other. The boards in turn appointed official positions of Aboriginal protectors (as well as sub-protectors and assistant protectors) who were responsible, through a chief protector, to the boards for the on-ground operations and application of the acts. The protectors were to live with the Aboriginal people on established reserves, organise their daily routines, learn their languages, promote Christianity and assimilate them into a 'civilised' British culture. Extra staff were employed to assist the protectors in their duties and a medical practitioner was appointed to oversee their health and physical wellbeing.

While there were specific objectives in the acts to regulate the Aboriginal communities, there was never total control over their application. Unless Aboriginal people had specific exemption, they were not to leave the reserves. However, the Aboriginal inmates frequently found ways of alluding the management. The historian Richard Broome writes that 'they secretly moved on and off reserves, maintained traditional values by hiding unauthorised kin in their houses, drank alcohol, gambled, refused to work for rations only, and refused at times to pay the rent'.[6] In almost all cases, the Aboriginal people on the reserves were subjected to the loss of their culture, which in turn led to the deterioration of psychological and physical health.

From their inception at various times in each colony, the protection acts were modified to meet the evolving perceptions of the day and the ideology of the governing bodies. Ultimately the acts produced a nationwide process of guardianship that resulted in the Aboriginal people becoming government wards. One of the worst results of these acts was the legal ability of the protectorates to remove young children from their families and culture.[7]

Management of Aboriginal people has existed in one form or another into the 21st century. A recent case in point occurred in 2007, when the then prime minister of Australia, John Howard, and the Indigenous affairs minister launched what was termed the Northern Territory Emergency Response (commonly termed the 'intervention') to curb a perceived rise in violence and family disruption in Aboriginal communities in the Northern Territory.[8] The response was instituted quickly, with little or no consultation, by deploying uniformed members of the Australian Defence Force into over 70 reserves and townships. The response included restrictions on alcohol, changes to welfare payments, acquisition of parcels of land, education, employment and health initiatives.[9] Once again, the lives of Aboriginal people were controlled by a government Act of Parliament. The intervention was modified in 2014, when a new federal government replaced the act with yet another, which is not due to expire until 2022.

The impacts of these acts in their various forms are still being felt today by many Indigenous families throughout Australia.

Deaths by Violence

This book is primarily concerned with the effect of introduced exotic diseases on the Aboriginal population of Australia and the resultant morbidity and mortality they incurred across the country. While the suffering and the deaths from these diseases were severe, they were not the only causes of the extensive population decline the Indigenous people suffered because of colonisation. Violence, between Aboriginal people and colonists, particularly on the colonial and pastoral frontiers,[10] accounted for thousands of deaths and untold suffering. This is the subject of ongoing studies into the colonial past of Australia and is not covered in this book. But, nevertheless, it should not go unrecognised as, together with the introduced diseases, violent deaths were a factor that radically altered forever the population and ancient cultures of this country.

Professor Lyndall Ryan, a historian who has devoted much of her academic career to frontier violence, has begun a rigorous analysis of historical documentation, revealing episodes and estimations of Aboriginal people killed on the colonial frontiers. She and her team have found evidence of over 12,000 Aboriginal people – male, female, young and old – who met their deaths by violence on the frontiers in central and eastern Australia alone. Most of the conflicts so far analysed took place along river systems and on land offering good pastoral prospects for the colonists. Bearing in mind that many of these deaths were carried out in secret, often under a code of silence to preserve the anonymity of the perpetrators, and that 'official figures' resulting from military actions were often understated, these 12,000 deaths should be considered as a minimal number.[11] There were many more deaths from violent action that were never recorded or the evidence for them has been lost or destroyed. The study by Ryan and her partners is an objective approach, bringing to light the violence inflicted on Aboriginal people during the colonial period of Australia's history. It is another part of our history that must be told.

The Diseases: History and Nature

It is now time to turn to the main concern of this book – the diseases that were introduced by the arrival of Europeans and that caused so much destruction to the Indigenous people of Australia. The primary focus is on the major infectious diseases – smallpox, measles, sexually transmitted diseases such as syphilis and gonorrhoea, and respiratory diseases such as epidemic influenza and tuberculosis. This small grouping of diseases was common in the populations of Europe at the time of Australian colonisation and was a major cause of morbidity and mortality.

In Europe and Asia these diseases were largely the result of the development of agriculture following the amelioration of the Ice Age (Pleistocene) to the warmer and wetter climatic conditions experienced today. This change, occurring slowly and in different areas over the last five to ten thousand years, led to a transformation for human populations from mobile hunter-gatherer economies to a more sedentary style of living in an agrarian economy. The result was that humans began to live in villages and, later, towns and cities with ever-increasing populations and a reliance on the domestication of plants and animals for their food sources. Domestication of animals such as pigs, sheep, horses and ungulates led to closer associations with these formally wild species and close association led to the transfer of pathogens from domesticate to humans. The end result was the emergence of new human pathogens (zoonoses) developing through genetic changes in animal hosts to invade human tissue and cause pathological responses.

In discussing the new diseases arising through domestication, Alfred W. Crosby wrote, 'When humans domesticated animals and gathered them to the human bosom – sometimes literally, as human mothers wet-nursed motherless animals – they created maladies their hunter and gatherer ancestors had rarely or never known.'[12] The virus causing influenza had its origins in horses, pigs and wild birds; the human tuberculosis bacteria came from cattle and pigs; smallpox had its origins in close association with cattle; the common cold was conveyed by horses; syphilis may have originated from monkeys; and the human measles virus is genetically associated with the domesticated bovine disease rinderpest. These diseases became well established in human populations and often flared up in epidemic forms inflicting high morbidity and mortality. Domestication of animals certainly had its advantages to more sedentary populations. They were reliable sources of food and held economic value for trading and clothing, but they had a severe downside that would permanently add to the human disease load.

Their pathogens, whether viral or bacterial, were very accomplished travellers, like their human hosts, and once entering Australia found a widespread Indigenous human population to infect and spread. They were the killer diseases. Their strategies (and yes, we can conceive of a bacterium or a virus having a survival strategy) were different. Some, like smallpox and measles, raged through the Indigenous populations causing an enormous number of deaths and debilitating sickness and then passed on, only to come back again to infect another generation. Others, like tuberculosis and syphilis, became established in the population, slowly but effectively and terribly killing their human hosts.

Before considering these epidemics, however, it must be noted that they were not the only foreign diseases that came into Australia on the ships from Europe. Others, such as poliomyelitis, typhoid, diphtheria, scarlet fever, mumps, cholera and viral hepatitis, to name just a few, entered and invaded Indigenous populations. But these diseases, while causing significant morbidity and mortality, were not on the same scale as the epidemics experienced in Europe. In many cases their presence among Indigenous people went unnoticed and unrecorded by European physicians and their impact may never be known with any certainty. Malaria, for one, was probably introduced multiple times into the northern tropical regions of Australia by seasonal fishermen coming from Malaya, where it was endemic. The disease is spread by the protozoan *Plasmodium* species carried by mosquitoes of the *Anopheles* genus, which inject the pathogen into the blood when biting a human. Australia has a species of *Anopheles* mosquito that may have in the past carried the disease locally among Aboriginal and Torres Strait Islander people. The disease was declared eradicated in its endemic form in 1981 but up to 600 cases on average are notified each year from travellers coming from tropical regions outside Australia.[13]

On the other hand, or the other side of the world from Europe, the Indigenous populations of Australia, who did not have a reliance on domesticated animals and, for the most part, did not live in crowded towns and cities, were not free from infectious diseases. They had their own suite of diseases, such as Murray River encephalitis, Barmah Forest infection, Ross River virus, Q fever, endemic typhus and a host of streptococcus and staphylococcus bacterial illnesses that caused sickness and could lead to death. These diseases were autochthonous (endemic) in Australia and may have been for centuries. There is also the distinct possibility that other diseases were active but have now disappeared – viruses and bacteria that formally caused a disease state but over time have either become extinct or have mutated to a form that no longer threatens the lives of their human hosts. The degree of morbidity and mortality these diseases might have had on Indigenous populations is unknown even today. But, in general, the diseases had achieved a form of biological balance with their human hosts and would rarely develop into epidemic killing diseases.[14]

Part 1

The Major Epidemic Diseases

Chapter 1

CONCEPTS AND CONSEQUENCES OF DISEASE

When Europeans began the colonisation of Australia in 1788 both they and the Indigenous people had well-established sets of beliefs regarding sickness and curing. Before beginning to examine the major epidemics brought into Australia, it is important to sketch the underlying concepts regarding disease and curing in both western Europe and Indigenous Australia to, at the very least, begin to understand their impact on Indigenous populations. Every human society is subject to illness in one form or another. Each in turn has evolved concepts that define the various physical and psychological conditions that affect personal wellbeing, explain the cause of illness and proffer cures. While the European and Indigenous medical systems, as they were in the late 18th century, differed in many respects, both were more socially than medically therapeutic. Neither could adequately cope with the morbidity and mortality of infectious diseases and neither could offer an effective cure to those infected.

Today, with the benefit of scientifically based medical knowledge, an infectious disease can be defined as the invasion and multiplication of a microorganism into the body tissues. If the invasion results in cellular injury or organ disfunction, an infectious disease is the result. The infectious agents (pathogens) capable of causing infectious disease range from minute and structurally simple viruses to more complex bacteria and large, structurally complex helminthic parasites. It is important to note, however, that infection by a specific pathogen does not necessarily result in disease. The progression from initial infection by an agent capable of causing pathogenic response in the host to the clinical symptoms of the disease depends on several intervening variables. These include the pathogenicity (ability to cause cellular destruction or disfunction) of the agent, the route of transmission of the agent to the host, and the ability of the host's immune system to combat the infectious agent. All these factors, in turn, are affected by the natural and social environments in which the agent and host juxtapose. In some cases, the environment may promote the transmission of the agent to the host, such as can occur in crowded and poor hygienic living conditions. In contrast, living in small groups with limited contact with other people and good hygienic conditions would reduce the risk of infection.

At the time of colonisation, the arriving European medical community largely subscribed to the long-standing humeral theories of sickness and health. These theories had been first advanced by Greek physician Hippocrates in the 5th century BCE, and later championed by another Greek physician, Galen of Pergamon, in the 2nd century AD, to such an extent that they became part of a quasi-religious medical dogma that lasted for almost two thousand years. The modern idea that minute organisms might be the cause of disease (the germ theory of today) had been postulated as early as the 2nd century but it had little impact on the medical establishment's conception of the causes of disease. It was not until the 19th-century breakthroughs of Louis Pasteur and Robert Koch espousing the germ theory that the role of microbes in the causation of disease began to be accepted. These theories did not go unchallenged in Europe, and the medical profession was slow to come to terms with the new ideas and the new ways of treatment. The new concepts were even slower to become accepted in the distant Australian colonies. The 'tyranny of distance', which so often influenced the political, social and commercial history of Australia in the 19th century,[1] also encumbered the dissemination of medical knowledge. So, at the beginning of the colonial period and well into the 19th century, the understanding of disease aetiology (the causes and manner of disease) and therapy was still based on the long-held theories of humeral causes.[2]

The theory held that four humours – blood, phlegm, white bile and black bile – present in the body coincided with the four elements that comprised the world – air, water, fire and earth. Each of the humours had qualities of hot or cold and wet or dry. The view held by Galen was that disease was not a discrete entity with a specific cause as we know it today, such as for tuberculosis, influenza, cancer and syphilis, but a holistic phenomenon caused by an imbalance of the four humours in the body. The various signs of a disease and the symptoms experienced were due to a large extent to the state and severity of the imbalance.[3]

As the theory passed through the centuries it became subtly altered and adorned with new connotations, but the core humoral concepts persisted. Illness in a previously healthy person was perceived to be the result of an imbalance between the bodily humours brought about by changing climatic or environmental factors. Most epidemic diseases were understood in much the same way. But some, for example smallpox, were seen to be rather different and appeared to result from a tangible contagion that was passed through the air from an infected person to others. This was the presumption underlying the development of variolation (injecting a small sample of smallpox scab into a person) and Edward Jenner's experiments with inoculation (injecting the milder cowpox virus into a person) as a safeguard against the smallpox virus. While the humoral thesis held sway, there was also an awareness that diseases could be contagious, passing from one person to another.

The underlying principle behind treating the ill and effecting a cure was to restore the balance of the humours. One of the most common practices up to the late 19th century was to bleed the patient to expel the corruption within and allow restoration of the humours. This practice (phlebotomy) may actually have been extremely deleterious to the health of the patient because it reduced the body's own ability to fight the infection by the loss of the very medium, the blood supply, that the immune system requires to combat the pathogen causing the disease. Another common method used to restore the bodily balance was to induce vigorous evacuation of the bowels (purgation). The drugs used for the treatment of diseases were, however, generally ineffective in combating the infectious agents and in most cases had only limited effect on the symptoms experienced by the unfortunate patient. For example, a range of drugs and concoctions was prescribed for the treatment of diarrhoea. Acute bacterial diarrhoea was a prevalent complaint of the times, mainly due to commonly poor hygienic conditions. Conversely, drugs purported to relieve constipation were used for almost all non-specific illnesses presenting with fevers, headaches, anxiety, rheumatism and so on. The added sufferings and loss of dignity these practices caused to the ill can only be imagined.

In many cases, drugs were prescribed to relieve pain symptoms. Before modern analgesics, the most effective were opium and its derivative, morphine, often causing problems of dependence and withdrawal symptoms when the drugs were no longer available. Other medicines were given for the relief of respiratory symptoms such as the common cold and coughs, and the effects of the more serious inflictions of bronchitis, influenza and tuberculosis. Perhaps the most dangerous form of chemotherapy of the time was the use of mercury, particularly in the treatment of syphilis symptoms. Until the introduction of arsenic-derivate treatments and the development of penicillin antibiotics in the 20th century, mercury chemotherapy had been the mainstay of treatment for syphilis for at least four hundred years. Despite such a long faith by the medical profession in its effectiveness, the drug had little effect on the symptoms of syphilis and was completely ineffective against the causative agent of the disease. But, if taken over a long period, as it customarily was by sufferers of chronic syphilis, it induced severe iatrogenic (caused by medical treatment) illnesses, the cause of which frequently went unrecognised by doctors and often resulted in the victims' ultimate demise. One particularly nasty and futile method was for the unfortunate sufferer to sit in a tub in a hot enclosed room and have a mercury-based ointment rubbed over the body, perhaps up to three times a day. Rub-a-dub-dub. The effects of such treatment on the patient and the person applying the ointment is left to the imagination.

Many of the drugs used in the 19th century were patent medicines (concoctions would be a better description) of little use in reducing the symptoms of infection. A highly popular concoction of the day was 'Holloway's Pills', reputed to cure gout, rheumatism, inveterate ulcers, sore breasts, sore heads, bad legs and so on. 'Doctor More's Indian Root Pills' was another invention that claimed to 'purify the blood' and to be a positive and permanent cure for 'biliousness, constipation, indigestion, headaches, kidney troubles, piles, pimples, and female ailments'.[4] Even as late as the turn of the 20th century, little effective treatment was available for most of the known infectious diseases, and doctors treating the ill were helpless because of their lack of knowledge of the true cause of the diseases.

In Indigenous Australia, the causes of illness, death and curing were multiple and complex, varying according to local beliefs and cultural regions across the continent. While there are differences in the way Aboriginal people perceived a healthy state of being to one of illness, there is an underlying commonality revolving around social and spiritual beliefs. These beliefs have been developed over a vast period of time leading up to British colonisation and to a large degree, despite the enormous cultural impact experienced, have been maintained up to the present in many Aboriginal societies.

The deaths of infants and the elderly were often considered to be the normal course of life's events and in most cases held no spiritual cause. Deaths and illnesses outside these age groups, however, may have had a supernatural cause, particularly in the event of a strange illness that appears to come from afar and affects many, causing excessive mortality. These events (including the introduced epidemics) were attributed to outside sorcery and blame often attributed to another neighbouring tribe or socio-economic group. Sound familiar? It is something like western European populations blaming different countries for an epidemic – 'French pox', 'Spanish flu' and so on.

Personal breaches of well-established social mores and/or taboos, it was believed, could lead to mild or serious illnesses. These beliefs, as noted in the

Introduction, are still held by some people and communities. Supernatural intervention from malevolent spirits was often seen as the cause of major disease episodes at the individual or group levels. Many diseases could come from secret-sacred sites or dangerous places where taboos restricted access for certain age or gender groups. The taboos usually had an ancient origin myth explaining their significance or were over a special ritual or ceremonial place where men's or women's business was held. Transgression into these places, whether deliberate or accidental, by the wrong people would have serious consequences. The resultant onset of illness for the transgressor was either a manifestation of the existing forces or power emanating from these places or meted out by a sorcerer as punishment. These were places to be avoided.

Traditional healers were usually especially skilled, adult initiated men but, in some cases, women also played an equal role. The healers were seen as possessing certain knowledge over and above that of the ordinary people in their society. Having such knowledge gave these people a special place in their society, a place of high esteem and trust. The knowledge they possessed, however, was usually acquired throughout their childhood and enlarged and refined into adulthood through special rituals over and above those required for the rest of the community. Once reaching adulthood most were able to practise their knowledge and skills among their community. Some individuals were seen to have the potential for special abilities early in their childhood and their role as a future doctor-sorcerer was set. The composite knowledge was often in the form of being able to understand and in some cases control the health and sickness of their people and the ability to cure illnesses. Sorcery was often an integral part of these abilities. They became the 'medicine men or women' or the 'clever men and women' of their society by curing the sick, assisting victims of outside sorcery or carrying out sorcery themselves.[5] James Dawson, a pastoralist and ethnographer, described one particular 'medicine man':

> When the white men came to Victoria, there was one doctor of great celebrity in the Western District, Tuurap Warneen, chief of the Mount Kolor Tribe. So celebrated was he for his supernatural powers, and for the cure of diseases, that people of various tribes came from great distances to consult him. He could speak many dialects. At Korroborees and great meetings he was distinguished from the common people by having his face painted red, with white streaks under the eyes, and his brow-band adorned with a quill feather of the turkey bustard, or with

> the crest of a white cockatoo. Tuurap Warneen was unfortunately shot by the manager of a station near Mount Kolor; and his death caused much grief to all the tribes far and near.[6]

Tuurap Warneen's widow, known as the 'White Lady', carried on the tradition as a supernatural healer.

When called upon to treat an ill person, the healers would attend the patient by touching or rubbing a painful area, or singing a ritual to remove the cause of the illness. Two of the most common diagnoses were the presence of foreign objects that had entered the body and caused the illness or that a specific organ had been compromised in some way. A common technique of curing was to suck or rub over the affected area to remove the foreign object. The object was believed to have been placed in the body by some supernatural intervention and so by evil influence caused the illness. The removal of the object from the patient by the healer would then result in a cure. The healer could also employ their particular skills by employing counter-sorcery to remove the evil influences causing illness.

Samuel Gason was a police officer stationed among the Dieri people around Lake Eyre and the lower Cooper Creek region of north-east South Australia in the 1860s. During his duties, mainly concerned with keeping the peace between the Dieri and the cattle graziers, he became familiar with the cultural beliefs, language, social systems and ceremonies of the Dieri. He wrote a small account of the Dieri medicine man attending to a sick person. His perception is not that of a trained anthropologist but is largely in accord with what was later observed by professional anthropologists.

> The 'Koonkie' is a native who has seen the devil when a child (the devil is called 'Kootchie') and is supposed to have received power from him to heal all sick.
>
> The way in which a man or woman becomes a doctor, is that if when young they have had the nightmare, or an unpleasant dream, and relate this to the camp, the inmates come to the conclusion that he or she has seen the devil. The males never practice until after circumcision, and in fact, are not deemed proficient till out of their teens.
>
> Whenever a person falls ill, the koonkie is requested to examine and cure him. The koonkie walks up to the invalid, feels the parts affected, and then commences rubbing them until he fancies, he has got hold of something, when he sucks the parts for a minute or two, and then goes out of the camp a few yards. He now picks up a piece of wood, about

> one or two inches long, and returns to the camp, where, procuring a red-hot coal, he rubs it in his hands to make them hot, and then feels the disordered parts again, and after a little manoeuvring, produces the stick which he had concealed in his hand, as if extracted from the patient's body, to the great surprise of all the natives, who conclude that this was the cause of the complaint.
>
> The imposter won't confess to his trickery, and, indeed, from constant practice, at least deludes himself into a belief of his skilful surgery, which all the other natives have implicit faith in. And, indeed, the force of imagination is so strong in some cases, that I have seen a native quite ill, and actually cry for the koonkie, who, after his humbugging, appeared quite recovered.
>
> Should the Koonkie fail in his effort to relieve the sick, he is prepared with a ready excuse – some koonkie of another tribe, possessing more skill, has stopped his power.[7]

If a healer was unavailable, refused for some reason to attend the patient or if the illness was considered to be mild, a vast range or medicinal cures in the local pharmacopeia could be applied or ingested by the patient or member of the community. In each region of Australia, from the tropical north to the central arid zones and the temperate southern regions, leaves, tree bark and sap, wild herbs, minerals and animal products (feathers, fur, tissue, fat and blood) were used as cures for specific illnesses. Treatment examples include liniment tree (*Melaleuca symphyocarpa*) for headaches;[8] tea trees (*Melaleuca* species) for coughs and colds; river red gum (*Eucalyptus camaldulensis*) bark for fevers; other species of eucalyptus bark for diarrhoea; paper bark tea trees (*Melaleuca* species) for binding wounds; northern black wattle (*Acacia auriculiformis*) for aches and pains; native hop (*Dodonaea viscosa*) for stings; and blackwood (*Acacia melanoxylon*) for rheumatism. The list goes on. The plants were prepared in a number of ways according to the ailment and particular knowledge of the most effective method. Drying, crushing, mixing with clays, burning for smoke inhalation or preparing powders mixed with wood ash were common practices. Applications made from the sap or bark of eucalyptus and acacia species were used for a number of ailments, including wounds and snake bites.

Many of these 'bush medicines' and healing practices are now being examined for their chemical properties and pharmaceutical benefits but undoubtably many were effective to various degrees, particularly those containing alkaloid compounds, which are synthetically produced for modern therapeutics today.[9]

A form of bloodletting (phlebotomy) was practised. Sub-Protector Le Souef observed one method:

> … they open a vein with a piece of sharp flint or shell; they often rub and knead with their knuckles the affected part.

Another method of faux bloodletting, on a 12-year-old boy, was also observed:

> A line made from the tail of an opossum was tightly tied round his waist. At a little distance the doctor sat with a portion of the line drawn through his mouth. Occasionally he spat blood from his cut lip into a billycan placed at a little distance further on. This blood was supposed to be drawn by the doctor from the body of the boy.[10]

While there was a strong association between illness and curing by supernatural means, there was also an awareness of the need to isolate the sick from the rest of the community. Dr W. H. Baylie, serving as a medical officer at the Goulburn River Aboriginal station in northern Victoria, noted in 1843:

> They are sensible of the infectious character of disease, and they use the precaution of removing their sick from the encampment by day to some distance, where on finding a shady place they erect a few brambles and form a shelter to the great comfort of the invalid.[11]

The Australian Indigenous pharmacopeia was quite adequate for dealing with the common wounds, burns, bites, stings, gastrointestinal ailments and body aches that were likely to occur in the daily life of any group. After all, the people had been using the natural remedies for 65,000 years. But there were no traditional remedies effective for the introduced European diseases such as tuberculosis, influenza and smallpox, those frightening diseases that caused so much anxiety, sickness and death after 1788. This is not to say that European medicine could cope any better with the same diseases. In reality, the European medical system could offer no cure and little relief from the major infections they brought with them to Australia.

The effects of an introduced infectious disease on an Indigenous population with no past experience of the disease (a virgin-soil population) and therefore little or no immunological protection (or herd immunity) could, and often has, resulted in excessive morbidity and mortality. The invading pathogen is highly infectious and virulent, and can spread rapidly through a population.[12] Herd immunity to an infectious disease within a population is acquired over time through continuous infection and recovery of individuals who have survived the disease and built up an immunity to the pathogen. These biomedical circumstances were present among the indigenous peoples of the Americas and the Pacific prior to the great expansion of Europe into the New World.

Much has been written about the effects of introduced diseases into the Americas following the expeditions of Columbus, beginning in 1492, and the spread of diseases brought into the populations. For the following three hundred years indigenous populations throughout the Caribbean and North, Central and South America suffered severe population losses, some at 85 to 90 per cent in different locations.[13] Smallpox first hit Hispaniola in epidemic form in 1518. Two years later the Aztec populations of Mexico were severely struck when Hernando Cortez (1519) and Pánfilo de Narváez (1520) invaded, introducing smallpox and killing up to two or three million. The destruction caused by smallpox enabled the Spanish conquistadors to take the Aztec capital of Tenochtitlán, even though greatly outnumbered. Smallpox then spread into Guatemala and south into the Inca domain. Vasco Núñez de Balboa (1524–27) invaded the Inca lands, resulting in 200,000 deaths and between 1515 and 1520 the Mayans of the Yucatán Peninsula suffered similar losses from smallpox. Indigenous populations in northern and southern America suffered severe population collapse. It is estimated that these outbreaks of smallpox killed off one-third of the populations. But more were to follow. In 1530–31 measles was introduced into Mexico and Peru, hard on the heels of the ravages caused by smallpox. In turn, the mosquito-borne diseases of malaria and yellow fever wreaked havoc on both the indigenous populations as well as the invading Europeans.[14] In 1558 influenza hit the virgin-soil populations of central America. This introduction may have been a new strain of the influenza virus as it was spreading through Europe around the same period.[15] Influenza is a great sea traveller, accompanying sailors around the world.

The epidemics in the Americas continued further north and south of their initial entry points. By the end of the 17th century epidemics had caused exceptional morbidity and mortality among the indigenous populations of California, ultimately resulting in a 90 per cent population collapse. This collapse and the comparative ease in which the Spanish, Portuguese, French and British managed to subdue the populations was not by the sword or the gun but by the pathogens the Europeans carried. Historian Alfred Crosby describes it as the '*Conquistador y Pestilencia*'.[16]

As ships from Europe brought their colonists into the Pacific, the cycle of epidemic diseases struck into South-east Asia and the Hawaiian Islands. On his third voyage into the Pacific, between 1776 and 1779, Captain James Cook,

RN, visited the Hawaiian Islands and the west coast of America, commanding HMS *Discovery*. Their visit to Hawaii was marked by the introduction of syphilis and gonorrhoea to the indigenous population. Over the next hundred years repeated visits by European ships introduced smallpox, measles, tuberculosis (most likely reintroduced into the Americas) and influenza, resulting in a collapse of 90 per cent of the Hawaiian population.[17]

These were the major introduced diseases that caused such severe loss of life, but diphtheria, mumps, malaria, dysentery, bubonic plague, yellow fever and possibly typhus also caused excessive losses.[18] However, it is difficult and most likely impossible to know or to grasp to any extent the true extent of morbidity and mortality the imported diseases caused, and the subsequent cultural and social changes incurred. But it is well agreed that they caused severe demographic collapse throughout. The effects – biological, social and cultural – of European colonisation in the New World resound to this very day. And, as will be seen, the impact on the Indigenous people of Australia has been another, later chapter of the same events.

But it was not always a one-way transmission of European diseases affecting indigenous populations. Along with the slave trade bringing Africans to the Caribbean and American colonies came an accidental stowaway – the mosquito genus *Aedes*, carrying the deadly yellow fever virus. Many of the slaves had developed an immunity to the virus in their African homelands and were not affected by the disease. For the European colonists and the indigenous people of the Americas, the disease was devastating and feared. Along with Africa, the Caribbean and American colonies gained the reputation of being dangerous postings for European diplomats, sailors and soldiers. Africa was known as the 'White Man's Grave' because of yellow fever and malaria, another African mosquito-borne disease, with death rates consistently exceeding 50 per cent. In the Americas, major outbreaks of yellow fever followed the steamboat routes along the Mississippi and spread north as far as Canada. In Philadelphia, an outbreak of the disease in 1793 forced President George Washington, and the government, to flee the city. When Napoleon sent an army to quell uprisings in the French colonies, he lost 35,000 to 45,000 troops, about one-third of the dispatchment on the island of Saint-Domingue. The loss of so many troops made Napoleon abandon French interests in the West Indies and turn to the conquest of Russia, where his troops faced devastation from the ravages of dysentery and typhus. Malaria had a profound effect on the American Civil War of 1861–65. It is estimated that over one million on both sides were infected, causing severe debilitation of the fighting troops and over 10,000 deaths. With the shortages of quinine by both sides, the effects on fighting abilities were profound. A Confederate surgeon, Dr W. J. Worsham, wrote from inside Vicksburg: 'The enemy shells annoyed us, but there was another foe we had to contend with more annoying than the enemy's shells – the mosquitoes, or, as our boys called them "gallinippers".'[19] These two mosquito-borne diseases imported from Africa had an influential impact on the history of America, the Caribbean and Europe.

An epidemic disease can also impact profoundly on a community. If the epidemic spreads through the community and imparts excessive morbidity and mortality, the effect could, and often does, lead to social disruption, permanently altering long-standing cultural practices even after the epidemic has passed on. One of the first responses when an epidemic begins to get a grip on a population is for the people to flee from the sickness and find a place of safety and sanctuary. It is a natural human response. In many cases, when the disease has an initial asymptomatic phase, the people can carry the infection with them and infect others, dissipating the disease even further. Author Daniel Defoe wrote about the mass migration from London city streets to the countryside during the bubonic plague epidemic of 1665, as people on horseback, on loaded carts or on foot tried to escape the sickness.[20]

Apportioning blame and finding a suitable scapegoat for the disease is another common response. The Aboriginal people of the southern coasts of Bass Strait between the mainland and the island of Tasmania considered the European sailors of the sealing ships as harbingers of the new diseases they began to experience.[21] When syphilis spread throughout Europe in the 16th century it was given several names according to the political relationships with neighbouring countries: for example, the French pox, the English pox, the Italian pox. We can still see this naming in the 20th century, such as for the Hong Kong flu pandemic of 1968. Even today some still refer erroneously to the 1918–19 influenza pandemic as the 'Spanish flu'. The term 'Spanish Flu' is commonly but erroneously used today for the 1918–19 influenza pandemic, even though it did not originate in Spain. (During the last years of the First World War, when the pandemic began, Spain was a neutral country and readily reported the effects of the pandemic, whereas the belligerent countries were secretive about its effects on the fighting troops.)

As an epidemic spreads and the morbidity and mortality rises, the ill are left behind. There is often no-one to care for them as they fight the disease. If they become immobile, which is often the case, then they cannot access food, water and warmth, basic requirements to enable the body's immune system to fight the disease. Many more die due to the lack of personal care. As the death toll rises bodies are left where they have died, with no-one around or willing to bury or dispose of the corpses. The usual rituals surrounding the death and disposal of a community member are abandoned. There is no time to grieve for the dead individual properly and appropriately, and this has an impact on the living. The soul of the dead person has not been properly treated according to the cultural lore, or has not been returned to their country for a final resting place, leaving a permanent emotional hole in the lives of the survivors. The bonds that hold a community together are severely impacted and in worst cases permanently lost.

In the case of the Indigenous populations of Australia, the diseases discussed in detail in this book had a profound result. With many people dying from infection during the epidemics and those who survived the initial mortality later dying from secondary causes, the most obvious effect on a society is the loss of lives, particularly of loved ones and relatives. In all of these diseases the loss of life was extensive. In fact, deaths among the Indigenous people, in many cases far ahead of the colonial borders, were never recorded. It must be assumed that they were incalculable but severe.

Along with the high death toll in the epidemics there comes the loss of culture. Cultural knowledge that has been embedded in the society and has survived for thousands of years by being passed down from the Elders to the younger initiates becomes another victim of epidemics. In an epidemic, mortality is generally high in the elderly and, with their deaths, knowledge and stories held in trust by the Elders is no longer passed down and is lost. Sometimes forever. Whole languages have been lost. It has been estimated that prior to European colonisation 250 languages, along with 800 dialects, were spoken across Australia. The Australian Institute of Aboriginal and Torres Strait Islander Studies (AIATSIS) has assessed that only 13 are now still acquired by children and approximately another 100 are spoken to various degrees by older generations, with many still at risk. Languages carry and transmit the cultural knowledge of a society, so the loss of a language invariable means a loss of culture and a loss of connection between the living and the ancestors. This loss of connection to people and to the stories of country have an impact on individual and group health and wellbeing, which can continue well into future generations.[22]

With population and language loss comes a disconnection between surviving groups and societies. A breakdown in the trade and reciprocity systems that have sustained the cultural and biological fabric of a population follows. The acquisition of valuable commodities and products that have been traded and exchanged, in many cases over long distances, are no longer available. There is a loss of contact with other social groups, contact that has sustained the kinship systems regulating marriage and social relations across the country. Epidemics not only kill people but can drastically alter, forever change and obliterate the very essence of a society.

What was the population of Australia prior to the arrival of Europeans in 1788? The short answer is we do not really know with any sense of precision. Over the years researchers have struggled with this problem and there has been considerable variation in the estimates. In 1930 anthropologist Arthur Radcliffe-Brown reviewed the available literature from explorers and government officials, which were based on observations and calculations in regional areas. Radcliffe-Brown determined the 1788 population across Australia to be at least 250,000 and possibly more than 300,000. But this figure is highly flawed and most certainly underestimated because it was based on concentrations of people who had been affected by frontier violence and multiple waves of epidemics incurring high mortality.

As a better understanding of Australia's Indigenous societies grew from archaeological, ecological and anthropological research and close reading of historical resources, it has been realised that the total population of Indigenous Australia being well over one million was far more likely to be the case. The most densely populated areas with food resources able to sustain the semi-sedentary population centres were the temperate south-east, the coastal areas in the north, parts of the south-west corner and western basalt plains, and along the Murray–Darling river system. Along the Murray River corridor, stretching from the western slopes of the Great Dividing Range, cutting through the extensive plains of New South Wales and Victoria, and through South Australia to the south coast, there is convincing evidence of large populations. Edward Eyre in 1845 wrote of seeing groups of 500 gathered at Lake Victoria on the Murray and 600 at Moorundie on the lower reaches of the river.[23] A further indication of high population density along the Murray comes from an analysis of skeletal remains. Pathological stress markers on recovered bones show a greater than normal occurrence here than in other populations examined in Australia. These markers are the result of nutritional and/or pathological conditions highly suggestive of sedentary populations living in close proximity and experiencing seasonal food shortages.[24] Whatever the total number may have been in January 1788 when a British flag was raised at Botany Bay on the eastern coast, it must be assumed that highly developed and dense population centres existed across the continent.[25]

Chapter 2

SMALLPOX

From its genesis in the distant past until it was officially eradicated in 1979,[1] smallpox had been an extremely infectious and serious systemic disease of humans, erupting in populations throughout the world in frightening epidemics. (The classic 1988 text on the subject, by Frank Fenner et al., is known as 'The Big Red Book' for its cover.) In 1983, Donald R. Hopkins, who witnessed the disease in Africa and Asia and later played a leading role in its eradication, wrote of smallpox: 'On the suddenness and unpredictability of its attack, the grotesque torture of its victims, the brutality of its lethal or disfiguring outcome, and the terror it inspired, smallpox is unique among human diseases.'[2]

The causative agent of smallpox, variola virus, now no longer occurs in its natural environment and exists officially in only two laboratories, one in the United States and the other in Russia. The last known case of naturally occurring smallpox was a three-year-old girl from Bangladesh. During her illness she was kept at home in well-guarded isolation until she was no longer infectious.[3]

The origin of smallpox is not clear. It most probably developed as a zoonosis (a disease caused by an animal pathogen that has crossed over to humans) during the Old World Neolithic period, when agricultural societies grew sufficiently large enough to provide a supporting human reservoir for the virus. An exclusively human disease with no known animal reservoir, smallpox, though devastating in its effect, required a large population to maintain itself and so almost certainly did not exist among the hunting and gathering peoples of the Palaeolithic.[4]

Descriptions of smallpox, or a disease of a similar nature, are known from China from 1122 BCE and, from around the same period,[5] one of the earliest known victims of the disease may have been Ramses V of Egypt, who died as a young man in 1157 BCE. His preserved mummy was medically examined in the 1980s and revealed a rash of elevated pustules on the lower face, neck and shoulders. Earlier photography showed that the rash was also prominent on the lower abdomen and scrotum. Dating back more than 3000 years, this is the earliest physical evidence of a skin condition that is consistent with smallpox. It then suggests that if such a royal and privileged person as a ruling king could contract and most likely die from smallpox then the disease may have been present and infecting the Nile population.[6]

A smallpox-like disease in devastating plague forms has been described by many observers throughout Europe, the Indian subcontinent and Asia since the death of Ramses V.[7] The Antonine Plague, which first flared up in 178 AD during the rule of the Roman emperor Marcus Aurelius, continued for over a decade, finally subsiding in the reign of his son Commodus. It was one of the most devastating epidemics of the Roman period. It appeared among the Roman army fighting in Mesopotamia, where it killed up to one in ten of the soldiers and incapacitated many more. It was brought back to Syria and Italy by returning soldiers in 164 AD, where it caused excessive morbidity and mortality in the population and weakened the military, as well as decimating the cultural life of the empire. Although the clinical features of the disease were somewhat inadequately described by the physician Galen, who observed the epidemic firsthand, a more recent critical examination of the texts strongly suggests that the disease was smallpox.[8]

As large centres of population developed in Europe, Asia and Africa, and movement of people increased, smallpox developed in step from the occasional epidemic outbreak to become a well-established endemic disease. For the last 1500 years smallpox has been known to be endemic in the densely populated agricultural settlements of the Ganges Plain.[9] The disease persisted there until it was finally eradicated in the latter part of the 20th century.

In 1241 smallpox reached Iceland. Although settled around the early 9th century, the disease had not reached the island in the past so the population in the 13th century, of about 70,000, like those native to the Americas (discussed in the previous chapter), had little or no immunity. It killed some 20,000 (29 per cent) of the island's people. Devastating to the population as it was, the disease returned in 1257 and yet again in1291, each time taking its toll on those who had not previously been exposed to the virus.[10] By the 18th century smallpox was present in most of the major towns and cities in Europe. It occurred regularly in epidemics sweeping through population centres, causing high mortality at a frightening level but always remaining as an endemic disease, with every newborn susceptible to infection. Although it was known by different names, smallpox became the most feared and recognised disease throughout Europe.

Its transoceanic spread began in the early 16th century, when it was carried across the Atlantic by Spanish expeditions to the New World. In late 1518 or early 1519, smallpox erupted for the first time on Hispaniola, 27 years after the Columbus expedition had landed on the island. It is not known for certain if the disease was brought by the Spanish sailors themselves or by the West African slaves the conquistadors had begun importing into the Caribbean Islands by 1503, but whatever the case the disease soon spread to Jamaica, Puerto Rico, Antigua, Martinique, Barbados and Cuba, then found its way into the continental populations of South and North America.[11] Mortality among these populations was extreme. Estimates of the death rate (case fatality rate, also known as the case–fatality ratio) vary from 25 per cent, which is severe in any population, right up to a staggering 50–75 per cent of those infected with the disease.[12] From 1775 to 1782 smallpox ravaged the indigenous populations of North America, killing more than a hundred thousand people from Mexico to the Great Lakes and beyond, maiming many more, leaving in its wake untold despair and forever changing the cultures and existences of those who survived and the future generations to come. Like its presence in the Old World populations of Europe, Asia and the Indian subcontinent, smallpox became well known and feared.

The first known introduction into the Western Pacific was to the Palau Islands in 1783. In 1853 smallpox ravaged the indigenous population of Hawaii; in the Carolinas it was responsible for the death of up 40 per cent; and on Guam 33 per cent. Other introductions were to Easter Island in 1863–64 and New Guinea some time before 1872 and later in 1893 and 1895. Quarantining of ships allowed Fiji to escape the introduction of smallpox and the disease killed only six in New Zealand, when two ships carrying active cases arrived in 1872.[13] Smallpox among the Aboriginal people of Australia was first recorded soon after the arrival of British colonists and that is where I will pick up the story of the destruction it wrought. But first it will help to know a little about the disease.

Biology of Smallpox

The causative agent of smallpox is variola virus. It gets its name from the Latin word, *varius*, meaning spotted or variegated, describing not the virus itself but the clinical progression of the disease on the human body. Variola virus belongs to the genus *Orthopoxvirus*, which includes similar viruses that can infect mammals, such as cowpox, horsepox, monkeypox and camelpox.[14]

In the world of viruses, the variola virus is a monster compared with other viruses. It is shaped like a brick, measuring 200nm wide and 250nm long, rather on the large size for a virus. But, unlike the clever, genetic shape-shifting influenza virus, the variola virus is rather dumb (excuse the anthropomorphism). Its core is made up of double-stranded DNA that is extremely stable when it comes to replication. It does not go through the rapid genetic mutations of the RNA influenza virus, which makes that pathogen particularly difficult for the human immune system to identify. It is this factor that gave its infected host the advantage of life-long immunity to smallpox disease (if, of course, the host was to survive), and was largely responsible for the scientific and medical community successfully eradicating it from its natural environment. A dumb but deadly giant all the same. Its 'dumbness' was increased because it could only exist and replicate in humans with no other host available to it. The clever influenza virus, for example, can exist in birds and pigs, and then genetically mutate to freely spill over and replicate in humans. And there is one other factor relating to the demise of variola and smallpox as a human disease: the virus could only be passed between its human hosts for a short time of two to three weeks after initial infection and could not be passed on after that period. Deadly and terrifying though it was, it was susceptible to successful eradication by modern science. But, while smallpox was the first human disease to be eradicated, it remains the only one so far.

All these factors aside, variola virus, or smallpox on the loose, was an acute killing disease that often led to a painful death within the first two weeks of infection and the appearance of clinical signs. Largely because a surviving human host was immune to further infection, smallpox could only become endemic within a population when there was a large reservoir of susceptible hosts. This was regularly achieved by new births within a population and immigration of susceptibles who had not been exposed to the disease. Once an epidemic of the disease had swept through a population, killing many and conferring immunity to the survivors, the disease would burn itself out, only to return in a few years when there were more susceptibles in the population.

Two main clinical-epidemiological varieties of smallpox have been recognised – variola major, the classic type of smallpox, and a milder form, variola minor. The two strains of variola virus differed quite significantly in their virulence to humans. Variola minor, as its name suggests, caused mild symptoms (known as alastrim) in its human host and had a case fatality rate in unvaccinated individuals ranging from 0.1 to 2.0 per cent. The more virulent variola major strain was the life-threatening disease known as smallpox. It often manifested severe symptoms and produced a much higher case fatality rate ranging up to (and in some cases above) 75 per cent.

The virus was transmitted mainly through the inhalation of respiratory droplets formed by coughing and sneezing by an infected person. Other means of transmission were: direct inoculation of the virus, as in variolation; inhalation of the sloughed-off skin lesions of patients; contact with material that had been contaminated by the virus; placental transmission; and airborne spread.[15] The period of communicability was greatest during the first week of initial infection and continued for approximately 21 days beyond that. Susceptibility to the disease was universal but long-term immunity usually followed recovery and second attacks were rare.

Research in the twentieth century identified several clinical manifestations and prognoses of variola major. Ordinary-type variola major was the most common. In typical cases of this type of infection an incubation stage ranged from 7 to 17 days but was usually between 10 and 14 days.[16] During this period of infection the virus replicated and spread throughout the body via the lymphoid organs (spleen, bone marrow and lymph nodes). The onset of clinical symptoms was often quite sudden. Fever, malaise, headache, severe backache, prostration and in some instances abdominal pain were the first to appear. These symptoms were easily confused with influenza, meningitis or pneumonia.[17] After two to four days the fever reduced, and the characteristic stages of the smallpox rash began, starting as small, flat, reddish spots on the skin (maculopapular rash), at first particularly in the mouth, throat and nasal passages and around the eyes. The rash then appeared on the trunk and extremities – the soles of the feet, the palms of the hands and forearms were focal points. The papules became vesicular (raised and containing fluid) within a day or two and then formed pus-filled blisters (pustules) within 48 hours. The fever often returned during this stage. By this time the patient was often in extreme pain and emitted a strong smell, which became characteristic of smallpox. The pustules dried and began forming scabs within eight to ten days of initial eruption. The matured lesions sometimes joined and became a continuous rash covering large sections of the skin and/or remained discrete. If the former occurred, then the patient had a high risk of dying. Finally, as the disease spread, the scabs fell off at the end of the third to fourth week if the patient had survived, leaving characteristic scarring. This type of variola major progress was documented as having high case fatality rates.[18]

The flat type of variola major, distinguished by lesions that projected little, if at all, above the surrounding skin surface, was relatively rare but had a case fatality rate reaching 98 per cent.[19] Equally as fatal was the haemorrhagic type, which caused, either late or early in its development, bleeding from the mouth, gums and nose (subconjunctival bleeding) and blood in the urine (haematuria). In this type of variola major, pregnant females were more susceptible than males and non-pregnant females. Variola minor and an abortive form of variola, in which the disease subsided usually without any eruption (variola sine eruptione), were rare and occurred principally in vaccinated individuals.[20]

The symptoms of variola minor were similar but much less severe and life threatening than variola major. Variola minor was often referred to as alastrim. The onset was, like variola major, sudden, with a fever, headache, backache and sometimes vomiting. The sequence of development and distribution of the skin lesions were also similar but their development was much more rapid. The eruptions became vesicular on the third day after the appearance of the papular stage and developed into pustules within 24 hours. The final crusting stage was established on the sixth or seventh day of the rash. The facial lesions were often sparser than in variola major and rarely reached the confluent stage. Secondary fever was rare, and the victims usually remained active and less affected during the disease.[21]

Smallpox among the European Population

In 1984 Professor Frank Fenner, writing on smallpox, stated that Australia has not loomed large in the global history of the disease.[22] Indeed, while there were several outbreaks of the disease among the European population of Australia, the mortality was never as severe as it was elsewhere and the disease often had only a slight effect on them. For this reason, perhaps, smallpox did not become established and endemic in Australia. Since the arrival of the First Fleet in 1788 there have been several outbreaks (opposed to epidemics) of smallpox among the Europeans. Table 2.1 shows the outbreaks that were considered serious enough by government and medical authorities in the 19th century.

All the outbreaks were due to importations by passengers arriving by ship. The 1881–82 outbreak, which spread throughout the port suburbs of Sydney, had the highest number of individual cases and a case fatality rate of 25 per cent. Most other cases were confined among the ship's passengers, who were quarantined. The containment of the outbreaks was largely due to the success of various colonial government bodies in emphasising a strategy of quarantine and vaccination of victims and contacts rather than the routine vaccination of children.[23] While this strategy was suited to a colonial population who had recently arrived from an endemic to a non-endemic country, where the major threat was the periodic importation of the disease by sea, it was not suited to the Aboriginal populations who had no previous experience with smallpox, no means of prevention and no means of controlling the disease in its epidemic form.

Table 2.1. Major smallpox outbreaks during the 19th century in the European population of Australia.[24]

Year/s	Region	Cases	Deaths	Case Fatality (%)
1857	Melbourne	16	4	25
1868–69	Melbourne	43	10	23
1871	Sydney, Melbourne	7	0	0
1881–82	Sydney	154	40	25
1884–86	Sydney, Melbourne, Adelaide	123	10	8
1887	Launceston	unknown	11	unknown
1893	Perth	52	9	17

Smallpox among Aboriginal Populations: The Epidemics

In great contrast to its limited presence among the European population, smallpox has had a lethal history in Aboriginal Australia. At least three (perhaps four) unconnected epidemics attributable to smallpox were recorded among the Aboriginal populations of Australia. The first began in March or April 1789.

A severe epidemic disease was seen by European colonists to be causing high mortality among the Aboriginal population living around the new settlement of Sydney in 1789. It appeared quickly and lasted in the Sydney region for a few weeks. Later historical evidence, however, suggests that, at the same time, it also occurred along the coastal populations north and south of Sydney and most likely among the inland populations along the river corridors.

Apart from a handful of written accounts by members of the First Fleet,[25] little is known about this epidemic, although much has been written about it by later historians. A few contemporary accounts survive, written by those who saw the disease active among the Aboriginal groups around Sydney Harbour, and its effects in surrounding groups. The First Fleeters attributed the disease they saw to smallpox, although this diagnosis has not always been accepted by historians.[26] Most writers, however, have accepted that the disease was indeed smallpox. Puzzling over the origin of the disease observed at Sydney Cove, several possibilities have been put forward by historians, including the accidental or deliberate release of variolous matter brought with the colonists of the First Fleet in January 1788; a visiting French squadron that arrived at Botany Bay; seasonal fishermen reaching northern Australia from Makassar, where the disease was endemic; and a type of 'native pox' presumed to be an endemic disease of Australia.[27] While many researchers have made articulate use of historical records, citing evidence for their particular case and in some cases speculating on evidence that does not exist, no one author or theory has in the end prevailed over the others. The question of origin of the 1779 smallpox epidemic among the Australian Aboriginal people has remained unresolved. The limiting factor in the debate has been the historical records themselves, which show no conclusive evidence either way.

To arrive at some understanding of this epidemic and the effect it had on the Aboriginal populations, it is far more relevant to examine the nature of the epidemic itself to establish the spatial and temporal extent, and the demographic and social effects it had than to deliberate eternally about its origin on evidence that does not sustain such an approach. And I would not hesitate to argue that such an approach goes for the other major epidemics that impacted on Australian Aboriginal populations.

The second epidemic occurred 40 years later, between 1828 and 1832, and was documented more extensively. It was first observed by European exploration parties on the river systems west of the Great Dividing Range in New South Wales, beyond the limits of the European settlements.[28] Later, as the frontiers extended, observations of Aboriginal people bearing smallpox scarring, and oral accounts from those who survived, revealed that the epidemic had extended further inland, along major river corridors to South Australia, and to the eastern coastline of the continent.

A third epidemic of smallpox was observed to be spreading among the Nawu, Wirangu, and Banggaria people along the western coast and inland regions of South Australia in 1866–67.[29] This epidemic was most likely the southern extent of an outbreak that was spreading among Aboriginal groups on the north and west coasts of Australia and through the centre during that time.

The First Epidemic: 1789

One year after the first European colonists established their settlement at Sydney Cove, they noticed a severe mortality among the Aboriginal groups seemingly caused by a disease. The few contemporary accounts referring to the incident describe it as an epidemic of smallpox. Aboriginal people at this time came to know it as 'galgala'.

The 1789 outbreak of smallpox among the Aboriginal people was the first epidemic in Australia to be recorded. It remains among the most poorly described. Potentially, the most informative sources on the epidemic would have been the medical journals of the First Fleet surgeons but, unfortunately, to a large extent these have not survived. The majority of surviving written records are by contemporary observers who had no medical education or background, and generally consist of accounts within official reports, personal memoirs and letters. Nevertheless, these diarists wrote accounts of the epidemic based on their visual observations and presumably on information they received from those who were medically trained. They should be accorded some credibility.

Since the arrival of the colonists in January 1788, it had been a common sight for those on the harbour waters to see Aboriginal people along the shorelines, fishing and camping among the coves and rock shelters of the harbour. The smoke from their numerous cooking fires rose among the low hills and bays of the harbour. Then, in April 1789, almost every ship and boat that sailed on the harbour going about the daily business of the colony began to see bodies lying about as if they had been abandoned where they had died. The smoke from the fires began to disappear. HMS *Sirius*, the former flagship of the First Fleet, was returning to the settlement from a voyage to the Cape of Good Hope. On board was William Bradley, naval officer and cartographer. Bradley had arrived in the colony the previous year with the First Fleet and had undertaken several surveys along the coast and in the hinterlands around the settlement at Sydney Cove. His main interest, however, was in the Aboriginal people he came across, some of whom he befriended, documenting these encounters in his diary. But sailing into Sydney Harbour on the *Sirius* that day he noticed 'a great number of dead Natives … in every part of the Harbour'. Later, Newton Fowell, another naval officer on board *Sirius*, commented that in some cases the bodies were found with the remains of small fires on either side of them and containers of water left within reach.[30] Bradley saw none of the Aboriginal fishing canoes that had previously been a common sight on the harbour. In fact, the waters and shores of Port Jackson appeared to Bradley and Fowell to be devoid of any living Aboriginal person.

David Collins, the colony's deputy judge advocate and lieutenant-governor, visited the harbour shorelines to investigate the observations for himself and reported:

> Early in the month, and throughout its continuance, the people whose business called them down the harbour daily reported, that they found, either in excavations of the rock, or lying upon the beaches and points of the different coves which they had been in, the bodies of many of the wretched natives of this country.[31]

The only Aboriginal people that were seen by Collins that day were the 'putrid bodies of those who had fallen victim to the disorder'.

At first the cause of the mortality was unknown but the repeated accounts of Aboriginal bodies about the settlement environs aroused the interest of the staff of the colony's hospital. A number of bodies were collected and brought into the settlement for the purpose of post-mortem examination.[32] No description of these post-mortems survive, so the results are unknown.

Watkin Tench, a young marine captain who accompanied Collins around the shorelines, gave a brief description of the symptoms in his account of the settlement:

> On inspection, it appeared that all the parties had died a natural death: pustules, similar to those occasioned by the small pox, were thickly spread on the bodies ...[33]

In mid-April, a small group of Aboriginal people was found suffering from the disease in a cove near to the settlement. The governor of the colony, Arthur Phillip, together with a surgeon, visited the shorelines. Tench again recorded in his account that:

> Here they found an old man stretched before a few lighted sticks, and a boy of nine or ten years old pouring water on his head, from a shell which he held in his hand: near them lay a female child dead, and a little farther off, its unfortunate mother ... eruptions covered the poor boy from head to foot; and the old man was so reduced, that he was with difficulty got into the boat.[34]

With Arthur Phillip's group was Arabanoo, a young Aboriginal man who had been captured at Manly on the last day of 1788 on the orders of Governor Phillip. Phillip had wanted to learn more about the people on whose land they had established their settlement. By this time the new colony, not yet a year old, was suffering a severe food shortage and Phillip wished to learn more from the Aboriginal people as to which native plants were edible. Arabanoo was first brought into the settlement as a prisoner in handcuffs but was later to become a favourite of the governor and a great source of information about his people and the neighbouring groups. But on this occasion he was extremely distressed to see his people suffering from this new and strange disease. Collins wrote of the sight:

> At that time, a native was living with us; and on taking him down to the harbour to look for his former companions, those who witnessed his expression and agony can never forget either. He looked anxiously around him in the different coves we visited; not a vestige on the sand was to be found of human foot … not a living person was anywhere to be met with. It seemed as if, flying from the contagion, they had left the dead to bury the dead. He lifted up his hands and eyes in silent agony for some time; at last he exclaimed, 'All dead! all dead!' and then hung his head in mournful silence.[35]

The old man and the boy were then brought back into the settlement and placed under the care of the surgeons. The old man lived only a few hours.

> By the encouragement of Arabanoo, who assured them of protection, and soothing behaviour of our medical gentlemen, they became at once reconciled to us and looked happy and grateful at the change of their situation. Sickness and hunger had, however, so much exhausted the old man, that little hope was entertained of his recovery. As he pointed frequently to his throat, at the instance of Arabanoo, he tried to wash it with a gargle which was given him; but the obstructed, tender state of the part rendered it impracticable.[36]

Despite being 'covered from head to foot' with eruptions when he was brought into the settlement, the young man survived the disease. Collins attributes his survival to the care he received from Surgeon White during the course of his illness. There is no surviving record by White of this incident.

Towards the end of April, Governor Phillip records that two more, an elderly man and a young female of ten or eleven years of age, were brought into the settlement suffering from smallpox.[37] Tench recorded them as 'a young man, and the other his sister, a girl of fourteen years old'.[38] Other accounts differ as to how many Aboriginal people were found suffering with the disease and were brought into the settlement. Collins reported that 'two elderly men, a boy, and a girl were brought up, and placed in a separate hut at the hospital';[39] and Hunter recorded that 'two children, a boy of six or seven years of age, and a girl about ten, were lately picked up labouring under the same disease; two old men; whom we had reason to believe were the fathers of the two children, were picked up at the same time, and much care taken of them'.[40] Whatever the number may have been, it is recorded by Tench, Collins and Phillip that, despite the care afforded them, the adults died of smallpox. Two children, however, showed signs of improvement soon after their arrival in the settlement and survived the disease.

Although there are no surviving descriptions of the symptoms by the surgeons who attended, it is possible to reconstruct, with some detail, the course of the symptoms from the diarists. Among the first group brought into the settlement in mid-April was the young male with eruptions covering most of his body. If this observation is accurate then the boy was past the initial symptoms of fever, malaise and prostration that would have occurred in the first two to four days of symptomatic onset. Tench's account is not clear as to which stage the 'eruptions' were at, but because he was able to sit up and offer some assistance to the adult male, and because they covered most of his body, we can assume that he was in an advanced stage of clinical signs, with the lesions reaching maturity, and was over the worst stages of the disease. No more is said of him in this respect other than that he recovered and was adopted into the family of the surgeon-general of the colony. The accompanying adult male may have been in about the fourth day of clinical signs, as Tench describes him in a condition of immobility and exhaustion when he was brought in. The next day his condition deteriorated, with the onset of secondary fever accompanied by periodic bouts of shivering. He remained prostrate and was unable to eat but drank water when it was offered. He remained conscious until he died. Of the second pair who were brought into hospital less is known. It can be assumed they were in an advanced stage of the disease, as Tench describes them both as being in 'a most deplorable state of wretchedness from the small-pox'. After three days the young male died and the female recovered, to be adopted into the family of a clergyman.[41]

When the ill were brought into the settlement, Arabanoo attended to them closely. He began to show signs of the disease on May 12th and died six days later. He was just 25 to 30 years old.[42] An incubation period of between 7 and 17 days, most commonly 10–12 days, before the onset of symptoms would suggest that Arabanoo caught the infection from the second couple to be brought in. According to Tench, Arabanoo had shown more sympathy and care for them than he had for the former group brought in, and most likely had more physical contact with them. A period of 6 or 8 days followed, during which the symptoms 'burst forth with irresistible fury' before he died:

> During his sickness he reposed entire confidence in us. Although a stranger to medicine, and nauseating the taste of it, he swallowed with patient submission innumerable drugs, which the hope of relief induced us to administer to him. The governor, who particularly regarded him, caused him to be buried in his own garden, and attended the funeral in person.[43]

The infection was limited almost entirely to the Aboriginal population. The only non-Aboriginal person to be infected was, according to Collins, 'a North-American Indian', a sailor belonging to the *Supply* who manifested symptoms on May 2nd and died a few days later.[44] The source of his infection is not known. Nothing is recorded of this man's movements in the days preceding his infection, or of his contact with the Aboriginal people within and outside the settlement. Nor is there record of the treatment he received during his illness or whether he was isolated from the rest of the community. But, even though the disease is highly communicable during the first week after the onset of symptoms, there is no record of the sailor transmitting the infection on board the *Supply* or within the settlement.

That the settlement escaped the epidemic was largely due to the low level of personal contact the Europeans had with the Aboriginal groups. Ironically, Governor Phillip had been concerned about the lack of friendly contact and rapport so far established. One of his tasks on establishing the settlement was to initiate a friendly relationship with the Aboriginal people, to conciliate their affections and to learn as much about them as he could for the benefit of the colony.[45] At first he was able to meet them on amicable terms but they remained generally aloof from the Europeans and avoided the settlement. No mutual understanding of their respective cultures developed and soon any good will, which had been tenuous at best, deteriorated into a series of violent skirmishes around the settlement lasting several years.[46] Because of this poor relationship Phillip had decided to capture one of the local people and bring him into the settlement in order to break down the communication barrier that had resulted and try once again to establish close association. Arabanoo, then, was the first of several whom Phillip captured.

Neither did the ill and suffering who were brought into the settlement hospital transmit smallpox further. They were immediately isolated in an unoccupied building next to the hospital. The colonists were well aware of the contagious nature of smallpox, as Collins commented:

> It was not a desirable circumstance to introduce a disorder into the colony which was raging with such fatal violence among the natives of the country.[47]

It is not known how many of the Europeans (about a thousand in all) were immune to smallpox, having either previously survived an infection or having been successfully inoculated against it. There was, however, one potentially susceptible group in the settlement – the children and infants who had been born either in the settlement or on the voyage out. There is no record of any inoculation procedure performed on them. Collins revealed:

> Notwithstanding the town of Sydney was at this time filled with children, many of whom visited the natives that were ill of this disorder, not one of them caught it.[48]

While the arrival of Aboriginal people in the settlement would have been the cause of great curiosity for adults and children alike, it is unlikely they would have risked, or been allowed, close contact with them when they clearly showed signs of a disease that was feared and known to be highly contagious.

The epidemic existed in the Sydney region during March and April 1789 and appears to have subsided by early May. Its extent, however, appears to have been far greater than the environs of Sydney. Two 20th-century scholars, J. H. L. Cumpston and Noel Butlin, refer to evidence of its existence far to the south-west in South Australia and to the north in the Hunter Valley region, but neither author indicates a source for these assertions.[49] The diarists of Sydney no longer report seeing active cases of smallpox among the Aboriginal people after May 1789, but the characteristic traces of the disease – facial and body scarring – were often seen in survivors.

In June 1789, two months after the outbreak at Sydney Cove, Governor Phillip led an exploration party to the mouth of the Hawkesbury River, 25km north of the settlement. They left their boat and crew at the northern end of Port Jackson and travelled first along the beaches and then overland, using the well-established Aboriginal trails to meet their boat again at Broken Bay. Collins writes that the path they followed 'was in many places covered with skeletons, and the same spectacles were met with in the hollows of the rocks of that harbour'.[50] Hunter, who also accompanied the party, recounts their meeting with a group who had been fishing in the waters of the bay. On seeing the boat approaching:

> ... they all made their escape, except this miserable girl, who had just recovered from the small-pox, and was very weak, and unable, from a swelling in one of her knees, to get off to any distance ... she appeared to be about 17 or 18 years of age, and had covered her debilitated and naked body with the wet grass, having no other means of hiding herself.[51]

Governor Phillip commented that they had seen the traces of smallpox wherever they had been.[52] Further to the north-west, in the Wellington Valley some 300km from Sydney and on the western side of the Great Dividing Range, John Mair, a military surgeon, reported seeing three old men with the characteristic scarring when he was investigating the second epidemic in 1830. Mair attributed them as being survivors of the 1789 epidemic.[53] Each claimed to have had the disease when they were young and each in turn was among the few who were not infected in this outbreak.

Well south of the Sydney and Botany Bay region, the situation was similar. In 1803 Lieutenant Grant, aboard the *Lady Nelson*, entered Jervis Bay, 160km south of the settlement. He remarked that many of the Aboriginal men and women he saw were marked with smallpox scars.[54] In February of the same year J. Flemming, of the *Cumberland*, was on a voyage of exploration between Sydney and King Island in Bass Strait. He landed at Port Phillip Bay on the south coast, where he met a group of 11 Aboriginal people, probably Woiworung. Two of them appeared to be marked with smallpox sequelae.[55] Although Flemming does not say so, the scarred individuals he saw were most likely adults and probably males, as they were carrying spears. If these reports are accurate, and there appears little reason for doubt, then these Aboriginal people would have been children when the 1789 smallpox epidemic reached the lower east and south coasts of Australia. It is highly likely then that they were the survivors of the 1789 epidemic.

If these observations at Broken Bay, Wellington Valley, Jervis Bay and Port Phillip are correct, then smallpox appears to have spread among the Aboriginal populations, at least as far inland as the Wellington Valley in the north and Port Phillip on the southern coast. Both points were well beyond the European frontier in 1789. Apart from Cumpston's assertion of the 1789 smallpox epidemic reaching South Australia,[56] there is no evidence to suggest that this epidemic broke out of the coast and highlands belt and penetrated the interior of the continent.[57]

The epidemic was severe for the Aboriginal groups living around the Sydney settlement. The First Fleet records leave a stark picture of high morbidity and mortality from the disease. Governor Phillip wrote:

> It is not possible to determine the number of natives who were carried off by this fatal disorder. It must be great; and judging from the information of the native now living with us … one half of those who inhabit this part of the country died.[58]

While this was a crude estimate by Phillip, it may not have been so inaccurate. If this were the first episode of epidemic smallpox among this population, then they would not have been immunologically protected against it and high morbidity and mortality would be expected. The effects of variola major among other unprotected and virgin-soil populations elsewhere in the world has resulted in extraordinarily high mortality.[59] In these circumstances the disease affects both sexes and all age groups of the population and case fatality rates ranging from 25 per cent up to 80 per cent can be expected.

How severe then was the mortality among the groups around the Sydney settlement? If Phillip's estimate of 50 per cent mortality is accepted, then how many deaths does this represent? In May 1788, just weeks after the settlement was established, Governor Phillip estimated the number of Aboriginal people living in the vicinity of Botany Bay, Port Jackson and Broken Bay, to be '... no less than one thousand five hundred'.[60] There is no way of knowing how accurate this was but, once again, Phillip may have been close in his estimate.[61] Other population estimates based on area and density calculations suggest a population of between two and three thousand people belonging to three main linguistic groups (Tharawal, Dharug and Kuring-gai) living between Jervis Bay in the south to Broken Bay in the north.[62] Other estimates have a population of between 2600 and 5200 for an area of 1300km^2 of coastal strip around the settlement.[63] While there are certainly inaccuracies in these estimates they point to a substantial number of people inhabiting the coastal plains and hinterland north and south of the Sydney settlement. With a postulated fatality rate of 50 per cent (similar to the Americas), a likely number of deaths from the smallpox epidemic would therefore lay somewhere between 700 and 2600).

The realisation that many had died in this epidemic remained with the European colonists. In 1822 a Russian visiting Sydney recorded:

> Many of those who had settled in close proximity to the English colonists became infected with smallpox and thousands died, several generations perished.[64]

Whatever the real extent of mortality may have been, it was certainly high, and alarming to the Aboriginal groups affected. Apart from seeing the many bodies around the shores of Port Jackson, the colonists had the accounts of the friendly Aboriginal people to rely on for an estimation of the severity of mortality.

> As a proof of the numbers of those miserable people who were carried off by this disorder, Bennillong [*sic*] told us, that his friend Cole-be's [*sic*] tribe being reduced by its effects to three persons.[65]

In April 1791, when the first exploration expeditions reached the Nepean River region some 50km inland from the settlement, they were informed by their two Aboriginal guides that 'this part of the country was inhabited by the Bidigals, but that most of the tribe were dead of the smallpox'.[66] By April 1791, just over three years since they had landed, the general opinion of the colonists was that the disease was rampant in the Aboriginal populations, causing a shocking mortality. The mortality in regions further away from the settlement was unrecorded and so remains unknown.

The response by the Aboriginal people to the epidemic by those who did not die immediately was to abandon the coastal regions near the settlement. Immediately after the epidemic was noticed by the Europeans, Port Jackson and the environs of the settlement appeared deserted by Aboriginal people. How far and to where they fled is unknown, but whatever the case it was not for long. Small groups of Aboriginal people were soon sporadically sighted around Sydney and Botany Bay by exploration groups travelling outside the settlement.[67] Some four to six weeks after the epidemic, Aboriginal people began to be seen again on the waters of Port Jackson. On June 2nd Bradley wrote in his journal:

> Twenty canoes passed Sydney Cove going down the Harbour; this was the first time any number of them had been seen together since the small Pox having been among them.[68]

In November Hunter again recorded a group of 20 to 30 on the shores. Later that month a group was met under friendly terms and two males, Bennelong and Colbee, were enticed back into the settlement. One year after the epidemic a group of three hundred Aboriginal people, including Bennelong and Colbee, who had since escaped from the settlement, was seen at Manly Cove, Port Jackson, feasting on a whale that had recently become stranded on the beach.[69] However high the mortality had been, it would appear that large numbers of Aboriginal people were again occupying the coastal regions of Port Jackson, as little as 12 to 18 months after the epidemic was first noticed.

The disease had burned itself out and had disappeared at least from around the European settlement of Sydney. But like the epidemics of old it was to return within two generations and again cause terror and death among the Aboriginal people.

A Second Epidemic: 1828–32

In early 1829 explorer Charles Sturt returned from an expedition into the north-west of New South Wales and brought back with him what was probably the first indication of a second epidemic of smallpox among the Aboriginal populations. He and his party had traced the course of the Macquarie River into the interior and had reached the Darling River near the present town of Bourke. On February 5th, while he was following the Darling southward, he encountered a group of 70 Aboriginal huts that appeared to Sturt to be permanent habitations. Further on he encountered a group of Barundji who he believed to be the inhabitants of the village. Sturt and his party were approached by an elderly male. Sturt recorded:

> As his tribe gathered around him, the old chief threw a melancholy glance upon them, and endeavoured, as much as he could, to explain the cause of that affliction which, as I had rightly judged, weighed heavily upon him. It appeared, then, that a violent cutaneous disease raged throughout the tribe, that was sweeping them off in great numbers. He called several young men to Mr. Hume and myself, who had been attacked by this singular malady.[70]

Four or five days later, while resting in camp, another group of about 70 approached Sturt's party. The women and children of the group passed the camp by, but Sturt noticed that several of the men who came nearer were afflicted with what he believed to be the same 'violent cutaneous eruptions' he had just recently seen. Sturt believed that this disease was smallpox. He was of the opinion that it was causing a severe decline in the population as the number of Barundji he saw on the Darling River bore no comparison to the size and number of the huts he had seen.

Further indications that a second epidemic of smallpox was occurring among the Aboriginal populations west of the Great Dividing Range, near Bathurst, were brought to the notice of the colonial government in 1830.[71] In August of that year five Wiradjuri were observed by a local pastoralist, Andrew Brown, suffering from what was thought to be smallpox. Two were described as being in the incipient stages of the disease and the other three in the more advanced stages. One of these was later seen with smallpox sequelae on his body, and when questioned he indicated that the others had died. Two months later, in October, the same symptoms, together with a high mortality, were again reported among the Wiradjuri. The disease was active until at least December. In August of 1831, the same symptoms were again witnessed by Brown in three Wiradjuri who had been in contact with others recently arrived from the Lachlan River to the south. The disease was reported to be causing high mortality among the Lachlan River Wiradjuri, many of whom were fleeing the region. A European family residing near Bathurst was struck with the infection. Four of the family showed eruptive and febrile symptoms and one, a two-year-old girl, died. The disease had arisen after the family had taken in a Wiradjuri child whose parents had died from a disease with similar symptoms, and who likewise later died of the same disease. Another European family living some 40km from Bathurst were infected and lost a child to the disease. The governor of New South Wales, on reading reports of the disease suspected of being smallpox, became concerned. He ordered an investigation and sent Dr John Mair, assistant surgeon to the 39th Regiment, to investigate.[72]

Mair was too late to witness firsthand the disease among the Wiradjuri but from accounts by eyewitnesses, whom he deemed to be credible observers, he pieced together the symptoms of the disease. While there appeared to be a variety of forms of the disease in different individuals, there were common signs and symptoms consistent with untreated smallpox infection. The initial pre-eruptive stages were characterised by a general malaise and fever lasting from two to eight days, accompanied by loss of appetite, headaches and chest and abdominal pains. The eruptive stage followed, with focal lesions of small 'red spots' (papules) resembling 'flea bites' commencing on the face and gradually spreading over the head, breast and extremities. Eruptions on the mucus surfaces (enanthema) occurred at this time, with lesions developing on the tongue and lips. The rash spread and in many instances the soles of the feet were observed to be studded with lesions. After the eruption had developed, usually observed to have occurred in 24 hours, the fever subsided. At this time, the patient experienced pain in the throat, most likely from enanthema on the pharynx, making it difficult to swallow solid foods. After three to eight days the red spots developed into raised vesicles containing a milky fluid in some and in others a 'yellowish' or 'straw-coloured' fluid. At their height, the lesions were the size of a 'small or large pea'. Scabs formed from the vesicles at different periods according to the length of time it took to reach maturation. These were occasionally confluent on the nose and cheeks and frequently left permanent scars or indurations on the skin. There appeared to be little doubt by the observers who witnessed the disease among the Aboriginal people that it was indeed smallpox. They were familiar with smallpox signs and symptoms, having seen it in England. While Mair did not see an active case of smallpox during his investigation, he did observe the telltale scarring on some of the survivors and stated they 'cannot be distinguished from the pits of Small Pox'. He was confident that the disease was smallpox and reported back to the colonial authorities. Aboriginal people from the Bathurst area called the disease 'boulol', and those from the Lachlan River and Wellington Valley region 'hunna hunna'.[73]

Mair's conclusions of a smallpox epidemic, however, did not go unchallenged. Dr George Busby had qualified as a surgeon at Edinburgh in 1824 and migrated to New South Wales, where he entered government service in 1828. He was put in charge of the convict hospital in Bathurst, where he resided for the rest of his life. In 1830 he was 'Johnny-on-the-spot' as far as the outbreak was concerned and was asked by the government for his opinion on the outbreak. In a report to the Sydney inspector of colonial hospitals, he concluded that the disease was varicella (chickenpox) and not smallpox.[74] Busby's observations, however, were not as extensive as Mair's. He saw only two Wiradjuri from the Bathurst district showing clinical symptoms but could not determine the nature of their affliction. He based his diagnosis solely on the symptoms he monitored in a European male, Tilman, who was confined in the Bathurst Hospital on August 6th 1831 under his care. Tilman was 40 years old and had been living in the same house as an Aboriginal person who had caught the disease and later died. He informed Busby that he had suffered from smallpox as a boy, being one of a family of six, all of whom had the disease at the same time. Tilman's symptoms were generally milder than those described by Mair in the Wiradjuri. Tilman complained of headache, pains in the back and limbs, lassitude, loss of appetite, nausea and fever. The primary fever was, however, severe and lasted until the eruptive phase, which was followed by secondary fever. The vesicles appeared earlier, achieved maturity quickly, covering most of the body, and were particularly numerous on the face, shoulders, back and lateral surfaces of the legs. As was often the case of a secondary bout of infection by smallpox virus Tilman's symptoms lasted for 14 days, terminating in his full recovery.[75]

Busby's view that the disease he had observed was not smallpox but varicella was based first on the modified nature of the symptoms he saw in Tilman and second on Tilman's previous infection with smallpox. In response to the prevailing epidemic among the Aboriginal population he concluded:

> I am, upon the whole, at present disposed to regard the eruptive disease lately prevalent among the black natives in this district as varicella, but possessing by no means a malignant character, nor likely, under ordinary circumstances of comfort and attention attainable in civilized society, to prove fatal in more than a few instances; the mortality it has occasioned among the blacks being sufficiently accounted for by the unfavourable circumstances in which they are placed.[76]

Mair, on the other hand, refuted Busby's diagnosis and stated that Tilman's infection was a case of secondary modified smallpox because it passed through the regular stages, albeit quickly, of ordinary smallpox. He also examined the patient about six weeks after his discharge from hospital. He described the skin on Tilman's face having a 'mottled appearance of red and white, burning scales were separating from it, and numerous small pits or depressions could be discerned', some recent and others older, which further strengthened his diagnosis.[77]

Busby's conclusion that the disease affecting the Wiradjuri was varicella was, however, supported by Inspector of Colonial Hospitals Dr James Bowman.[78] Bowman, a naval surgeon, had first arrived in New South Wales in 1816. He was later appointed as principal surgeon to the colony, where he made improvements to the nursing staff and dietary regime of the Sydney hospital wards. However, he blotted his copybook with the governor when involved in some shady deals with cattle and sheep sales.[79] In his role as inspector of colonial hospitals, Bowman chose to dispute and dismiss Mair's diagnosis of smallpox and cast doubts on the reliability and integrity of his witnesses. Writing to the colonial secretary, he claimed that Mair was incorrect in his diagnosis and had formed his opinions that the disease was smallpox from information he received from persons incapable of determining 'so important a point', despite Mair's assertions to the contrary. Bowman also suggested the disease among the Wiradjuri was not smallpox but varicella, which while common in the colony at that time was of little threat. He called it 'native pock' (incorrectly believed by some to be a local form of varicella). It was a convenient conclusion (albeit incorrect) by Bowman. The authorities were more comfortable with the assumption that the disease was a mild outbreak of varicella, which would cause no panic or disruption to the colony, as would the terrible spectre of smallpox raging through the population.

Bowman presented these arguments to the governor and members of the executive council of the colony in December 1831. The council readily agreed with Bowman and passed over the whole matter of the epidemic apart from recommending a government notice should be published stating that suspicion had arisen as to the current prevalence of smallpox. They recommended that voluntary vaccination could be obtained from any of the colonial surgeons. They also agreed that measures should be taken 'generally to induce the Aboriginal Natives also to submit to vaccination'.[80]

Mair had spent several days riding around the region collecting evidence from those who had observed the disease. He reported on varied clinical symptoms among the Aboriginal populations. Among those in the Wellington Valley, where a missionary station had recently been established by the Christian Mission Society, Mair reported that the vesicles began to coalesce on the face during the eruptive stage, to be followed in a day or two by excessive salivation. An escaped convict who had lived among these people before and during the epidemic described 'water pouring from the mouth as they lay on the ground'. About the 10th or 12th day after the initial symptoms were noticed, many patients were seen to experience convulsions and the fluid discharge from the mouth became more bloody and viscid in appearance. The bloody discharge from the mouth and its late onset may be indicative of bleeding from the oral mucous membranes, a symptom of the more fatal haemorrhagic type of variola major.[81]

Among the Wiradjuri living on the Lachlan River and Wellington Valley regions, death generally resulted after the third day of the eruptive stage. Mair reported that secondary fever was seldom observed among these groups and, when it did occur, he suggested it was due to local low ambient temperatures. The rarity of secondary fever, which usually begins on the seventh or eighth days in severe cases, can be explained by the early fatality of most of the victims. Many were reported to have died at the very onset of the disease, before the beginning of the eruptive stage.

Most of the eyewitnesses consulted by Mair remarked that the disease proved chiefly fatal to adults and the elderly but seldom to children, even though their length of exposure to infected individuals was the same. However, it was reported to Mair by several of the observers that many adults who bore pockmarks on their skin, evidence of a previous exposure to smallpox, escaped the disease altogether.[82]

The usual duration of the disease was stated to be between 14 and 21 days in cases where the patient survived and was restored to health. Many patients who did survive were unable to walk for a considerable time due to the separation of the epidermis from the soles of the feet. In other survivors more of the characteristic forms of smallpox sequelae were present. Severe keratitis and/or corneal ulcerations were reported in several victims who recovered from the infection. Andrew Brown, one of Mair's trusted observers who had seen the disease firsthand stated to Mair:

> … I found one middle aged woman who had lost her sight altogether by it, one who had lost an eye, and two children male and female who had each been deprived of an eye by it.[83]

In others, secondary infections left the sufferer with ulcerations in different parts of the body where the smallpox lesions had occurred.

Among those who escaped infection it was observed that some had been exposed to smallpox before. Brown informed Mair that it extended to most of the Aboriginal people he saw. He did, however, see three old men with 'evident marks', who informed him that they had been infected by the same disease when very young. Others had been vaccinated (or variolated) by European settlers several years prior to the epidemic. During the epidemic Mair vaccinated many of the Aboriginal people he encountered. He met with little opposition among them, most of whom had come to realise the benefits that the simple procedure conferred in the face of the serious morbidity and mortality caused by the epidemic. After his return to Sydney, Mair sent supplies of recent and dried vaccine lymph to the colonial assistant surgeon at Bathurst for future use.

The disease was not limited to the Aboriginal communities around Bathurst. Government surveyor and explorer Thomas Mitchell also observed Aboriginal people suffering from the epidemic. On December 5th 1831 Mitchell and his expedition crossed the Liverpool Range, north of Bathurst, which at that time divided the settled areas from the unexplored districts of the colony. He recorded:

> We reached at length, a water-course called 'Currungai' and encamped upon its bank, beside the natives from Dart Brook, who had crossed the range before us, apparently to join some of their tribe, who lay at this place extremely ill, being affected with a virulent kind of small-pox. We found the helpless creatures, stretched on their backs, beside the water, under the shade of the wattle or mimosa trees, to avoid the intense heat of the sun. We gave them from our stock some medicine; and the wretched sufferers seemed to place the utmost confidence in its efficacy.[84]

According to Mitchell these people he saw were from another region as they had little knowledge of the countryside they were now in. Mitchell continued his journey to the north, reaching the Gwyder River, but made no further mention of smallpox among the Aboriginal groups he encountered.

From these districts the epidemic spread along the river systems far in front of the colonial frontiers. Firsthand observations of the epidemic by Europeans were now no longer possible. From the upper Darling it spread downstream. In 1835 Mitchell was again exploring beyond the frontier, following the southerly course of the Darling River. On May 28th, while at his base camp at Bourke, he was visited by a group of Aboriginal people. They consisted of four adult males, seven females and children. Mitchell remarked that most of them had visible smallpox scarring 'but the marks were not larger than pin heads'.[85] From Bourke, Mitchell and his expedition continued along the Darling River as far as Menindee, 190km above its junction with the River

Murray. He turned back on July 12th after an affray with the Barkindji. He had seen smallpox scarring on many of the Aboriginal people during the journey. At Menindee he recorded:

> These natives, as well as most others seen by us on the river, bore strong marks of the small-pox, or some such disease, which appeared to have been very destructive among them. The marks appeared chiefly on the nose, and did not exactly resemble those of the small-pox with us, inasmuch as the deep scars and grooves left the original surface and skin in isolated specks on these people, whereas the effects of small-pox with us appear in little isolated hollows, no parts of the higher surface being detached like islands, as they appeared on the noses of these natives.[86]

Mitchell may have observed the sequelae of confluent-type smallpox. He was of the opinion (correct) that the disease had been severe and had caused a great mortality among the groups living along the Darling River.

The epidemic did not reach the Murray River populations until at least the second half of 1830. In January of that year Charles Sturt, on his second expedition of exploration, began a journey down the Murrumbidgee and Murray rivers. He arrived at the termination of the river systems at Lake Alexandrina, in what was to be the colony of South Australia, on February 9th, passing the Darling River junction on his way. Sturt was an astute observer and documenter, describing the landscape, geology, the people and their state of health in some detail.[87] Along the Murray he noted that 'the most violent cutaneous eruptions' were affecting many of the Aboriginal people he encountered and remarked on their 'miserable state of disease and infirmity', Sturt was in two minds as to what the disease actually was, describing it in one instance as leprosy and in another as syphilis. He made no suggestion, however, that it was due to smallpox, a disease he was surely familiar with among Europeans in Britain and had seen just one year before among the Aboriginal populations of the upper Darling. Neither did he mention seeing any Aboriginal people with smallpox-like sequelae that would have indicated a previous epidemic. Sturt returned the way he had come, along the Murray and Murrumbidgee system, arriving back in Sydney in late May.

In 1830 the middle and lower Murray River corridor was well beyond the European frontier and the spread of smallpox went unobserved, and hence unrecorded, by Europeans. There is, however, some indication that the epidemic had reached the populations of the lower Murray well before the first European settlement was established on the Adelaide plains in 1836. In February 1838 Joseph Hawdon and Charles Bonney overlanded the first herd of cattle along the Murray to the newly established settlement of Adelaide.[88] Hawdon and Bonney were to be the first of several overlanders to drive cattle and sheep along the Murray and Darling route to Adelaide. On February 11th Hawdon set camp near the present town of Swan Hill on the Murray and met up with a group of Wadi Wadi people.

> In the evening some of the Blacks came to Swan Hill, where we were encamped. After holding a little conversation with us across the river, they swam over to us. They were fine, well-made men about five feet eleven inches in height. Their faces were nearly all marked with smallpox, but otherwise their features were pleasing.[89]

The next day Hawdon saw 52 men, accompanied by women and children, and described them as 'not a good-looking set of men' and many of them 'blind in one eye'. Hawdon makes no further mention of smallpox sequelae although he met several more large groups along his way.

Hawdon's observations of smallpox sequelae alone could not be accepted as being reliable evidence of a former smallpox epidemic. However, later the same year (1838) Charles Sturt followed Hawdon's trail along the Murray corridor, also bringing cattle to the colonists at Adelaide.[90] His observations of smallpox sequelae support Hawdon's. Approximately five kilometres below the junction of the Murray and Murrumbidgee rivers he came across a large group of Aboriginal people.

> ... in the course of the forenoon we were joined by various parties from different quarters that when united formed a considerable body of athletic and well proportioned men. They came with the most peaceable intentions and several of them assisted us in our work. I observed many of them as if pitted by the Small Pox, or that would appear as the disease which was having such a fearful effect upon them when I was on the banks of the Darling in 1828 and the Hume [the Murray above the junction of the Darling] in 1829. It must have committed dreadful havoc amongst them, since on this journey I did not see hundreds to the thousands I saw on my former expeditions.[91]

Smallpox was present on the eastern coast by late 1831. In October of that year two Aboriginal men brought an ill convict, Richard Scarme, to the European settlement at Port Macquarie. Scarme had escaped from the penal settlement at Moreton Bay, in what is now Queensland, some time before and had been living with a group of Dainggatti people near the mouth of the

Macleay River at Trial Bay, 60km north of Port Macquarie. He stated that he had seen more than 50 ill with smallpox, a disease he had seen in England before he was transported. The military officer in command of Port Macquarie, Captain Smyth, stated that Scarme was recovering from a disease that bore a 'striking resemblance to the Smallpox'. Scarme was held in custody and later sent to Sydney, where he was seen by Dr Mair and Dr Imlay. They examined him and reported that his skin bore unequivocal marks of the recent epidemic of smallpox. Scarme said he had not previously suffered from smallpox or cowpox and he bore no vaccination scar.[92]

Six weeks after they had brought Scarme into Port Macquarie, the same two Aboriginal men returned to the settlement. Captain Smyth described them as covered from 'head to foot' with the disease. By late December, the Dainggatti living around the Port Macquarie settlement were in turn infected. Many of the worst cases recovered but five died, all of whom were young and had previously been in good health. The disease did not affect the European population. Smyth isolated the Dainggatti by keeping them on the opposite bank of the river that flowed through the settlement.

As the European frontiers expanded in later years, many of the settlers noted smallpox scarring among Aboriginal people with whom they had frequent contact. Peter Beveridge, a squatter who held a property on the Murray River below Swan Hill for 23 years from 1845, and who acquired an extensive knowledge of the Aboriginal people, commented on the smallpox epidemic and its timing:

> All the very old aboriginals in the Colony [Victoria] show very distinct traces of small-pox, and in speaking of the scourge which has so indelibly left the marks of its foul presence, they say that it came with the waters, that is it followed down the rivers in the early flood season (about July or August), laying its death-clutch on every tribe in its progress.[93]

Further evidence of the epidemic spreading along the Murray comes from accounts by Aboriginal survivors. In South Australia, a survivor of the epidemic, a Ngarrindjeri woman from the Lower Murray and Coorong region named Clulwuwyrie (Jenny Pougie), died in 1911. She remembered the first visit by Sturt to the Murray in 1830 when she was a child and related that the disease, which left her with pockmarks and carried off many of her people, came soon after Sturt had gone.[94] Another woman, Kontinyeri (Louisa Karpeny), possibly the niece of Clulwuwyrie, could also recount her experience of the epidemic. She lived most of her life on the southern shore of Lake Alexandrina and as a small child could remember her first sight of Europeans, soldiers arriving at the lake at the time the colony of South Australia was established, in 1836. She was interviewed by Edward Stirling, a consulting surgeon in Adelaide but whose main interest was Aboriginal anthropology. Stirling was the medical officer and anthropologist with the Horn expedition, which, in 1894, made a comprehensive survey of the arid regions of South Australia between Oodnadatta and the MacDonnell Ranges. He was the author of the anthropological section published as part of the four volumes that recorded the expedition's discoveries. Clulwuwyrie described to Stirling the coming of the sickness, which was several years before the arrival of the soldiers:

> The old black spoke of the coming of a strong West wind which made the reeds all tremble, and this, she said, was taken as a sure sign that the sickness was coming ... She described how the faces of those affected with the disease came out all over [with] spots, and how that many died of it, including many children.[95]

Another survivor, an old man named Malo, who lived at Moorundie on the lower Murray, related that when he was a small boy there was a sickness among his people that killed many and left him with scarring on his face. Dr De Lisle, of the 96th Regiment, examined the scarring on Malo many years later and concluded that he had undoubtedly suffered from smallpox.[96] Three old Aboriginal men from nearby Swanport often spoke to Europeans about a great sickness that came along the Murray causing a great number of deaths. Such was the scale of mortality that the living could not cope with disposal of the dead. They described that those who were inflicted by the disease broke out in spots all over their bodies. Another account comes from a 35-year-old male from Lake Alexandrina who bore smallpox sequelae on his face. He related to Stirling that as a small boy a 'big one wind' came from the east, carrying the sickness, and caused the marks on his face.[97]

George Augustus Robinson, Aboriginal protector for Port Phillip (Victoria) noted the presence of smallpox sequelae during a journey through the southern highlands. In 1844 he spent three days among a group of 300 Aboriginal people near the present town of Yass. He noted that 'the virulent effects of Variola or Small Pox was apparent'. Near Gundagai he reported that the Aboriginal populations in the Murrumbidgee valley and surrounding highlands were 'strongly marked with smallpox'. Robinson does not give the ages of the individuals he saw bearing smallpox sequelae but as his sightings came a decade after the last epidemic, as opposed to 55 years since the first, the former occurrence of the disease would most likely have been the cause.[98]

As the European frontiers extended north into Queensland, many of the colonists saw the telltale sequelae on the faces of the survivors. During the 1850s and 1860s pockmarked Aboriginal people were regularly seen and reported along the coastal regions as far as the Gulf of Carpentaria. Inland the extent of the pockmarking was seen north of the Darling, along its tributaries and near Cloncurry.

There is little evidence of the severity and extent of the epidemic south of the Murray River and its Victorian tributaries. There is no evidence at all that the 1830s epidemic reached the Kurnai people living in the Gippsland ranges in eastern Victoria, and indeed this region appears to have escaped altogether.[99] Prior to European occupation, distinct social, political, linguistic and economic boundaries existed between the Kurnai groups of Gippsland and surrounding populations, resulting in exclusion and mutual hostility. This disjunction of the Gippsland populations from their neighbours would most likely have acted as a deterrent to other Aboriginal groups fleeing the epidemic to enter Kurnai territories and so acted as a barrier to the transmission of smallpox.

The epidemic also seems to have missed the groups living in South Australia's Mallee districts south of the River Murray valley. Unlike inland New South Wales, no active cases of smallpox were seen by the early settlers in Victoria. This is not surprising, as the European settlement was only permanently established in 1834 at Port Phillip Bay (Melbourne), well after the epidemic was at its peak. A few of the settlers do, however, report seeing Aboriginal people bearing the characteristic sequelae that would be expected if there had been a previous severe epidemic of smallpox.

Before this settlement there had been a failed attempt to establish a southern outpost of the colony of New South Wales in September 1803 at Port Phillip Bay. William Buckley, a convict at this settlement, escaped in that same year and lived with the Wathaurong near the present city of Geelong for 32 years. After his return to European life he became known as the 'wild white man'. He recollected:

> I never observed any European contagious disease prevalent in the least degree; and this I thought strange. There was at one time however, I now recollect, a complaint which spread through the country, occasioning the loss of many lives, attacking generally the healthiest and strongest, whom it appeared to fix upon in preference to the more weakly. It was a dreadful swelling of the feet, so that they were unable to move about, being also afflicted with ulcers of a very painful kind.[100]

Buckley's description of the disease is vague. Although there is no other evidence for it, he may be referring to an epidemic that had preceded his association with the Wathaurong and that he had heard about through their recollections. Smallpox does affect the soles of the feet and, if secondary bacterial infection occurs, could cause the ulceration and swelling that Buckley describes. Such symptoms, two among the many of smallpox, may be all that Buckley was informed of, or all that he could recollect being told. But there are other problems with Buckley's account. Buckley was largely illiterate and the record of his life among the Wathaurong was written for him, after his return to the European colonists, by John Morgan, who had interviewed Buckley at length. It is impossible to discern just how much Morgan's impressions and conceptions misconstrue Buckley's reminiscences. Therefore, any diagnosis of smallpox made on this evidence can only be uncertain at best. Yet it is still intriguing that Buckley did not identify the disease as smallpox.

Several of the early colonists of Victoria do refer to smallpox south of the river systems. James Dawson, a pastoralist and amateur ethnologist, spent much time with the Aboriginal people of south-western Victoria. He learned the local dialects and in 1881 published a book on their languages and customs. He briefly discussed smallpox and thought the epidemic had caused high mortality on the south coast, particularly on the coastal dunes to the east of Port Fairy.[101] It was, however, a common misconception of the time that many of the extensive Aboriginal burial areas in the coastal and riverine dune systems, often with exposed skeletons, contained the victims of smallpox and were a direct consequence of the high mortality wrought by the epidemic. Radiocarbon dates from several of these burial sites have since shown an extended antiquity, in some cases dating back into the late Pleistocene, indicative of a long and consistent use for burial purposes.[102] Edward Curr, another Victorian pastoralist, compiled two volumes on Australian Aboriginal people in 1886. He discussed smallpox among the Aboriginal populations but cited no strong evidence for the 1830s epidemic in Victoria and relied mainly on secondary evidence from New South Wales and the Murray River corridor for his information.[103]

As well as leaving marks on the faces of the survivors, the epidemic left its traces in the oral traditions of Aboriginal people. Among the Aboriginal groups affected by the epidemic, smallpox was given many names. In the river districts of central and western New South Wales, where the epidemic was first recorded, it was called 'booert', and on the Darling River, where the first active cases were seen by Sturt, it was called 'mungga'. North of the Darling, among the Muruwari of the Narran River region, it was called 'dunnerh-dunnerh'. The Wiradjuri from the Wellington Valley referred to the disease as 'danna-danna' and to the sequelae as 'gulgog-gulgog'. In the western districts of Victoria, the epidemic was called 'meen warann', and among the Dhiari of northern South Australia it was called 'moora moora'. Years after the event a song or chant, known as 'Mallae Mallae' in Victoria and 'Nguyapalti' in South Australia, was performed by many groups in remembrance of the epidemic and the many who died from it throughout south-eastern Australia.[104]

James Dawson wrote:

> They called it Meen warann – 'chopped root.' They have still a very vivid recollection of its ravages, and of the great numbers cut off by it in the Western District. In remembrance of it they still chant a wail called Mallae mallaeae, which was composed in New South Wales, where the disease first broke out and is known to all the tribes between Sydney, Melbourne, and Adelaide. The malady spread with rapidity from tribe to tribe, in consequence of the infection being carried by the messengers who were sent forward to communicate the sad new of its ravages. It was considered to be so infectious and deadly, that when anyone sickened and refused food, and when pustules appeared on the body, the tribal doctor gave them up at once, and the friends deserted them, leaving beside them in the wurun a vessel of water to drink. When they died, the body was allowed to decay where it was; and, long afterwards, when all infection was supposed to be gone, and nothing left but bones, some of the relatives returned, and burned the wurun and the remains. If a mother was affected by the disease, her child was immediately removed and given to female relatives to rear, while the mother was left to die. The aborigines say that the Meen warann came from the west in form of a dense mist; and that the chief places of mortality were round the Moyne lagoon, and on the sand hummocks to the east of Port Fairy.[105]

The assignment of blame for the epidemic by the Aboriginal people was attributed in some instances to the Europeans, in others to the malevolent magic of neighbouring tribes or to mythical entities. Like the other major diseases of syphilis, gonorrhoea, influenza and tuberculosis that had severe effects on the Aboriginal people, they often saw the occurrence of smallpox as a direct result of the arrival of Europeans among them. Sturt was blamed by the Wiradjuri of the Wellington Valley. He and his expedition passed through that region in 1828, just as the smallpox epidemic was advancing along the river systems. Others in the same region placed the blame for the epidemic on Darrawirgal, a mythical entity who lived far to the west of Wellington. They believed that Darrawirgal was angry for the want of a tomahawk and so sent the disease among them. When the epidemic subsided, they assumed that he had finally obtained one and the disease would therefore not return. The malignant power of the Rainbow Serpent Mindye, was believed to be the source of the disease in Victoria. Ahead of the colonial frontiers, where Aboriginal groups were yet to have direct contact with Europeans, the blame was apportioned to neighbours. Among the Muruwari, traditional enemies were claimed to have sent the disease on the winds, which hung it on trees over camps to drop on to its victims.[106] Clulwuwyrie, the Ngarrindjeri survivor from the lower Murray, often spoke of a peculiar wind-like noise immediately preceding the arrival of smallpox, which came among her people from the east.[107]

This epidemic may have been present among the Aboriginal groups on the west and north coasts. One settler, who described himself as 'An Old Australian', recollected:

> While residing at Swan River [Perth] for 12 years from 1840 I knew several old natives who were deeply pitted [scarred] with what we believed to be small-pox, which they had suffered from long prior to the settlement of the colony in 1829.I remember joining in a discussion on the subject between Governor Hutt and Dr. Harris, the colonial surgeon, when the latter expressed his conviction that the marks had been occasioned by small-pox, and thought it might have been introduced by the French towards the end of the last century, or possibly by some whaler.[108]

Vague though it is (and likely incorrect as to its origin) this may be the first indication of smallpox among Aboriginal people in the Western Australian colony. There were no recorded outbreaks among Aboriginal populations in the 1830s, when the colony was being established, and the Benedictine missionary, Bishop Rosendo Salvado, who established an Aboriginal mission at New Norcia in 1846, stated after two years that smallpox was 'quite unknown to the Australian native'.[109]

A Third Epidemic: 1850s–1860s

German-born Paul Foelsche was the first inspector of police in the Northern Territory. He arrived in Darwin in 1870, when conflict between the Aboriginal people and the settlers was becoming widespread. Five years after his arrival he sent a police party to pursue Aboriginal people who had attacked a telegraph station on the Roper River, south of Darwin, killing the station master. His orders were to capture any who could be identified as the attackers 'dead or alive' and that 'prompt action' should be taken to prevent any who escaped. 'I cannot give you orders to shoot all natives you come across,' he wrote, 'but circumstances may occur for which I cannot provide definite instructions.'[110] Despite his willingness to condone violence against Aboriginal people, he later made an effort to establish an interest in their culture and customs. In 1881 he wrote an authoritative paper, *Notes on the Aborigines of North Australia*, which was read to the Royal Society of South Australia.[111]

Foelsche interviewed a 25-year-old Aboriginal man, named Mangminone (or 'Mr Knight', as he was known among the Europeans), whose face was deeply pitted by smallpox scarring. Mangminone told of an epidemic that occurred when he was about five years of age, called 'goowimnah' by the people around Port Darwin. The disease began in the northern dry season, May to August, when the people burned the grasslands. Mangminone recounts that old and young alike were stricken with the disease and that the deaths were so many that it was impossible to carry out proper burial customs, with the dead left lying about. Many of those who survived were permanently scarred and blinded. The epidemic lasted through the dry season and by the onset of the wet season in November it had disappeared. Aboriginal people around the Port Darwin settlement were sure it had come from neighbouring groups from the Alligator River, 170km to the east, where it travelled westward along the coast.[112]

The epidemic almost certainly reached into the inland populations, as Foelsche states that 'pock-marked' Aborigines, survivors of the epidemic, were still to be found long distances from the coast. Another of Foelsche's informants, an Aboriginal male given the European name of 'Jack Davis' who was able to converse fluently in English and the Malay dialect of the seasonally arriving trepang fishers, told him that elders remembered a disease they named 'meeha-meeha' had swept through the coastal populations of the north and 'killed plenty blackfellows' and that, 'by-and-by Meeha-Meeha will come again' when he is an old man. It is uncertain what time is being referred to here but, if it was prior to European settlement on the east coast in 1788, these people may well have been the first recorded Indigenous deaths from smallpox in Australia.[113]

Foelsche continued:

> The position of the Port Essington natives of the appearance of Small-pox in their tribes is very similar to that of the Darwin natives. Some of the

> Port Essington tribes called it Yi'arick; also Unallah, now numbering about thirty all told, who had the disease, are still alive, and from information gathered from them, it leaves no doubt that the malady raged there the time and year it was at Port Darwin. They state it was a long time ago, and after the soldiers had left (the old settlement was abandoned in December, 1849), and came one year, shortly after the Malay Prahus had started back for Mocassar [*sic*] (bout the end of May), and when the grass was burnt it came to the tribes to the eastward of them, and went on to the Alligator and other tribes to the west of them. Plenty of old and young (and even dogs) [?] died, but by the time the rain came on (about October or November), the disease had disappeared.[114]

Foelsche and his Aboriginal informant Jack Davis were mistaken in thinking that the dogs were dying of the same disease. Smallpox was a disease specific to humans.

The remedy used by the Aboriginal people of the area was the thick milky exudate taken from the leafless stems of caustic bush (*Sarcostemna astrale*), found along the northern coastline. They called it 'gaoloowurrah'. The stems were snapped open and the white sap spread on to the smallpox pustules until they formed scabs, then washed off. The remedy was thought to be a sure cure for smallpox by the Aboriginal people but could in some cases result in the loss of eyesight.

Foelsche was quite adamant that the disease was smallpox and was brought into the coastal populations by Makassan fishermen on the north coast. Makassans (or Macassans) was a general term used for the crews of fishing fleets that regularly came to the north coast of Australia from South Sulawesi, in what is now Indonesia. Makassar held a strong influence over trade markets in the eastern Indonesian archipelago and would regularly send fleets of fishing prahus to the northern coastline of Australia to collect trepang, turtle shells and pearl shells. The links with the north coast of Australia began around the middle 1700s and continued until 1907, when the South Australian government, which administered the Northern Territory at the time, passed legislation to ban the Makassan fleets in a bid to control the trade. The crews of the prahus were an ethnic mix of Makassans, Bugis, Papua-New Guineans, Javanese, Sumba and Badjuese. They would follow the monsoon winds, usually in December, and make the trip from their Indonesian archipelago in 10 to 15 days. In December 1802, Matthew Flinders, making his way in the *Investigator* charting the northern coastline, encountered traces of their activities on the Sir Edward

Pellew islands in the Gulf of Carpentaria. He found earthen jars, trees cut with metal axes, 'remnants of bamboo lattice work, palm leaves sewed with cotton thread into the form of such hats as are worn by the Chinese, and the remains of blue cotton trowsers [*sic*], of the fashion called moormans'. But what puzzled him most was a line of stones forming a low wall forming 'compartments' and the charcoal remains of fires in each.[115] What Flinders did not know at the time was that he had found the remnants of a Makassan fishing and processing camp abandoned from a previous season. In February 1803 Flinders encountered a fleet of six boats off the coast of north-eastern Arnhem Land. And five more were to arrive while he was at anchor. He met the fleet commander, an elderly man named Pobassoo, who informed him that a fleet of 60 boats with over a thousand men were presently working along the northern coast.[116] A few months later the French commander, Nicholas Baudin, encountered more along the Kimberley coast far to the west.[117] The crew of the fishing fleets set up camps, in some cases numbering up to two hundred men, catching the trepang and drying them for transport back to Indonesia and ultimately to markets in China. The fleets would stay on the north coast until April then leave to follow the monsoon winds back home. While on the north coast of Australia they had regular contact with Aboriginal communities, who would assist them with their catches and trade goods with them. Associating closely with the Aboriginal people during the five to six months of their stay, regular introduction of pathogens was inevitable. Smallpox was endemic throughout much of South-east Asia at the time and, with its infectious period up to 21 days from initial infection, it is quite reasonable to conclude that the disease could have entered Australia a number of times, carried by the fishing fleets.

Foelsche wrote:

> Malay Prahus, about 30 in number, visit the coast eastward from Port Essington to Blue Mud Bay, in the Gulf of Carpentaria, every year in search of Beche-de-mer, and have done so in all probability for centuries past. They arrive from Mocassar at the beginning of January, and leave again at the end of May. During the time they are here, they employ all the coast tribes trepanging for them, and they all live close together, and I think there can be doubt as to the small-pox having been brought to the shores by them, and on the last occasion by a Prahu that visited the Gulf, for they leave as soon as the South-east Monsoon has fairly set in, and shortly after the Prahus had left, the disease appeared, coming up the coast with the S.E. winds, as stated by the natives, and travelled

> through all the tribes to the westward. Is it not likely that this terrible disease, 'The Small-pox', was introduced here by these trepang fishers some hundreds of years ago, and then spread gradually all over the Continent?[118]

Smallpox made its appearance again in epidemic form in late 1866. It was recorded during a six-month period among Aboriginal people living on the arid west coast of South Australia, on the periphery of European settlement, and into the inland regions. The first reports of this third outbreak were made by police in the remote regions of Streaky Bay and Venus in late October and early November of 1866. They noted an epidemic disease among the Wirangu and Nawu that was causing damaging skin eruptions on many who regularly visited the settlements.

When informed, the initial reaction of the medical authorities in Adelaide was that it was just another outbreak of the 'native pock' and therefore of little concern to the colonists. (Native pock was a contemporary euphemism given to impetigo contagiosa, a staphylococcal disease of the skin common among Aboriginal people and, while sometimes confused with smallpox, has no relationship with the latter.) The Vaccination Board of South Australia was, however, more cautious. Its primary concern was to protect the colony from any outbreak of smallpox that may occur, through a program of vaccination aimed at rendering the whole population immune. Any outbreak of smallpox in the colony, whether among the European or Aboriginal communities, was therefore to be given immediate attention. The board instructed a government medical officer, Dr Robert Gething, to leave at the earliest opportunity to investigate the outbreak and carry out a vaccination program among the European and Aboriginal populations.

Gething spent 21 days travelling the coastal regions between the two bays, meeting Aboriginal groups and vaccinating as many as he could. On January 12th 1867, approximately 50km from Streaky Bay, Gething met a group of Wirangu suffering from the disease

> … which had all the characteristics of having been pure variola; but which in these cases seemed to have been singularly mild, as there could be only three or four deaths distinctly traced to that cause.[119]

Although his report to the Vaccination Board did not describe clinical signs, Gething was in no doubt that the disease he saw in these people was smallpox and not 'native pock'. His initial diagnosis of smallpox was soon strengthened:

> The next day the natives I had seen the previous day came down to me at the Bay, bringing with them others who had had the disease somewhat more recently, thereby enabling me to see it in another phase. This strengthened my opinion as to the nature of the disease, which was confirmed on an after occasion.[120]

Gething vaccinated as many Wirangu as he could and then proceeded south to Venus Bay. There he met a group of Nawu suffering from the disease, one of whom was a young female in the stages of secondary fever 'suffering unmistakably from pure variola'. This particular case was probably exhibiting the earliest stages of smallpox that Gething had so far encountered.

The extent of the smallpox epidemic may have extended further than the bay regions visited by Gething. To the west of Streaky Bay, and at the limit of European occupation, a hut-keeper at Fowlers Bay wrote to *The South Australian Register* informing them that the Wirangu there were 'very much diseased' and that many of them had died.[121] He queried why Gething, who had attended at Streaky Bay, had not made his way further west to treat the Aboriginal people with smallpox.

More observations of the extent of the epidemic came from the Aboriginal sub-protector responsible for a large portion of central and northern South Australia. Sub-Protector Buttfield, a former Methodist minister, had only recently taken up his position and had travelled extensively, meeting many of the Aboriginal groups living in regions remote from European settlements. On the south-east coast of Eyre Peninsula, he reported that during the first six months of 1867 the Nawu in the region of Port Lincoln had been suffering from the same disease as that previously notified by Gething near Streaky Bay. In the Mount Remarkable region, near the present town of Port Augusta, Buttfield reported to the acting protector that Aboriginal people (Nukunu) were suffering from an eruptive skin disease 'resembling in some of its characteristics, smallpox'. Buttfield reported no deaths from this disease and those infected were convalescent. Buttfield was not a medical practitioner and was not entirely sure that the disease was indeed smallpox. He thought it may have been a skin disease caught from dogs 'covered with loathsome sores and vermin'. The timing and locality of Buttfield's observation, while not strongly supporting a presence of smallpox, do give some indication to the probable extent of the epidemic.[122]

This epidemic was almost certainly associated with simultaneous outbreaks of smallpox among Aboriginal populations in the north and west of Australia.[123] Throughout central Australia and on the north coast, periodic outbreaks of smallpox infected Aboriginal populations between 1860 and 1869.[124] In 1984, Heather Goodall, an anthropologist working among the Pitjantjatjara and Yankunytjatjara in the Central Desert region, noted that a number of people could recall their parents or grandparents talking about an illness of plague-like proportions that may have been smallpox. Goodall states, however, that it was extremely difficult to follow up these indirect statements.[125]

The origin of these outbreaks has been attributed to the visiting Makassan fishing fleets. Other sightings of active smallpox and facial scarring have been reported on the central west coast and in the central arid regions north and south of the present town of Alice Springs between 1865 and 1870.[126] During the same period Aboriginal people on the west coast of Australia, between Geraldton and the Gascoyne River, along with several European settlers, were severely affected by smallpox.[127]

But how did this epidemic, presumably originating from an entry on the north coast of the continent, travel the vast distance to the southern coast – a distance of over 2600km (as the crow flies but much further as the virus made its way through the populations)? Examining the journals of the first European explorers who travelled through the northern, central and southern regions of the continent can provide an idea.

In 1844 Charles Sturt and his expedition party, leaving from Adelaide, reached the remote Cooper Creek in what is now known as Sturt's Stony Desert. The area lies in the far north-east corner of South Australia and is bordered by the Simpson Desert to the west and the Strzelecki Desert to the south-east. The region is an arid ecosystem marked by ephemeral surface water and low annual rainfall. On the way Sturt contacted several Aboriginal groups and was led by them through the sand dunes. Reaching the summit of one dune complex, Sturt was confronted with a view he did not expect. He wrote in his journal:

> … we reached the hill soon after the natives had gone over it, and on gaining the summit were hailed with a deafening shout by 3 or 400 natives, who had assembled on the flat below … I had never before come so suddenly upon so large a party. The scene was of the most animated description. And was rendered still more striking from the circumference of the native huts. At which there were a number of women and children, occupying the whole crest of a long piece of rising ground at the opposite side of the flat.[128]

Sturt and his party had been following distinctive Aboriginal-made trails through the landscape in use for many years. Sturt remarked:

> ... the paths of the natives became wider and wider as we advanced. They were now as broad as a footpath in England, by a roadside, and were well trodden; numerous huts of boughs also line the creek, so that it was evident we were advancing into a well peopled country.[129]

These trails were part of the major trade and exchange networks that criss-crossed not only the arid regions on north and central Australia but most of the continent. For example, the Diyari (or Dieri) of Cooper Creek were at the centre of a long trade route stretching from the Flinders Ranges in the south to the Gulf of Carpentaria in the north, covering more than half a million square kilometres. They formed a chain of connection linking the different socio-linguistic groups through ceremony and exchange, often through long-distance expeditions by groups of men honouring and maintaining trade obligations. From the north came the narcotic drug pituri and stone axes mined by hand from basalt outcrops; from the south came red ochre used for ceremonial purposes and artwork and grindstones, also mined by hand, from sandstone outcrops. These valuable items were passed hand by hand through ceremonial exchange north and south over long distances.[130] Baler shells (*Melo diadema*) from the tropical coastal waters of Cape York in the far north made their way south via ceremonial exchange networks through the centre of the continent to South Australia. There they were prized as sacred objects used in ceremonies.[131] These networks, or 'songlines', were the cultural, economic, ceremonial and genetic conduits that linked the people north to south and east to west. Large groups would gather, perform the ceremonies, exchange the goods and form marriage partnerships. And through this chain from person to person came smallpox.

Sturt also encountered what he called villages where 'huts were built in rows, the front of one hut being at the back of the other, and it appeared to be a singular but universal custom to erect a small hut at no great distance from the large ones'.

> We passed several native huts shortly after leaving the creek that were differently constructed from any we had seen. They were all arched elliptically by bending the bough of a tree at a certain height from the ground, and resting the other end on a forked stick at the opposite side of the arch. A thick layer of boughs was then put over the roof and back, on which there was also a thick coating of red clay, so that the hut was impervious to wind or heat. These huts were of considerable size, and close to each there was a smaller one equally well made as the larger. Both were left in perfect repair, and had apparently been swept prior to the departure of their inmates.

Some ten years later, in 1861, the South Australian surveyor general, George Goyder, travelling into the north of the colony and at times following in Sturt's wake, came across the same structures. At Lake Blanche he remarked that at least one was a large structure in a 'settlement ... constructed in a similar manner to those described by Captain Sturt, and very warm and comfortable, the largest capable of holding thirty or forty people'.[132] In 1874–75, J. W. Lewis surveyed an area to the east of Lake Eyre and along the Warburton and Cooper catchments following good rains. There had been little penetration of Europeans into the area and Lewis came across many large Aboriginal camps capable of housing several hundred. He estimated that the total population along the waterways would have been several thousand. At one camp he encountered 40 huts, each capable of accommodating six or seven people. Lewis considered that following the rains, when the surface water began to dry up, the people would break up and disperse.[133] In the same year, John McKinlay was chosen by the South Australian Government to lead an expedition in central Australia to look for traces of the doomed Burke and Wills expedition. He began his search concentrating on the lakes and river systems north of Lake Eyre and made his way to the Gulf of Carpentaria on the north coast. While in the middle of the Cooper Basin he recorded seeing groups of 200 at Lake Perigundi, more than 300 at Hamilton Creek, 200 to 300 south of Coongie Lake and 150 at Lake Blanche.[134]

From the early 1980s Australian archaeologists conducted intense research into the human occupation of the deserts and dryland areas of the continent. Site surveys and excavations of rock shelters and open sites focused on the tropical north, the central deserts, ranges and coastal regions. It has resulted in a quantum growth in the understanding of settlement and movement patterns extending back into the deep past and up to more recent times. Canberra archaeologist Mike Smith reviewed the data from many of the research projects in his book *The Archaeology of Australia's Deserts*.[135] This research shows an increase of sites in the last 5000 years, and an increase in the number of tool inventories and density of artefacts and rock art in sites, as well as shifts in settlement patterns, particularly an increase in the use of marginal and outlying areas as they became seasonally accessible. The last 1500 years shows a more intense increase in site use. An unavoidable interpretation of this change in the archaeological evidence is that the population of the desert and arid areas increased. The direct cause of the population increase is still the subject of debate, whether from an amelioration of climatic conditions enabling a more direct management of resources, a more established social and economic system employed by the occupants or both. But whatever the cause the archaeological evidence collected over the years points to larger and more active population centres throughout the arid and desert regions.

In 1995 Elizabeth Williams studied the archaeology of the lake systems in the Cooper Basin near Innamincka. She states that the groups occupying the region appear to have been relatively fluid, with large gatherings of 150 or more taking advantage of the flush of food resources that appeared as the freshwater lakes filled. As they dried out the people followed the water to other lakes or split into smaller groups. Other areas in the basin, such as the saline lakes, where food sources were less abundant, were used primarily by small mobile groups using the lakes as navigation aids while moving through the surrounding dune systems.[136] Other archaeological research aimed at establishing settlement patterns in the arid central regions have revealed a rise in population beginning around 5000 years ago and increasing in the last 1000 years. Discussing the settlement of arid Australia, archaeologist Harry Lourandos stated:

> After about 5,000 years ago, Aboriginal settlement spread throughout arid Australia even into the driest of areas, the harsh sandy deserts. Archaeological signs of occupation of all desert regions, and of individual sites, increase dramatically after this time. The implication here is of an increase in both the size and density of Aboriginal populations …[137]

Lourandos suggests that important economic activities by Aboriginal people shifted towards more use of grasslands and seed production. Long-standing social networks were further developed with increased permanence of residence.

What is noticeable about the arid inland of the continent at the time of first contact is the areas of high density and in some cases permanent or semi-permanent residential sites, large social gatherings, particularly when water and food resources became abundant, together with regular movement between settlements following water sources. All this adds up to a population dynamic suited to the transmission and translocation of an epidemic pathogen.

What is of concern here is that the spread of smallpox from an origin on the north coast of Australia could indeed penetrate into the interior and then into the southern areas of the continent as it progressed from person to person along the defined pathways and through the ceremonial trade networks where large groups gathered.

The degree of morbidity and mortality from the epidemic is impossible to estimate. Gething's report suggests, however, that morbidity was high among the Nawu and Wirangu along the south-west coast of South Australia. After the disease first came to the attention of the police stationed at Streaky Bay, in October and November 1867, it was estimated that at least 30 to 40 Aboriginal people showed active smallpox at any one time. By January of the next year, when Gething was investigating the disease, between 200 and 300 had been infected at Streaky Bay and between 60 and 70 at Venus Bay – a range of between 260 and 370.[138] The number of Nawu and Wirangu living in the area at this time cannot be calculated with any accuracy and so no estimates of relative population loss from the epidemic can be made. Given the previous history of smallpox epidemics and the resultant mortality, however, it would be reasonable to assume that the case fatality rate was high.

Gething reported a young male and female living on a property between the two bays were the only Europeans recorded with smallpox during this epidemic. The effect of the disease was mild and both survived, having been previously vaccinated. In each case the disease left only a few scars on the neck and face of each.

The mortality among the populations along the coast and those inland, beyond the frontier of European occupation, remains largely obscure. Gething had little idea of the mortality caused by the disease and could account for only six to eight deaths. For an epidemic of smallpox among a population who had not been vaccinated regularly, if at all, such a figure would appear to be a gross underestimate. In all likelihood it was. Gething had spent only 21 days on the west coast and most of that in a restricted region between Streaky Bay and Venus Bay. He had not gone beyond the borders of European occupation. Unless he had travelled further, he would have had no knowledge of the extent and severity of the disease in the interior, nor would any of the European settlers he used as informants. Further, he had observed the epidemic only in its earliest stages, during January. According to Sub-Protector Buttfield the epidemic lasted for a further five months among the Nawu in the Port Lincoln region alone, and it was his opinion that the disease had 'threatened destruction to the native population' in that region. The mortality would almost certainly have been more than that reported by Gething.

The 1860s epidemic appears to have been widespread, reaching into the north, centre and west of Australia. As the fledgling colony of Western Australia progressed during the 1830s, the local authorities became concerned about the entry of smallpox with the increase of shipping from the east, arrivals from overseas and the presence of fishing fleets on the north-west coast. They were acutely aware of the presence of smallpox among the populations of the Indonesian archipelago and the possibility of the disease infiltrating the Aboriginal groups of the north and making its way into the European settlements. With this constant threat in mind, a campaign to inoculate Aboriginal people in contact with the Europeans was suggested in 1854 by H. Burnham Bryan a surgeon of Busselton, in the settled south-east of the colony, writing to the Guardian of Natives in Perth. But it was not to be effective in keeping the dreaded disease away. By 1860 smallpox appears to have been established on the north coast, the likely entry via the large Malay fishing fleets that regularly stayed during the dry seasons.

Alexander Robert Richardson, a grazier from Victoria, saw opportunities of acquiring land in the northern areas of Western Australia. He, along with a brother and cousin, established the Pyramid grazing station on the George River some 40km south-east of Roebourne around 1865. Richardson stayed there until 1876. In his memoirs, written in 1909, Richardson recorded:

> That deadly epidemic smallpox, which about the year 1867, coming down the coast from perhaps Camden Harbour where Malays in search of beche-de-mer [trepang] visiting the coast had inoculated [here meaning infected] them with the disease, carried them off in hundreds if not thousands.[139]

It is unclear whether Richardson actually saw active smallpox among Aboriginal people he met with or that he was just repeating what he had heard or, indeed, whether he had personally observed the smallpox scarring in those fortunate enough to have survived.

One person who spent almost a lifetime with Aboriginal people was anthropologist and welfare worker Daisy Bates. Known to the Aboriginal people of the north-west as Kabbarli, meaning grandmotherly person, she first began her work among the clans of the Roebuck Plains and Broome region in 1900. She was to record much of the language, culture and social life of the people of the north-west and in her later years those on the edge of the Nullarbor Plain in the south. Daisy Bates recognised the smallpox scarring on Aboriginal people she met at the Trappist mission at Beagle Bay, south of Camden Harbour, and in the Roebuck area, when she lived for a short time with her husband on a cattle station where Aboriginal people from Broome resided. She recorded in her personal papers:

> In 1865–6, an outbreak of small-pox occurred in the Nor' West probably introduced by the Malays. Great numbers of the Ngoorla and Ngallooma tribes died of the malady. The natives said it came from the eastward – 'weerajoo' (east), and they became so terrified of this horrible and unknown disease that they fled from those of their tribe and family who

> contracted it, and for many months after this epidemic had run its course, bleached skeletons might be found in many of the deserted camps.[140]

Bates also interviewed Jubyche, an Aboriginal man from the colony's south-west, asking him about a smallpox epidemic.

> Ngorrart (scab) was the name given by the southern natives to smallpox. Jubyche says his mother told him that this disease carried off very many blacks and he saw many marked with the disease, but it had passed over the country before his time. His mother told him it came from the north inland over the ranges. None of the present day natives have any marks from this disease. Jubyche states that his mother was a young woman when the disease passed through her tribe. Her two brothers died of the disease. Jubyche's mother was very old when she died.[141]

Disproving the Doubters

Despite the varied nature of the surviving historical documents, there is strong evidence that the three epidemics were indeed smallpox. This conclusion has been challenged by both contemporary and modern writers, particularly for the first epidemic, in 1789. The little evidence that pertains to the 1789 epidemic in the Sydney region has left some historians and medical writers with doubts as to whether it was smallpox. Chickenpox (varicella) has been proposed as the main alternative to smallpox, with others suggesting that it was cowpox, a form of 'native pox' or some other fatal disease not specified. All these scenarios can be eliminated from serious contention on several lines of evidence that lead to the conclusion that it was indeed smallpox.

First, the First Fleet recorders of 1789 who reported on the disease were unanimous in their opinions that it was smallpox. Some saw it firsthand, others did not. Those who did not were in all probability basing their comments on the general opinion of the settlement that smallpox was the disease infecting the Aboriginal people. Most, if not all, the recorders would have had experience with the disease, known of its effects and been familiar with its signs, as it was the most widespread and fatal disease throughout the British Isles in the 18th century.

Second, although none of the journals or diaries from the First Fleet surgeons survived, it can be surmised with confidence that they were involved with the epidemic, and their opinions were known to the colony. This is indicated by accounts that describe Aboriginal people being brought into the settlement and being treated for the disease in the hospital by the medical staff. Indeed, one of the child survivors was later accepted into the household of Chief Surgeon White. There appears to be little doubt that the medical staff had other experiences with those suffering from the epidemic. When it was first brought to the attention of Governor Phillip in April 1789 that Aboriginal people were dying among the coves of Port Jackson, he immediately left the settlement with a small party, including a surgeon, to investigate. They saw firsthand the effects of the disease in the living and the dead. It can then be stated with equal confidence that, when Governor Phillip reported back to London that the disease affecting the Aboriginal people was smallpox, he had been advised so by his medical staff.

A third line of evidence that strongly links the epidemic to smallpox is the sighting of Aboriginal people bearing visible smallpox-like sequelae, both facial scarring and blindness, after the epidemic had passed. The epidermal damage done by smallpox infection can be severe, and residual scarring is common – up to 85 per cent in unvaccinated variola major cases.[142] In chickenpox, the epidermal damage is more superficial and, in most cases, quickly repaired after infection, with facial scarring rare. The reporting of residual scarring attributed to smallpox among Aboriginal people was widespread after each of the three epidemics. After the 1789 epidemic, sightings were seen to the north and inland of the Sydney settlement and in the coastal regions to the south at Jervis Bay and Port Phillip Bay. The recorded sightings after the second epidemic are more profuse. Explorers travelling beyond the frontiers of European settlement and colonists establishing new grazing lands commented on seeing Aboriginal people bearing facial scarring that they attributed to a previous epidemic of smallpox. The sightings were spread over a large area of south-eastern Australia following the major river systems and their tributaries.

With a low rate of residual scarring, chickenpox would be an unlikely candidate for the epidemics. The observations by Dr Mair, a qualified medical practitioner, are more reliable. Mair was in no doubt that the scarring he saw on Aboriginal people 'of very advanced age' corresponded 'with the pits left by the Small Pox' and that it was a result of the 1789 epidemic.

The evidence for smallpox is more cogent for the second and third epidemics. Both outbreaks were investigated by qualified medical practitioners who would have been familiar with the disease, if not from practical experience, then most likely from their medical training. From the clinical descriptions and the behaviour of the 1830s disease provided by Mair, there can be little doubt that it was an epidemic of smallpox and not varicella (despite the opposition of Inspector of Colonial Hospitals Dr James Bowman) or another disease displaying similar symptoms. After his investigation Mair concluded that the 'eruptive febrile disease' that had so affected the Aboriginal people 'approached more nearly in its symptoms to the character of Small Pox, than any other disease'. The descriptions of the symptoms by those who observed the active disease, later compiled by Mair, closely match the progress and clinical features of ordinary-type confluent and semi-confluent variola major. The symptoms suffered by the European male, Tilman, on the other hand, are more indicative of a secondary infection of variola major in a person who had been either previously vaccinated or infected with variola minor. It would appear by his own account of a previous childhood infection, and Mair's observation of old and recent sequelae resembling pockmarks, that the latter was the case.

Gething, who saw active smallpox among South Australian Aboriginal people in 1866–67, gave no clinical description of the disease. Nevertheless, he was in no doubt himself that what he observed was an outbreak of smallpox, and not chickenpox or some another non-specified eruptive (exanthematous) disease. According to his report, he saw on three separate occasions Aboriginal people suffering with what he described as the unmistakable symptoms of the disease in its various clinical stages. The residual sequelae from this outbreak were still noticeable on surviving Aboriginal people some 15 years later. The Royal Society of South Australia was informed at its meeting in June 1882 that the outbreak had passed through the Wirangu people living near Streaky Bay and Fowlers Bay, leaving 'a great number of them dying', and that a few of the survivors were 'very much pitted, more especially an old lubra who was blind'.[143] Sightings of Aboriginal people pockmarked by this epidemic were common throughout the centre of the continent when the overland telegraph line was being constructed and further north on the coast during the settlement of Port Essington and Darwin.

The three epidemics, although differing in their geographic and temporal aspects, had common characteristics, each compatible with the epidemic behaviour of smallpox in a virgin-soil population. They were highly transmissible. Accounts of all three epidemics report that the disease spread rapidly from person to person. This was later confirmed when observers noted that exposure to a sufferer could result in infection. For example, Arabanoo caught the same disease as those whom he attended and a European family suffered the same symptoms as an Aboriginal child after they cared for her within their home.

The epidemics were almost entirely confined to the Aboriginal communities. In all three epidemics the disease was first noted to be spreading among the Aboriginal communities either on the periphery of the European settlements or ahead of the frontier. Despite the spread of European settlements and their ever-increasing population, particularly after the first epidemic, very few Europeans were infected during the epidemics. The reason can be seen in the separation of the two groups. From the beginning of the first settlement in 1788, the social and cultural restraints particular to the two groups largely ensured that European and Aboriginal people lived in separate domiciles with physical proximity restricted to a few individuals. Infection by smallpox is usually a result of close contact such as would be expected of individuals living in the same household. The disease is rarely spread by fomites, such as contaminated clothing or bedding, or by limited exposure to airborne agents. Only in exceptional cases did epidemiological conditions enable the spread of smallpox freely between the two societies. In most of the recorded cases of non-Aboriginal people acquiring the disease, there had been close and sustained contact with infected Aboriginal people.

The extent of each of the epidemics followed a course through regions where Aboriginal population density was high and European settlement low, or where there were well-established exchange and ceremonial networks crossing the landscape. The evidence surviving for the first epidemic indicates that it was largely confined to the coastal and hinterland regions on the eastern side of the continent and did not extend far inland. The second epidemic followed the courses of the inland river systems forming the vast catchment area (1,036,000km^2) of eastern Australia that terminates at the mouth of the Murray River on the southern coast of South Australia. It appears to have bypassed the region of Victoria below the Murray and most of the coastal populations. The regions affected by the epidemics were resource-rich coastal and riverine environments and carried high population densities. The geographical extent of the third epidemic has been documented over a large area of Australia from the northern and western coasts through the arid centre to the southern coast.[144] In south-eastern Australia, however, it was confined to the coastal and central-inland regions where, during the 1860s, the major remnant populations of Aboriginal people lived. In an 1861 census in South Australia, the Western, Northern and North Eastern Pastoral Districts accounted for 2761 Aboriginal people, or 58.9 percent of the total population included for the state. These groups bore the major impact of the epidemic. The smaller population groups living on the fringes of the European settlements and along the River Murray largely escaped.

The three epidemics caused severe mortality, attested to by recurring and stark observations by all recorders as to the high mortality among the Aboriginal populations inflicted with smallpox. Just how high then was the mortality? The immediate answer, using the historical descriptions of each of the epidemics, is that the mortality was severe – but just how severe?

Throughout its historic association with humans, smallpox has had a high case fatality rate, particularly among those who had not been protected from the disease either by previous infection or by inoculation. Case fatality rates from smallpox among unprotected populations vary according to the clinical type, but in most cases are severe, ranging up to 90 per cent of the population infected. The young, the elderly and pregnant women were the most likely to die from smallpox. The lethal nature of smallpox became graphically apparent when the disease was introduced from Europe into the New World in 1518. The effect of variola major among the unprotected and virgin-soil populations in the Americas resulted in extraordinarily high mortality, with estimates ranging from 25 to 90 per cent or more. In just two decades from the introduction of smallpox in the north-east of United States, the indigenous populations were severely reduced by a factor estimated to be between 65 and 95 per cent.

The surviving clinical descriptions for the first and third smallpox epidemics do not allow discrimination of precisely which types of variola major were present, although the discrete type would be favoured because of the high mortalities indicated by the reporters and diarists. Governor Phillip estimated that the 1789 smallpox epidemic killed 50 per cent of the Aboriginal people living around the Sydney settlement. However, the descriptions of smallpox by Mair during the second epidemic, and later by Mitchell describing the smallpox sequelae of the Barkindji on the Darling River, indicate symptoms that accord with confluent and semi-confluent clinical types. Mortality was estimated by Mair to vary from one in three (33 per cent) to one in five or six (17–20 per cent) of infected cases. He thought, somewhat wishfully, that it could have been lower if the victims had been able to access medical care and shelter.

Although the general tone of the majority of reporting on the epidemics strongly implies high mortality, caution is required in accepting any mortality estimate categorically for all populations in the path of an epidemic. In the cases of all three smallpox epidemics, several unknown factors relate to the prevalence of the disease and mortality. In all three epidemics, regional variation in the number of people infected would be expected. Some groups would have had a high proportion infected and a resulting high mortality, while other nearby groups seem to have managed to avoid contact with carriers and so escaped the epidemic. Within the infected groups there would have been a degree of differential resistance to infection. A number of individuals would have had an active immunity to the disease in which the body reacts specifically to the pathogen and is able to survive the course of the symptoms. This would depend chiefly on the amount of exposure to the virus, the current health of the individual and the ability of the immune system to combat the spread of the virus. Also, a genetically inherited nonspecific resistance to the virus by some groups cannot be discounted.

Finally, and as a word of caution, there is no way of determining the number of individuals who were infected by smallpox and the number who managed to escape infection. It is one thing to consider the various case fatality rates of smallpox and another to equate those rates with mortality in one entire community or region. In all epidemics a number of individuals, families and groups manage to escape infection entirely. This can happen due to fortuitous circumstances, such as living away from others who became infected or active avoidance of the disease by gaining prior knowledge of its presence and fleeing its path. It is simply not known what this number may have been for any of the epidemics, or in any of the regions they occurred. When using case fatality rates to estimate population loss, the number of cases of infection must first be known, or reasonably estimated. For the three epidemics I can see no way of estimating a reasonably accurate number of infected cases. Therefore, any estimation of Aboriginal population loss incurred by the three smallpox epidemics of south-east Australia based on case fatality rates must be treated with caution.

What cannot be denied, in my estimation, is that three major epidemics of smallpox swept through Aboriginal populations across the continent: the first starting in 1789, a second in the 1830s and a third in the 1860s. But smallpox was a disease that, until it was finally eradicated by modern medical science, did not always go away after a fierce epidemic. In Europe and Asia, it was a common disease of the young, always present in an endemic form, and when there were enough susceptibles it flared up into local or even widespread epidemics. This was likely the case among the Aboriginal populations throughout Australia. Smallpox never really went away after the 1860s epidemic.

Coda: Securing the Future of the Colonies?

Did the 1789 epidemic of smallpox ensure the future of the European colony? Stephen Gapps, author of *The Sydney Wars*, tends to think so.[145] Violence was just weeks away from the establishment of the settlement at Sydney Cove in 1788. The first clash using firearms against Aboriginal people occurred when they attempted to take a spade and axe from an island near to the Sydney Cove settlement. A garden was being established on the island by the crew members of HMS *Sirius*. As the Aboriginal people were leaving with the equipment, the marines on guard were ordered to fire at their legs using small shot. The first shots in anger had been fired, all for the sake of an axe and a spade. The axe was recovered but not the spade. It was the beginning of a long history of violent confrontation that was to last for many decades across Australia.

More violence was to occur. On May 30th 1788, two men employed to collect rushes for thatching did not return and were later found dead. One man was found with four spears in his body. One spear had been thrown with enough force to pass clean through. The other man was found some distance away without any apparent injury. Governor Phillip wrote in his despatches back to Britain:

> [I] am sorry to say that the natives now attack any straggler they meet unarmed; and though the strictest orders have been given to keep the convicts within bounds, neither the fear of death or punishment prevents their going out in night; and one has been killed since the Sirius sailed.[146]

Receiving a report on the rushcutters' demise, Governor Phillip went out with an armed party of 12 to find out why the men were killed. They landed where the event had taken place and then went south to the northern shore of Botany Bay without meeting any Aboriginal people. On their return the next day they came across a large group of 'two hundred and twelve men' with women and children nearby. There was wariness and mistrust between the two groups. Phillip was extremely anxious not to cause trouble, being well outnumbered, but this time cordial, though perhaps not so friendly, relationships prevailed and the groups parted. Relations were, however, to deteriorate further.

The convicts had soon found a way to make a lucrative business by collecting Aboriginal artefacts. Spears and equipment left by the local Aboriginal people on the beaches or in their huts while they were fishing from their canoes became desired items for convicts. They would venture out from the settlement, collect the artefacts and take them back to sell to the crews of the transports. The artefacts would fetch a neat price to collectors in Britain when the ships returned. But the convicts, and no doubt the military and free settlers, were taking Aboriginal possessions without honouring or even knowing about Aboriginal traditions surrounding exchange and reciprocity. It caused further distrust and anger. Phillip continued:

> The natives, as I have observed, revenge themselves on any they meet unarmed …

> The natives still refuse to come amongst us, and those who are supposed to have murdered several of the convicts have removed from Botany Bay, where they have always been more troublesome than in any other part. I now doubt whether it will be possible to get any of those people to remain with us, in order to get their language, without using force; they see no advantage that can arise from us that may make amends for the loss of that part of the harbour in which we occasionally employ the boats in fishing.[147]

More clashes were to follow, more guns fired and more spears thrown, as relationships between the British and the Aboriginal groups along the shores and inland began to deteriorate. In these early days, the settlement could best be described as a military post where Governor Phillip strived to maintain a military routine and discipline, not only to keep the convicts in order but to protect the settlement from incursion from the outside. The new colonists were soon to find the Aboriginal people to be more aggressive than they expected. Within the confines of the settlement, regular demonstrations of firearms and military manoeuvres by the marine contingent were staged to display their might and superiority for any watching from outside. Regular armed patrols were conducted. It was believed that such displays of military might would instil a sense of caution among the Aboriginal people.

By the end of the first year the settlement was in jeopardy. Food and supplies were becoming scarce and what had been brought with the First Fleet had to be cautiously rationed. Establishing garden and grazing areas outside the military compound became hazardous, with continual clashes between the colonists and the Aboriginal people, who by now had become to realise that the newcomers were not going away. The colonists would often see large groups of a hundred or more Aboriginal men near the settlement. It was a tense period for the colonists and the military. The colonists saw themselves in danger of venturing outside the settlement without armed support and under constant threat of attacks on the settlement by a large force. The Aboriginal people saw the colonists as violent interlopers who were taking over traditional land and exploiting their fisheries and food resources – all without asking.

The situation was soon to change in favour of the colonists. It is not known with any certainty if the Aboriginal groups planned to attack the settlement with a united force and rid themselves of the problem they faced. The colony itself was in distress and the military capacity for defence was at a low point, making them extremely vulnerable to attack from a force with superior numbers. But an outright attack never eventuated, despite the situation. The deciding factor could well have been smallpox.[148]

As has been seen, the epidemic swept through the surrounding Aboriginal groups with devastating morbidity and mortality. The death rate could well have accounted for 60 to 80 per cent of the population around the Sydney Cove settlement. The dead were laying around the harbour in great numbers and suddenly, after months of seeing groups of Aboriginal people around the settlement, there were none. The patrols that went out into the hinterlands reported seeing the dead laying along once well-used paths and huts abandoned with only dead inside. Smallpox had swept ahead of the military campaigns in the Americas, causing great destruction and allowing complete domination of the indigenous populations by the Europeans. And so too the situation on the shores of Sydney Cove in 1789 may have been a deciding factor in the initial success of the colony. Any combined retaliatory response from the Aboriginal people had died along with their numbers succumbing to the unseen, galgala.

Chapter 3

MEASLES

In 1830 Robert Dawson, a company agent, pastoralist and explorer who had spent over 30 years in association with Aboriginal people, mainly in the Port Stephens district of New South Wales, stated: 'Neither smallpox, measles nor hooping [*sic*] cough are known amongst them, nor do these diseases exist among the white children in Australia, whether European or native.'[1] Dawson was wrong about smallpox, as there had already been a serious epidemic among the Aboriginal groups back in 1789. It would seem that the memory of that disastrous epidemic had faded from colonial history, at least as far as Dawson, in his experience, was concerned. The memory had faded probably because the outbreak had little or no presence among the European population and was not seen as a defining point in the biological history of Euro-Australians.

He may, however, have been correct about measles. Measles had most likely entered the New South Wales colony in 1834, but the first definite record of its presence in the colonies was not until 1838, when the *Bussorah Merchant*, a passenger ship carrying emigrants from Ireland, arrived in Hobart. Of 133 passengers, 4 women and 64 children died during the voyage, most of smallpox and measles.[2] The passengers were quarantined in Hobart on arrival and measles appears not to have subsequently caused a serious problem for the colonists, but whether the disease reached the Aboriginal communities, a virgin-soil population to the measles virus, is unknown.

Measles is a highly contagious viral disease caused by the measles virus (genus *Morbillivirus*). Humans are its natural hosts. The disease is characterised by a rash that develops on the skin and spreads rapidly over much of the body. Prior to modern vaccination development and widespread applications, measles was a common disease of childhood, frequently occurring between the ages of five and ten years. Recovery from the infection confers lifelong protection and the disease in adults occurs infrequently. At the time of Australian colonisation, the disease was endemic in Europe, with high rates of infection in the young but with low mortality.[3]

Complications developing from infection by the virus largely result from secondary bacterial infections, often as a consequence of compromised immune systems, poor diet and poverty. Pulmonary infections are common, leading to pneumonia as a cause of death when untreated. In the colonial period, causes of death among Aboriginal people (particularly adults) diagnosed as being from respiratory illnesses may often have been a result of an unidentified infection by the measles virus. Another complication of untreated infection was inflammation of the inner ear (otitis media), leading to deafness.

The measles virus is another great traveller. It followed the paths of European explorers around the world, causing great devastation among indigenous, virgin-soil populations with minimal immunity to a newly introduced disease.[4] Mortality rates as high as, or higher than, 25 per cent were not uncommon in the populations of the Americas in the 16th century following the arrival of Europeans. Measles was particularly destructive in Mesoamerica and the Andes in the 1530s[5] and later during the European colonial expansion into the Pacific. When the virus was introduced to Fiji during the first four to six months of 1875, measles was estimated to have killed between 27,000 and 40,00 people comprising 20 to 30 per cent of the population.[6] During the last quarter of 1848 and early 1849, deadly epidemics of measles, combined with whooping cough and influenza, struck the indigenous population of Hawaii. An estimated 10,000 died, more than 10 per cent of the population.[7] In 1900 the 'Great Sickness', a combination of measles and influenza, struck western Alaskan indigenous communities, losing 25 to 50 per cent of their members, and with an estimated total loss of a quarter of western Alaska's population.[8]

It was then almost inevitable that the virus would eventually find its way to the Australian colonies and inflict severe morbidity, mortality and suffering on the Indigenous populations, who also had no previous exposure to or immunological defence against the virus. Table 3.1 shows the years of outbreaks in the 19th century.

Measles among Aboriginal Populations

There are few historical accounts of measles among Aboriginal people for the first half of the 19th century. The first record of the disease among Aboriginal populations is from the Reverend Threlkeld at the Lake Macquarie mission (Newcastle). Its origin was most likely the 1834 outbreak in Sydney (Table 3.1). In his 1835 annual report the Reverend Threlkeld commented on its presence:

Table 3.1. Epidemic years of measles in the 19th century in the European population of Australia by colonies.

NSW	Vic	Tas	SA	Qld	WA
1834	–	1835	–	–	–
–	1853–54	1854	–	–	–
1860	1860	1861	1861–62	1860	1860
1867	1866–67	–	1868	–	1865
1874–75	1874–75	1874–75	1875	1875	–
1880–81	1880	1881	1881	1882–83	–
1883–84	1884	1885	1884	–	1883–84
1888	–	–	–	–	–
1893	1893	1893	1893	1893	1893
1898	1898	1898	1898	1898	1898

Source: J. H. L. Cumpstson, *The History of Diphtheria, Scarlet Fever, Measles and Whooping Cough in Australia* (Canberra: Government Printer, 1927), p. 248.

> During the present year the Measles have been very prevalent among the Aborigines, and have carried off many of the natives, from whom Mrs. Threlkeld and our nine children caught the complaint and were laid up at one time.[9]

The epidemic was not confined to the Aboriginal people living on the settlement. Threlkeld's report alludes to high mortality from measles and respiratory disorders causing extreme mortality among inland populations:

> … the Measles, the Hooping [*sic*] cough, and the Influenza, have stretched the Black victims in hundreds on the earth, until, in some places, scarcely a Tribe can be found. Of one large Tribe in the interior, four years since, there were 164 persons, there are now only three individuals alive.[10]

Threlkeld's observations of population loss following the measles epidemic are supported by official returns of Aboriginal people enumerated at annual distributions of government-issued blankets. Table 3.2 shows a sharp fall of 511 (24 per cent) in the enumerated population of the settled districts of New South Wales between 1835 and 1837.

Table 3.2. Official returns of estimated number of Aboriginal people in the settled districts of New South Wales between 1835 and 1837 enumerated during government blanket distributions.

Year	Male	Female	Total	% Decrease
1835	1195	898	2093	
1836	952	630	1582	24.4
1837	930	601	1531	3.2

Source: Peter J Dowling, '"A Great Deal of Sickness". Introduced Diseases Among the Aboriginal People of Colonial Southeast Australia 1788-1900', PhD thesis, Australian National University, 1997, p. 230, https://openresearch-repository.anu.edu.au/handle/1885/7529 accessed 16 December 2020.

From Threlkeld's report it is unclear whether measles or influenza was the main cause of mortality. However, in January 1836, Charles Darwin, on the return voyage of HMS *Beagle*, visited the colony of New South Wales and travelled inland into the Great Dividing Range as far as Bathurst. He commented on the decrease in the Aboriginal population, attributing it in part to measles. Darwin also noted that the introduction of alcohol into the Aboriginal populations added to the decrease in population:

> This decrease no doubt, must be partly owing to the introduction of spirits, to European diseases (even the milder ones of which, such as the measles, prove very destructive).[11]

Threlkeld's missionary attempts had to be eventually abandoned due to the steadily falling population in the district, and by 1841 the mission closed. While neither measles nor indeed whooping cough and influenza can be held entirely responsible for such a population loss (Aboriginal deaths had also resulted from acts of aggression by European colonists) it was probably a major factor. Threlkeld was of the opinion that many had died from the 'Act of God' during the measles epidemic.[12]

The next known epidemic, 1853–54, was restricted mainly to Victoria and Tasmania and little is known of its effects on Aboriginal populations in those colonies. There is, however, evidence of measles breaking out among Aboriginal people and settlers in South Australia. In August 1854 Surgeon Clindening reported on an outbreak of measles among Aboriginal employees at the Encounter Bay Fishery on Fleurieu Peninsula.

> … measles have made their appearance in the district – both the settlers and aboriginal natives are alike suffering from the disease. Up to the present time there has been no mortality from measles, with the exception of one of the natives who died yesterday at Encounter Bay Fishery. The natives will not take medicine, and I have no doubt, from exposure to the inclemency of the weather there will be great sufferings from the disease.[13]

If the outbreak was indeed measles, and there is little reason to doubt Clindening's diagnosis, it is most likely the first record of the disease attacking both European settlers and Aboriginal people in the South Australian colony. The outbreak was most likely a localised event, the infection arriving by sea from ports in either Victoria or Tasmania.

Two outbreaks of measles causing severe mortality were reported among the Ngunawal and Ngambri people of the southern highlands in what is now the Australian Capital Territory, in 1858 and 1862.[14] There was no recorded epidemic in the surrounding European population of New South Wales during the 1850s but there was among the European population in Victoria in 1853–54 (Table 3.1). If the 1858 outbreak among the Ngunawal was measles, it may have come from the south in Victoria, along with the annual movement of Aboriginal groups to the highlands to collect aestivating moths.[15] Large groups of Aboriginal people gathering in the highlands were recorded until 1890, almost 60 years after the first arrival of Europeans.[16] Alternatively, it may have been a localised epidemic brought into the district by the movement of European settlers. The second outbreak, in 1862, was most likely associated with the general epidemic throughout the colonies in the early years of the 1860s.

During the Tasmanian epidemic in 1860 Surgeon Smith reported one woman transferred from the Oyster Cove Aboriginal settlement to Hobart under treatment for measles.[17] She survived the infection and was returned to the settlement seven weeks later. This is the only mention of measles by Smith, who attended the inmates of the settlement for a period of ten years. During 1860 four deaths were recorded, but none from primary measles infection or secondary complications. Although the Oyster Cove people were subject to many ailments, measles was never reported to be a serious cause of morbidity.[18]

In Western Australia a measles outbreak was recorded by anthropologists in the Elder Exploring Expedition in 1865. It was reportedly affecting the Aboriginal groups inhabiting the coastal districts from Geraldton in the mid-west to Albany in the south. The outbreak appears to have been severe, as the population was reported to have been reduced to half its former number following the outbreak.[19] How much further along the coast and inland the outbreak spread among the Aboriginal population is uncertain.

The 1866–68 measles epidemic was widespread throughout Victoria. Surgeon James Gibson administered to the Aboriginal people living on the Coranderrk settlement between 1865 and 1875. He mistakenly reported the epidemic as 'intermittent fever', a contemporary medical term for recurrent fevers and chills often associated with malaria.[20] The disease was affecting the Aboriginal residents as well as Gibson and his family.[21] In March he noted 7 out of 105 suffering while several others were recovering from the infection. He returned in April and reported one death, a male 22 years of age, and a further 16 under treatment, 4 adults, 5 in their teens and the remainder ranging between 2 and 10 years of age. Many were leaving the settlement to avoid the epidemic. By June the general health of the residents had improved, with only 4 convalescing, and by August the epidemic had burned itself out. There is no evidence to the fate of those who left the settlement during the height of the epidemic and the presence of measles among Aboriginal people living off the settlements is unknown.

The 1874–75 Epidemic

The evidence for the 1874–75 measles epidemic is more substantial in terms of its occurrence among Aboriginal people. This epidemic was one of the more severe episodes of measles in the 19th century, occurring throughout the European settled regions of south-eastern Australia. The crude mortality rate of Euro-Australians in South Australia alone reached 144 and 136 per 100,000 in males and females respectively.[22]

The epidemic was also severe among the Aboriginal populations elsewhere in south-eastern Australia. The epidemic extended into several of the mission settlements, causing high morbidity among European and Aboriginal residents alike and in some cases exceedingly high mortality among Aboriginal people. Other Aboriginal settlements experienced high morbidity but recorded few deaths. Some Aboriginal populations in regional centres and settlements escaped the epidemic completely.

The first reports of the epidemic among Aboriginal people began in Victoria. On December 20th 1873 Gibson noted an 'eruptive disease' among Aboriginal people on the Coranderrk settlement. He had not seen any Aboriginal people displaying the primary stages of clinical symptoms but only the 'marks left on a few cases'.[23] He diagnosed it as a species of *Papulae viccae* and reported that there was no danger from it. Whether these were the first cases of measles and Gibson was mistaken in his diagnosis is uncertain, but by February 20th the following year measles was spreading through the settlement, with 15 cases treated out of a population of 142. By March 20th, apart from a few of the elderly people, who may have developed immunity in a previous epidemic, all of the 142 residents had been attacked by the disease. Gibson noted that none of the cases was severe and, with a little care, he anticipated a satisfactory result.[24]

Gibson's optimistic prognosis was grossly incorrect. By the end of 1875 measles had caused extreme morbidity and excessive mortality among the Aboriginal residents. So high was the mortality that it came to the notice and concern of the Victorian Parliament. The report to the Legislative Assembly by Chief Medical Officer W. McCrea is worthy of repeating at some length:

> ... in 1875, with a population of about 150 people, 31 deaths took place – one out of every five human beings in one year perishing from disease. This awful mortality was doubtless exceptional, an epidemic of measles having been prevalent in the early part of the year; but this epidemic prevailed all over the colony, causing a considerable increase in the general mortality; yet when the mortality of the whole colony, about 17 per 1,000 is compared with that of [the Aboriginal residents of] Coranderrk, the discrepancy is appalling, the latter amounting to 193 per 1,000, or in other words, for every person out of the general population who died, 11 deaths [Aboriginal] occurred at Coranderrk.[25]

McCrea's assessment of the crude mortality rate at 193 per 1000 is based on all the recorded deaths on Coranderrk settlement for 1875 and from a population that he estimated at 150. His estimate was close. An examination of the settlement's register of births, deaths and marriages[26] shows 27 deaths that could be attributed to the measles epidemic, 7 from measles directly, 11 caused by pleuro-pneumonia and 4 others caused by respiratory disorders and dysentery. Three other deaths, of children under one year old, were attributed to 'thrush', a possible misdiagnosis for the initial (prodromal) stage of measles, and the cause of another, a two-year-old male, given as 'disease of the ear affecting the brain', possibly post-measles otitis media developing into encephalitis. The population of the settlement just prior to and during the epidemic was 142, counted during Gibson's visits. The crude death rate from measles at Coranderrk would then be 190 per 1000.

Other settlements in Victoria were affected by the epidemic, although not to the same extent as Coranderrk. On December 9th 1874 Surgeon Brewer[27] observed an 'exanthematous disease' causing some illness and sore throats at the Lake Condah settlement. He reported the disease as scarlet fever. After his visit most of the children of the settlement, including the superintendent's own children, were attacked by measles. The disease was at first seen as mild, causing no great stress to the Aboriginal children. By January 3rd, however, measles had spread to most of the population (numbering around 86) with 24 showing the signs.

> I found nearly all the adults down with the measles. They were much more severely affected than the children had been – two had severe pneumonia, three severe bronchitis, two diarrhoea, one constantly recurring haemorrhage from the nose, one woman just recovered from confinement had severe bronchitis.[28]

The children who had initially been infected had recovered, with just two in a low febrile condition and pneumonia. The remainder of the establishment Brewer found in bed or lying around in various symptomatic stages. Three deaths were recorded by Brewer, two elderly females, one of whom died from post-measles complications after recovery from the initial infection, and a 14-year-old. All other victims gradually recovered. By the end of April, the disease had passed the Lake Condah settlement.

In the Framlingham settlement, in south-east Victoria, Surgeon Jamieson[29] reported measles affecting approximately 20 out of a population of 58. The disease had been brought to the settlement by returning Aboriginal men who had been working in the immediate district where measles was prevalent among the European population. By April 30th Jamieson reported all residents had recovered from their symptoms. No further cases were reported.

Table 3.3 shows the Aboriginal mortality statistics from measles or post-measles complications during this epidemic, which were reported to the Victorian Parliament by the Aboriginal Protection Board. The deaths were all recorded on Aboriginal settlements and do not include Aboriginal people who may have died away from the settlement, for example, when fleeing from the epidemic, or those who were attached to European rural properties or residences.

The differential rate of death from measles ranged from 0 to 20 (percentages are revealed in the above table). The two Gippsland settlements of Lake Wellington and Lake Tyers, located on the east coast, escaped the epidemic with no reported deaths, although the surrounding European population was affected. Separation of the Aboriginal residents from the European population, particularly during the period of the epidemic, most likely saved these two settlements from infection. Reverend Hagenauer, superintendent of Lake Wellington, reported:

> Different diseases have been about in the district, such as scarlet fever and measles, and not one of our natives have had them though the measles were within two miles of the place.[30]

The settlements to the west were, however, involved in the epidemic, with varying degrees of mortality reported. A similar spatial pattern of differential mortality during measles epidemics occurred during the epidemic of 1867 among the European population of Sydney[31] and in the islands of Fiji in 1875.[32]

Table 3.3. Recorded number of Aboriginal deaths in Victorian Aboriginal settlements attributable to the 1874–75 measles epidemic.

Settlement	Deaths Attributed to Measles	Approximate Average Population	%
Coranderrk	27	142	19.0
Lake Condah	4	86	4.7
Framlingham	6	58	10.3
Lake Hindmarsh	16	78	20.6
Lake Wellington	0	68	0.0
Lake Tyers	0	73	0.0

Source: Compiled from *Twelfth Report of the Board for the Protection of the Aborigines in the Colony of Victoria*, Papers Presented to Parliament. Legislative Assembly, Victorian Parliamentary Papers, No. 25, 1876.

Following the outbreaks in Victoria, measles appeared among Aboriginal people in South Australia.

In his annual report on the state of the Aboriginal groups, E. L. Hamilton, the sub-protector for the colony of South Australia (including what is now the Northern Territory), wrote:

> The tendency of the aborigines to succumb to disease when exposed to the influences of the unfavourable side of civilization, has been exhibited to a very marked extent during the year by an exceptionally high rate of mortality; 52 births and 140 deaths have been recorded, being an excess of 88 deaths over births. The causes of death include 38 from consumption, and 55 from measles ... The epidemic of measles is stated to have first attacked the whites, and afterwards spread among the blacks ...[33]

This exceptional mortality rate for 1875 can be broken down to indicate 39 per cent of the deaths were from the measles epidemic, 27 per cent from tuberculosis-related causes and the remainder from other non-specified causes. These figures, however, can only be seen as rough estimates and almost certainly just represent the tip of an iceberg of exceptional mortality for that year, particularly in the more remote arid regions of central Australia, where official enumeration was challenging and often non-existent. Hamilton went on to report:

> Probably these figures can only be accepted as approximate, for perfect accuracy in records of this nature is almost impossible when dealing with native tribes in circumstances such as those of the aborigines.

In the northern districts, along the Flinders Ranges, the sub-protector reported from Blinman of the epidemic in February 1875:

> I am sorry to record the fact that in common with the settlers here and elsewhere the Aborigines have suffered extensively from measles. At the Sliding Rock [near Beltana] during one of my visits I found many suffering and instructed Mr. Powell the surgeon to attend to those in the neighbourhood of the mine professionally. Two of the Blacks – a man and woman have died in this neighbourhood [Blinman] and I have been informed that several aged Blacks at Beltana and at Numdowadana succumbed to the disorder named.[34]

The epidemic had probably been present among these communities since at least December 1874. The epidemic first appeared among the Europeans in the Flinders Ranges settlements and afterwards spread among the Aboriginal groups, who suffered severely.[35]

Although official evidence of the epidemic is understandably sparse in the more remote areas, to a certain extent, some insight into its effect can be gauged from another major epidemic in these areas, reported some 70 years later. Leading up to this time Aboriginal groups were experiencing a period of intensifying intrusion from missionaries, mining companies and pastoral activities. In 1948 the Ernabella Mission, located in the Musgrave Ranges in the far north-west corner of South Australia, suffered a most devastating measles outbreak complicated by bronchial pneumonia. This epidemic was reported to have killed at least 50 people on the mission and countless others in the surrounding area.

Sister Melba Turner, who attended the people during the epidemic, wrote:

> Within a week or two, seven people had died, three out in the bush and four at Ernabella; but in the succeeding days we had more deaths. Ten of the very old people died, and five babies, and some of the younger folk. They would move their camps every few days, and we would have the greatest of trouble to even find them again, to give them the necessary treatment. Some went 'off bush' and became ill, and returned starved and emaciated beyond recognition. There is no food in the bush for sick people, the native foods are excellent to keep people alive, if they are strong enough to digest them, but once ill and unable to fend for themselves, the outlook is pretty grim. No milk, no bread even, only water and their half-cooked animal food; the mothers would lose their milk, and the babies would suffer in consequence. One baby was brought in too starved to cope with, it was helped by another mother for a time, but the foster mother failed and they didn't let me know; others hid their babies under blankets, until so ill that it was almost impossible to do anything; some of the parents were afraid we would stick needles into their children, or would force medicine down their throats, and it was difficult to find out who was sick and who wasn't.[36]

The epidemic was then reported to have moved into the western districts of the colony. Traditional ceremonial and trading routes linked the small population groups in the remote areas[37] and most likely facilitated the spread of the epidemic from person to person. Hamilton reported that information passed to him indicated that measles made its first appearance among the groups inhabiting the Gawler Ranges and from there spread west along the coast near the settlements at Venus Bay, Streaky Bay and Fowlers Bay, and to southern Eyre Peninsula, where it infected almost all the residents living on Poonindie Mission. One resident of Fowlers Bay wrote to Sub-Protector Hamilton:

> The epidemic (measles) carried away some twenty old and young. It first made its appearance at Streaky Bay, and I hear, was brought there from Adelaide by Europeans. Some of the Fowlers Bay natives were there at the time, and caught it, bringing the disease here, and that I feel sure, was caught from the blacks.[38]

Measles was also reported among the Aboriginal communities at Guichen Bay in the colony's south-east. Police Trooper Morris reported to Sub-Protector Hamilton:

> There has been much sickness among them than usual, owing to the prevailing epidemic, measles and scarlatina [scarlet fever]; but they have all without exception got over it favourably; it has necessitated me issuing them extra blankets and medical comforts. The two deaths which have occurred here have been caused by disease of the lungs, by which they all seem more or less affected.[39]

Little could be done for those infected. Hamilton supplied the Aboriginal depots in the infected areas with 'medicines specially prepared, and medical comforts'[40] but with little effect. Some accepted the limited treatment and help from those Europeans settlers who offered it to them, but in many cases the Aboriginal people refused treatment, preferring their own traditional healers and methods. Only one was treated for measles in the Adelaide Hospital in 1875, a one-year-old female who was admitted for treatment on November 30th.[41]

The measles epidemic bypassed the Point McLeay mission (Raukkan) on the lower Murray River and the community living in the Port Augusta region at the head of Spencer Gulf. George Taplin was superintendent of the Point McLeay mission on the lower Murray River from 1859 until his death in 1879. Following the measles epidemic in the immediate region he wrote:

> We never had the measles on the Station at all altho [*sic*] settlers had them within two miles of us and they raged violently at Milang and Meningie. Altho a large number of natives were gathered in camps at a sheep shearing and some of them, mostly half castes had measles, yet they did not spread generally. This is surprising since absolutely no care was taken to prevent infection.[42]

In his half-yearly report on the Aboriginal people at Port Augusta, Police Sergeant O'Shanahan stated quite specifically that they had 'not suffered in any way from measles'.[43]

The failure of the epidemic to affect the Point McLeay settlement and the Aboriginal population of Port Augusta, even though no measures were taken to prevent infection, may indicate that many had been exposed to the virus during an earlier outbreak and had gained immunity to the present epidemic. The epidemics of 1861–62 and 1868, which reached South Australia, may then have been the source of original exposure and protection from the 1874–75 epidemic. Although there is little evidence to support this, Taplin, in the same report, does state that measles had been 'very prevalent' at some time in the past.[44]

Although most sources reporting on measles indicate severe morbidity and many deaths, a few statistics are available that can give some impression of the degree of mortality but, again, these enumerations should be taken with care. Sub-Protector Hamilton stated that 39 per cent of 140 Aboriginal deaths reported in the colony for 1875 had been from measles. He also reported an exceptionally high death rate on the Poonindie Mission, with 75 cases of measles reported and 10 deaths (a case fatality rate of 13.3) in a population of approximately 90[45] and at Fowlers Bay 20 deaths of people both old and young.[46]

Following the 1875 epidemic five more epidemics or major outbreaks of measles occurred in Australia during the 19th century. Apart from just a handful of reports mentioning measles, there is little other evidence of the disease affecting the Aboriginal people. In 1883, during a royal commission into the treatment of Aboriginal people in Western Australia, members of the inquiry board visited the Rottnest Island Aboriginal prison, where 148 prisoners were held. They found that 'nearly all the natives were ill with measles'. The commission found that the 'cells are too small for the number in them, and only 140 cubic feet is at present allowed for a native; and, as the cells are also generally badly ventilated, it is not nearly sufficient'.[47] In most cases four or five prisoners were held in an 18 x 40 foot cell (5.5 x 12.2 metres) – ideal conditions for the spread of measles in the prison. Measles was most likely carried to the island by infected and ill prisoners transported from the mainland and spread throughout the prison by the customary exchange of clothing between the prisoners. This custom of exchanging clothes was regularly practised by the Aboriginal prisoners in a ceremony after the issue of a meal in which a large number of prisoners participated.

In 1887, at Lake Wellington Aboriginal settlement,[48] in Victoria's Gippsland district, Reverend Hagenauer reported just one case of measles, which did not spread to the rest of the community.

During the epidemic period of 1893–94, measles was reported among the communities on the north coast of New South Wales:

> There are now fifty Aborigines in residence at the [Aboriginal] 'Home' near Grafton. The health generally has been good during the year. Measles and influenza went through the settlement, but all the patients recovered, though several died of the same complaints in camps in other parts of the Clarence district.[49]

Measles, accompanied by respiratory disease, was also reported in the New South Wales southern highlands at Tumut[50] and on the Point McLeay mission in South Australia in 1894:

> The epidemics of influenza and measles have been prevalent at the [Point McLeay] station, and this cause may have attributed, to a certain degree the comparatively heavy mortality over the year.[51]

The extent of mortality from these epidemics is unclear. There were 19 deaths recorded among the Aboriginal people in the South Australian colony for 1894: 7 children, 2 youths, and 10 elderly. Eight of these appear on the register of births and deaths for Point McLeay mission and one for Point Pearce mission, but measles as a cause of death was not attributed to any.

This last epidemic of the 19th century reached into the remaining Aboriginal groups living traditional lifestyles in central Australia, 23 years after the 1875 blight that had caused excessive suffering and mortality. This outbreak of measles appears to have had much the same effect. Sub-Protector Francis Gillen, an anthropologist, described the epidemic:

> The general health of the Aborigines was good until the month of December, when measles, first appearing at Oodnadatta, rapidly spread through the tribes, causing much suffering and a number of deaths, chiefly among the old people. Only such deaths as have occurred at or near, the depots have been recorded, and it is therefore reasonable to suppose that the mortality in outside districts, where the aborigines have no opportunity of getting medical treatment or advice, was much heavier. The disease, which is often complicated by pleurisy, is still raging, and will doubtless spread from tribe to tribe throughout the continent. Where the sufferers have access to a waterhole their favourite method of treatment is to plunge into the water for the purpose of cooling their bodies, and this very often proves fatal.[52]

Although this last epidemic in the 19th century occurred in the European populations in all the colonies of Australia, the extent of its presence among other Aboriginal population centres is unknown. The records of death in Aboriginal settlements in Victoria and South Australia have no mortality from measles, nor do they report its presence among the residents. Even though measles was present among the groups in central Australia, it would appear that the Aboriginal populations in Victoria and South Australia escaped the epidemic for that year.

The beginning of the 20th century did not of course mark the end of fatal measles outbreaks among Aboriginal populations. In the more remote areas of northern, western and central Australia, Aboriginal settlements were being established under the coercive protectionist and assimilation policies of the state governments.

At the Carrollup Aboriginal mission near Katanning, in Western Australia's south-west, measles broke out in the winter of 1900. Daisy Bates, who was caring for the Aboriginal people in the area, recalled:

> There were some fourteen family shelters at the camp, besides two bachelors' huts, a total of inhabitants being between forty and fifty occupants. Togur and Daddel had come to my camp the morning after the visit to the pictures … It was the last merry day at the camp.
>
> The second morning after the visit to the pictures, they came to tell me that Togur and Daddel were sick, and would I come over to see them. I went over, and knowing that measles was rife in Katanning, I turned down their lips – the easiest way to tell when a native has got measles – and found of course what I looked for. It seemed to me a case of doctor and hospital, so I sent a messenger post-haste to town, and on the heels of the messenger came the doctor.
>
> 'Yes, it's measles,' he announced, 'and Daddel has got it rather badly.'
>
> 'When will it be convenient to take them to the hospital, Doctor?'
>
> 'Can't do it. The hospital is full to overflowing with measles and other patients; they'll have to remain in camp, and I'll come out daily to see them. You'll have to do the best you can, and I hope it won't spread amongst them. Give them gruel, milk, soup, tea, any liquid food for a few days,' and the busy doctor hurried away, leaving me stranded with two measles patients.

Bates began to offer care and 'gruel'. By her own admission she was a poor cook and at first did not know how to cook gruel, but she managed to provide nutrition to the ill people. She did not mention any form of medication.

> … Togur and Daddel became convalescent, and just when I was in sight of a little rest from nursing and cooking, Daddel's own mother, and his 'second' mother, and his seven brothers and sisters all caught the infection … Baiungan, the older wife, got the measles very badly and lay absolutely helpless for days. Her little baby, Muilyian, was also very ill, and not having been weaned, there was the added trouble of special baby food. Baiungan and her five children occupied her half of a beehive shelter, a space not more than five feet [1.5 metres] in diameter holding the family! They lay with their heads within the shelter, their feet towards the open fire-place between the two huts, and to reach one I had to lean over the others, who were huddled up at either side. They

were like peas in a rounded pod, in that dreadful hut, with the smoke blowing in upon them at every gust of wind.

Dillungan, the younger mother, whose attack was not nearly so severe as Baiungan's, did nothing but grunt and groan, and open her mouth to be fed, and resume her groaning. Her two little children, the baby and his brother, howled and roared, and refused to take nourishment and medicine without endless coaxing. Their mother, scarcely more than seventeen years old, paid no heed whatever to them. She suckled her baby by fits and starts, but the disease had dried both her breasts and Baiungan and the poor little children suffered greatly from the sudden stoppage of their natural food.

... Before Baiungan and Dillungan and their families had got rid of the measles, Mungail's wife, Warinyan, and her two children were down with it but they were good little patients and gave not trouble. Then Kaiar, his wife Wirijan, and their four grandchildren, Wenyil, Genujan, Florrie and Bobbie, caught the infection, and after them came Derdingburt, his woman, Yoolbian, and their little adopted child Win-ngur-man. All these at once, and in the rain and cold they claimed my services.

I believe it was about this time that all of them got it into their heads that it was good to have the measles and have their mother, sister, auntie, granny or whatever relation I was to each one, to wait upon them, and bring them their food in nice clean mugs and cup and saucers and plates ... The older patients would laugh with me when I announced fresh cases, and the new ones would settle themselves comfortably to go through the ordeal, taking medicine and food with equal readiness. Barderuk ... Yiner, and their son Roy, wandered from sick camp to sick camp, seeking infection. They caught it at last, to their great delight, and I used to see Barderuk, when she got better, go over to the other camps and play cards and talk gossip, until she saw me coming over with a meal, when she would return to her camp and pretend she had never left it, lying down, and assuming all the airs of the pampered invalid.

And those awful huts! How we all escaped fever I don't know. They lived, ate, slept in, and never moved out of these huts for days, and in all that stench one had to lean over to the patients, who might be huddled in their farthest corners, and inhale the germs of every filth-producing disease. Bending over them to cleanse them and give them food, I was so sorry for them that I would not be sick.[53]

Daisy Bates's impression 'that it was good to have measles', was borne from the belief that once infected by measles the person would acquire immunity (immunomodulation) to the disease for life – a belief not entirely false and one that has persisted into the present. However, infection by measles can often result in immunosuppression, predisposing the former patient to opportunistic infections for periods up to several weeks or months. It is not known how the Aboriginal people under Daisy Bates's care fared after their bouts with measles.

Many Aboriginal groups maintained traditional lifestyles, following long-held cultural and economic practices of moving from place to place, but still far away from European control. On Cape York, in the Mitchell River area, for example, an outbreak occurred in 1944. The disease was brought into the mission settlement by an Aboriginal stockman returning by plane after holidaying at Normanton. Measles spread throughout the settlement, causing at least 21 deaths. Within four to six weeks the disease had spread by an overland route through the widely separated bush camps carried by the regular traditional movement of people throughout the area. It was further reported to have spread north by a coastal lugger to Mapoon on the northern tip of Cape York. Measles returned again in 1953, this time breaking out in the Aurukun mission settlement on the Gulf of Carpentaria coast of York Peninsula and 100km further north at the Weipa settlement. Both these outbreaks were brought in by residents returning via mission launch from x-ray check-ups on Thursday Island.[54] A similar situation occurred in central Australia in 1948 at Ernabella mission station, as earlier mentioned. Measles outbreaks followed both the traditional movements and the government-controlled movements of Aboriginal people, causing severe morbidity and mortality.

* * *

Little of substance can be said on the extent of Aboriginal mortality due to measles epidemics prior to 1874–75. The historical documentation presented here shows that the disease was present among the Aboriginal populations in south-eastern Australia during the three major epidemic periods of 1835, 1853–54 and 1867. Just what the levels of morbidity and mortality were, and the extent of their spatial distribution in these early epidemics, is a matter of conjecture. Most of the Aboriginal deaths from measles went unrecorded or unnoticed by European observers and only indirect and anecdotal evidence survives.

However, in a population that had no previous experience with measles and no herd immunity to it, high morbidity and high mortality are to be expected.[55] In this early stage of colonisation the Aboriginal populations of south-eastern Australia had not been fully institutionalised and confined to designated settlements. Traditional lifestyles and economies were still present among many groups living away from major European centres and beyond the frontiers of colonial settlement. While these groups could not sustain measles endemically, it is quite possible that they may have facilitated a chain of infection enabling dissemination of measles and the relocation of epidemic centres throughout regions beyond the European frontiers.

It is also quite likely that some groups felt the full force of the epidemic, experiencing severe morbidity and mortality, others less so and some escaped the infection entirely. Linguistic and socio-cultural differences between groups would have acted as permeable or inviolable barriers restricting the spatial dissemination of the virus. Physical obstacles such as rivers, lakes and mountain ranges would also have affected the spread of the disease, again acting as barriers to slow, shape or even stop the process of diffusion. Those groups that escaped one epidemic would then, however, have been equally susceptible to the next. Whatever the case may have been, it would be expected that the dissemination of the outbreaks was wide, and severe population loss would have been experienced in the regions affected by the first three major epidemics leading up to 1874–75.

By the second half of the 19th century, Aboriginal population centres were not large enough, or closely associated enough, to keep the measles chain of infection going, enabling it to spread throughout most of south-eastern Australia and remain endemic. However, during at least the 1875 epidemic, the Aboriginal populations did not need to be large to sustain an epidemic. The chain of infection was easily supported by the European population, which, with its high numbers of immunologically susceptible individuals, maintained the active disease at low incidence levels, peaking periodically into epidemics. It is safe to assume then that, because of the highly communicable nature of the virus and the associations between Europeans and Aboriginal people, the disease would have crossed repeatedly from the former population to the latter. It is most likely that the disease spread in this way throughout most of the Aboriginal populations of Australia.

However, a clearer picture of the effects of measles for the 1874–75 epidemic can be obtained. In the second half of the 19th century Aboriginal settlements and mission stations had been established and local causes of death were recorded. Table 3.4 compares the estimates of the crude death rate from Aboriginal settlements in Victoria and South Australia with those from Methodist Church centres in Fiji[56] following the 1975 epidemic. The Fijian epidemic can be considered a trans-Pacific extension of the 1874–75 epidemic experience in south-eastern Australia. While the crude death rates for Australian Aboriginal people are in most cases lower than those in Fiji, they share a similar pattern of widely varying mortality between one population centre and another.

Table 3.4. Estimated crude death rate (CDR) from the 1874–75 measles epidemic among Fijians and Aboriginal Australians.

Centre in Australia	CDR	*n*
Point McLeay	0	0
Lake Condah	47	4
Framlingham	103	6
Poonindie	111	10
Coranderrk	190	27
Ebenezer	205	16

Centre in Fiji	CDR	*n*
Totoya	137	75
Komo	192	20
Matuku	229	162
Lakemba	258	210
Moala	259	205
Fulaga	342	107
Kabara	363	107
Moce	383	59
Namuka	435	54
Oneata	755	120

Note: The crude death rate is the number of deaths occurring among the population during a given period, per 1000 population, calculated as (Total deaths in centre / Total population in centre) x 100,000; *n* = Total deaths attributed to measles.

Source: P. Dowling, '"A Great Deal of Sickness": Introduced Diseases among the Aboriginal People of Colonial Southeast Australia 1788–1900' (Canberra: PhD thesis, Australian National University, 1997), https://digitalcollections.anu.edu.au/handle/1885/7529 (accessed July 2016).

Two significant epidemiological points arising from the figures in Table 3.4 must be considered. The first is that the crude death rates among the local Fijian populations are generally all higher than those of the Australian Aboriginal populations included. The exceptions are Coranderrk (CDR 190) and Ebenezer (CDR 205), which have higher crude death rates than those of Totoya (CDR 137).

Two explanations may be offered for this. First, the local populations are smaller for Australia and the crude death rates may be influenced by a small sample size. If this were the case, however, it would be expected that the bias would show random death rates both above and below that of Fiji. This does not occur. A second explanation, and one that goes towards addressing the former problem, is that the low crude death rates among the Australian Aboriginal populations, when compared with the Fijian samples, does indeed reflect the true nature of the epidemic. Prior to this epidemic, Aboriginal people in Victoria and South Australia had been exposed to three previous epidemics, 20 years, 15 years and 8–10 years before. An unknown number of Aboriginal people living through the 1874–75 epidemic had presumably been infected in one of the previous epidemics, survived and developed immunity to the virus, and so did not fall to the disease on its return in 1874–75. A small herd immunity to the disease would then have then existed in the older community members. This was not the case for Fiji in 1875. This epidemic was the first experience the Fijians had with measles. Measles had spread from Australia into the Pacific in 1854, when it reached Tahiti and the Cook Islands (probably from an American ship on its way from Newcastle in New South Wales), but it did not reach Fiji.[57] The Fijians can be considered an island population with no herd immunity to measles in 1874–75, whereas in Australia for the same period there was at least some degree, albeit unknown, of herd immunity to the virus. The differences in the crude death rates between the two populations are then explained.

This explanation then raises further questions. If, as I believe can be safely assumed, there was no endemic measles in Australia prior to European settlement, and if the first recorded epidemic in 1834 was the initial exposure to the virus for the Aboriginal populations, was the crude death rate in 1834 much higher than in 1874–75, and was it as high as seen for some areas in Fiji? There are, of course, no solid answers to these questions, but epidemiological inference, in this case, allows speculation that for the subsequent measles epidemics the mortality rate in Australia was similar. When a second epidemic of measles was introduced into Fiji in 1903, there was a much reduced mortality. Although there are no official records on the timing or extent of this epidemic, the estimated number of deaths was between 1800 and 2000.[58] Based on a higher-than-average crude death rate for all deaths for Fiji in 1903, demographer Norma McArthur has estimated the crude death rate from a subsequent epidemic of measles for that year at approximately 20 per thousand.[59] The reason for this much-reduced figure from the 1875 epidemic can be explained by a higher herd immunity at the time of the population's second exposure to the virus. The majority of the population who survived the first epidemic would have acquired an immunological protection from the virus and would have escaped the symptoms of the disease. The section of the population at risk to measles in 1903 comprised those born after the 1875 epidemic; that is, those under the age of 27. A substantially reduced number of susceptible individuals would then account for the reduced crude death rate. There is, of course, nothing new in this. It follows the well-known epidemiological pattern of measles epidemics occurring throughout the world and their effect among virgin-soil populations.[60]

It can then, I believe, be assumed by analogy with Fiji that the initial epidemics of measles among the Aboriginal people of south-eastern Australia were responsible for a much higher case fatality rate than those calculated for the 1874–75 epidemic. This assumption can be strengthened further by taking into consideration the supportive care available to Aboriginal people living in missionary and government settlements during the 1874–75 epidemic, and the lack of it among those infected in previous epidemics. Whether a person dies from measles largely depends on the availability of supportive care and the quality of hygiene and nutrition maintained throughout the course of the primary and secondary illnesses.[61] It is therefore important that the ill person receives care from those not infected or not immobilised from the disease.

In a virgin-soil population with all susceptible to the infection, typically, many individuals of all ages are sick at once, and there is often no-one to provide for the basic needs (food, water, comfort) of the sick or attend to basic hygiene. Such a situation was almost certainly the case among Aboriginal groups living beyond the European frontiers when they experienced the first epidemics of measles. The mortality from measles during the 1874–75 epidemic would thus have been reduced by the supportive care offered to the Aboriginal people then living in settlements by those who were not incapacitated by the disease. The lower crude death rates from the 1874–75 epidemic are then from localised populations, many of whom had developed a measure of herd immunity to the disease and who had access to supportive care, food and water during the epidemic, all of which would have reduced mortality from measles.

The second epidemiological point involving the local crude death rates presented in Table 3.4 is their irregularity and, by inference, the irregularity of the attack rates of the virus. Several factors operating in conjunction are responsible. Unlike the influenza virus, which undergoes regular and major genetic changes, the measles virus is a stable myxovirus.[62] Therefore, on the basis of present virological knowledge, it can be accepted that the measles virus attacking a population centre during an epidemic is genetically the same as that which attacks another centre. The same can be said for epidemics several decades apart. For the same reason, lifelong immunity to the virus is gained after the first infection. Further, the virus has a simple transmission mechanism, primarily from one human to another, requiring no intermediate host or vector to intercede. Attack rates then depend on the amount of exposure each individual has to the virus and on their personal immunological immunity to the virus.

The mortality rate is also dependent on the ability of the immune system to fight the virus effectively. Those with impaired immune systems due to other infectious agents, particularly chronic infections such as syphilis or tuberculosis, lose the ability to combat the measles virus effectively and are prone to more severe and debilitating primary symptoms. These same individuals are more susceptible to post-measles secondary invasion by other pathogens. Further, the irregular pattern of crude death rates also relates to the effectiveness of local supportive health care available during an attack.

* * *

The history of measles in colonial Australia can be seen as a series of recurring epidemic events beginning in 1834. Although there is little evidence available regarding the morbidity or mortality among the Aboriginal populations during the epidemics before 1874–75, there is evidence to suggest a similar pattern in when they happened and how long they lasted (timing and periodicity) between the Aboriginal populations and the European populations in south-eastern Australia. Excessive morbidity and mortality during these early epidemics in immunologically vulnerable Aboriginal populations could be expected. The few surviving reports referring to these early epidemics suggest that this is the case.

The 1874–75 epidemic in south-eastern Australia was a part of a world pandemic of measles. Records of this epidemic provide the best evidence regarding the morbidity and mortality of measles among Aboriginal populations.

Historical accounts show that this epidemic spread throughout many Aboriginal population centres living both in and away from established settlements. Two of the hardest hit settlements in terms of mortality were the Lake Hindmarsh settlement, which lost 20.6 per cent of its population, and Coranderrk, which lost 19 per cent. Other population centres were bypassed by the epidemic. The settlements of Lake Wellington and Lake Tyers on the east coast of Victoria, Point McLeay in South Australia and the population living in the European town of Port Augusta escaped the epidemic with no recorded morbidity or mortality.

The crude death rates from the 1874–75 epidemic, while indicating excessive mortality from measles, are much lower than those from Fiji for its epidemic. The experience of previous epidemics among Australian Aboriginal populations, providing a substantial number of immunologically protected people, can account for the lower mortality in south-eastern Australia and in turn suggests greater severity of the earlier, largely unrecorded, epidemics.

Records from Aboriginal settlements in south-eastern Australia after the 1874–75 epidemic suggest that measles was no longer a major lethal disease. The records of mortality from settlements in Victoria and South Australia between 1876 and 1900 show just four deaths in young children and two over the age of 15 years.[63] An exception was the 1898 epidemic, which penetrated the northern, western and central arid regions of Australia following pastoral expansion. This was the last epidemic of the 19th century to seriously affect an Aboriginal population.

Coda: Immunisation in the 21st Century

In April 2014, Australia was officially declared to be measles-free. Beginning in the late 1960s–70s, a comprehensive vaccination program was instituted by the Australian Government aimed specifically at children. The result of this program, which incorporated vaccinations for measles, mumps and rubella (MMR), was to see a dramatic fall in childhood and adult measles across the country. No longer would measles be accepted as an inevitable disease of childhood that had to be endured in order to obtain lifelong immunity. The 2014 declaration was verified by an international panel of infectious-disease experts and was based on reporting of the disease showing that the MMR program had been able to interrupt the endemic measles virus transmission for a period of at least 36 months.[64]

Caution must be taken here, however. Eradicating measles, or any infectious disease for that matter, as an endemic disease that continually infects the younger age groups in a population is a highly significant achievement, and that was what the MMR vaccination program achieved. But it does not mean that measles has entirely disappeared from Australia for good. Ironically, in the months preceding the measles-free statement, more than 15 people caught the highly infectious disease after attending a dance competition in Sydney. A Filipino competitor had contracted the virus in the Philippines, where the disease was still present, and carried it to the competition. In the same year, 11 cases of measles were confirmed in Queensland, 6 of which were initially acquired in the Philippines, one in Vietnam and one in Papua New Guinea. These introduced cases were acquired and carried by unimmunised individuals, and transmitted to similarly unimmunised people locally. Nevertheless, fewer cases may now enter Australia because of mass vaccination campaigns being undertaken in the Western Pacific region alone. Since 2009 more that 230 million children in the region have been immunised against measles. The reported cases of measles plummeted from 12,100 in 2000 to around 2000 in 2012. However, measles is still around. In 2019 the World Health Organization indicated that there were more measles cases worldwide than in any other year since 2006.[65]

What has the MMR vaccination program achieved for Australia's Indigenous population? In short, the program has been highly successful. The Australian Department of Health has reported that between 2007 and 2010, prior to the measles-free declaration, the rate of measles reporting in Aboriginal and Torres Strait Islander populations is below that for the rest of Australia for all age groups.[66] In terms of introduced diseases among the Indigenous populations of Australia that can only be good news, for measles at least. Nevertheless, the spectre of new outbreaks remains. Further introduction of the virus carried from overseas remains a possibility, especially by air travellers entering Australia. While there is a high and constant level of immunised people, particularly the young, then the virus is not likely to pose a major problem. But this depends on the willingness of Australians to participate in MMR vaccination programs. Also, the possibility of drug-resistant varieties of the measles virus emerging and making their way into Australian populations and causing serious outbreaks remains. The spectre of the 1874–75 epidemic and the havoc it incurred on Aboriginal populations should not be forgotten or ignored.

Part 2

Sexually Transmitted Disease

Chapter 4

SYPHILIS BEYOND THE COLONIAL BOUNDARIES

In 1829, New South Wales Governor Ralph Darling asked Captain Charles Sturt to lead an expedition into the interior of the colony. The aim was to ascertain the nature of the country and the course of the rivers flowing west into the unexplored regions. In 1813 the Great Dividing Range, which had dominated and formally enclosed the coastal settlements, had been crossed and agricultural land areas were being opened up. Darling saw the need to extend the colony further west, beyond the mountains and into the unknown interior. Sturt, who had been appointed military secretary to the governor, was a good choice to head up an exploration. He had little interest in the politics of the colony but was greatly intrigued by the mysterious and unknown geography of the lands beyond the colonial settlements. He had already led an expedition to the west of the settlements along the Macquarie River, reaching the Darling River, which he named after the governor.[1]

In November 1829 Sturt, along with the son of Colonial Secretary George McLeay and 12 others, set off. They made their way west along the Murrumbidgee River, reaching the extent of the known settlements near present-day Jugiong. In January 1830 Sturt decided to break up the group and, with McLeay and 5 others, embarked in a whaleboat on the waters of the Murrumbidgee River. Their travel downstream was swift. On January 13th they entered the Murray River and nine days later came to the junction with the Darling River. They followed the Murray to its termination in Lake Alexandrina and on February 11th Sturt and McLeay stood on the sand dunes overlooking Encounter Bay on the southern coast of Australia. The expedition then turned back and made its way upstream, into the Murrumbidgee again, reaching the colonial settlements around Yass. On May 25th, after an absence of six months, Sturt returned to Sydney with much to tell Governor Darling.[2]

What Charles Sturt Saw in 1830

During his exploratory expedition along the inland river systems Charles Sturt[3] reported the presence of a disease severely affecting many of the Aboriginal people he encountered. The day following his entry to the Murray River, Sturt and his party were met by a group of 83 Aboriginal men, women and children (either Latje or Kureinj) whose appearance he described as being 'extremely picturesque and singular'.[4] Two days later, after setting camp, Sturt was approached by another group, of 35. He recorded:

> The most loathsome diseases prevailed among them. Several were disabled by leprosy, or some similar disorder and two or three had entirely lost their sight.[5]

Further downstream Sturt was again struck by the appearance of a disease, this time among the Barkindji. He saw many more affected by it:

> The most loathsome diseases prevailed throughout the tribes, nor were the youngest infants exempt from them. Indeed, so young were some, whose condition was truly disgusting, that I cannot but suppose they must have been born in a state of disease; but I am uncertain whether it is fatal or not in its result, though, most probably it hurries many to a premature grave. How these diseases originated it is impossible to say. Certainly not from the colony since the midland tribes alone were infected. Syphilis raged amongst them with fearful violence; many had lost their noses, and all glandular parts were considerably affected. I distributed some Turner's cerate to the women, but left Fraser to superintend its application. It could do no good, of course, but it convinced the natives we intended well towards them and, on that account, it was politic to give it, setting aside any humane feeling.[6]

Crossing what is now the border between Victoria and South Australia and into the territory of the Meru, Sturt and his party were in daily contact with larger groups, now numbering up to 200 or more per day.

> Their sameness of appearance, the disgusting diseases that raged among them, their abominable filth … combined to estrange us from these people, and to make their presence disagreeable.[7]
>
> … Some were blind and had difficulty in walking.[8]

Sturt and his party continued to observe the presence of this same state of disease among Aboriginal people during their progress downstream towards Lake Alexandrina. Finally, he commented on the Ngarrindjeri people he met on the lower Murray:

> It would disgust my readers were I to describe the miserable state of disease and infirmity to which these tribes were reduced. Leprosy of the most loathsome description, the most violent cutaneous eruptions, and glandular affections, absolutely raged through the whole of them.[9]

From Sturt's observation there can be little doubt that the Aboriginal people he met were indeed suffering from some form of debilitating disease, but what disease (or diseases) was it? Sturt alternately attributed the signs he saw to leprosy and syphilis. His confusion is understandable when the regions of the body displaying leprosy lesions are compared with those affected by syphilis. Leprosy affects the cooler parts of the body, with infection involving the nasal mucosa, upper respiratory tract and anterior segments of the eyes leaving the victim with nodular-like distortions of the face that can be confused with syphilitic destruction in the same areas.[10] The testes can also be affected, giving the misleading presentation of a sexually transmitted disease to the inexperienced observer. Because of their similar clinical features, leprosy and syphilis have often been confused by early writers.

Leprosy, however, can be ruled out. While this disease was later a problem among Aboriginal people in northern Australia, where it became endemic, no clinical or palaeopathological evidence for this disease has come from Aboriginal people in the southern half of Australia.[11] The disease described by Sturt appears to be of very high prevalence, affecting all ages. Leprosy, however, has a low attack rate and a long incubation period, ranging on average from three to six years, making its communicability low and clinical consequences presenting in just a few individuals.[12] Leprosy does not fit the description put by Sturt.

Was the disease Sturt observed in 1830 smallpox? An epidemic has been postulated as the cause for the destructive skin diseases described by Sturt along the Murray River.[13] However, the visible signs Sturt described in 1830 are not consistent with the characteristic rash, pustular stages and sequelae of smallpox.[14] An epidemic of this disease does appear to have swept along the Murray River corridor in the second half of the 1830s, several years after Sturt's journey by boat along the river. He had previously observed and recognised the disease among Aboriginal groups of the upper Darling River in

1828 and was familiar with the visible lesions and subsequent scarring of the disease.[15] Yet, he makes no mention of smallpox along the Murray during his 1830s Murray River expedition.[16]

What then of syphilis? Sturt was an astute and methodical observer and recorder during his expeditions but his descriptions of the disease he saw are those of a layperson. Sturt's education was not in medicine but in classics, mathematics and the natural sciences, from which he developed a 'superior dilettante acquaintance with botany, ornithology, zoology and geology'.[17] We have little way of knowing how experienced he was in identifying the clinical signs of diseases, although, like others of his time, he would have had at least a passing knowledge of syphilis and its symptoms, having lived in England where it was a common disease of children and adults.[18]

Nevertheless, Sturt's use of the term 'syphilis' alone cannot be seen as a firm indicator that the disease existed among the people he saw along the Murray. But, looking more closely at his comments in an aetiological and epidemiological context, several points emerge that support an epidemic disease, most likely syphilis, spreading along the Murray River populations at the time Sturt and his party were exploring the river. The infected Aboriginal people Sturt observed were living in a region then far removed from any colonial settlements in a land largely unexplored by Europeans. From Sturt's observations and descriptions, the diseased state was active between a point upstream of the Murray–Darling junction (between the present towns of Robinvale and Mildura) and the mouth of the Murray at Lake Alexandrina. The prevalence of infection was high among the groups, affecting both sexes and all age groups, including infants, strongly suggesting a congenital presence. The areas of the body involved, from Sturt's observations, included integument tissue (skin, hair and nails) over much of the torso, and soft tissue and bone destruction of the nasal region. Sturt also commented on blindness and lameness in some individuals he met.

The disease state of the Aboriginal groups Sturt described along the middle and lower Murray is indicative of an active epidemic of syphilis (caused by bacteria of the genus *Treponema*, which also causes endemic syphilis, pinta and yaws). Destruction of the peri-nasal soft tissue and bone would indicate that the disease was in its tertiary stage in some of the individuals. The blindness seen by Sturt may have been the result of tertiary syphilis of the central nervous system (neurosyphilis) or interstitial keratitis, a condition of late congenital infection affecting mainly an age group of 4 to 30 years.[19] The dissemination of skin lesions is consistent with the primary and secondary stages of untreated syphilis. Foetal involvement also seems to be represented, with infants displaying lesions to the surface of the body similar to adults.

Bioarchaeological Evidence

The presence of a treponemal infection along the Murray River corridor was diagnosed in osteological collections excavated from burial sites adjacent to the river in the 1900s.[20] However, physical anthropological research into past Australian Aboriginal populations using the osteological collections from around the continent has undergone a major change (and most likely a permanent change) since the late 1980s and 1990s. Prior to this time the osteological collections held by institutions had been freely available to legitimate researchers: early work was done on dental variations and wear; further work on these collections, particularly aimed at an understanding of the origins of Australian Aboriginal people, was done using a variety of techniques, including morphological variations; later work included examinations of trace elements and stable isotope analyses of bone samples, non-metric genetic variations and paleopathology.[21] However, since the 1990s much of this work was severely curtailed, with legislative controls over the housing of human skeletal collections, and the repatriation and reburial of large collections by Aboriginal custodians. Further study of the existing collections by researchers required permission from the various Aboriginal cultural communities.[22]

The effects of these changes, in regard to physical anthropological research in Australia, still resound today. Anthropologists have turned to re-examining previously collected data and applying new techniques or utilising cultural, historical or literature sources to extend their understanding of past Aboriginal populations.[23] Limited paleopathology examinations have occurred but primarily on single individuals excavated during specific archaeological digs. In these cases, the skeletal elements are either examined on-site or temporarily loaned to be examined under laboratory conditions. In both cases the remains are reinterred at the earliest opportunity, at the request of the Aboriginal custodians.[24]

In terms of examining the past populations along the Murray River corridor, the Roonka Bioarchaeology Research Project in South Australia took a step forward in continuing research on one of the remaining available collections, before running out of funding. This long-term collaborative project addressed pre-contact Aboriginal social and biological complexity along the Murray using the Roonka Flat archaeological and osteological[25] collections, as well as examining variations in cultural practices of existing Aboriginal burials and cemeteries.[26]

The Roonka Research Project aside, the result of the repatriation and subsequent loss of access to skeletal collections has resulted in the inability of many of the previously described skeletal pathological changes to be reinterpreted using new techniques. The osteological evidence of treponemal infection in the past populations along the Murray River that Sturt observed must therefore rely on examinations done prior to the repatriation process.

A comprehensive investigation of bone pathology using archaeological skeletal samples collected over a period of several decades from most of Australia's geographic and climatic regions was carried out when these collections were held in museums.[27] A substantial part of the investigation involved collections from the upper, middle and lower Murray River regions. A second study of archaeological skeletal samples, focused specifically on the middle and lower Murray River regions, was conducted by this author in 1997.[28] Both these studies agreed that the Murray River populations had a high prevalence of treponemal bone lesions.

Table 4.1. Treponemal infection in undated Australian Aboriginal crania.

Area	*n*	Cases	%
Murray River corridor	1374	94	6.8
South coast	263	7	2.7
Desert	183	9	4.9
Tropical	154	6	3.9
Coastal	219	4	1.8

Note: *n* = number of samples examined.

Source: S. Webb, *Palaeopathology of Aboriginal Australians: Health and Disease across a Hunter-Gatherer Continent* (Cambridge: Cambridge University Press, 1995).

Several important questions now arise. What type of treponemal infection had affected these skeletal samples? Was it venereal syphilis, a form of non-venereal syphilis or yaws? Was it introduced or was it occurring naturally among Aboriginal populations? How long had it been present when Sturt reported on it and how long did it last among the Murray River people? Why was the disease restricted to the middle and lower Murray populations and absent from those further east, as Sturt's records imply?

Both studies further agreed that the disease Sturt observed was indeed a form of treponemal disease but could not determine whether it was introduced venereal syphilis or an endemic form of the disease transmitted by non-venereal means. The inability to resolve the nature of the disease stemmed from two main considerations. First, while the diagnostic criteria for treponemal lesions in dry bone have been well determined,[29] the discrimination between venereal syphilis, non-venereal (or endemic) syphilis and yaws has not.[30]

Current understanding of treponematoses has now shown that the disease is caused by four closely related spirochetes: *Treponema pallidum pallidum* causes venereal syphilis, *T. pallidum pertenue*, *T. pallidum endemicum* and *T. pallidum carateum* are the agents of yaws, bejel (or endemic syphilis) and pinta respectively.[31] While these disease states can be isolated to the specific causative agents in living-tissue and soft-tissue examinations, apart from pinta, each can under particular circumstances affect living bone. The bone lesions left by the pathogens in dry samples (archaeological bone) can be similar and as such can be exceedingly difficult to diagnose to a particular causative agent.[32]

The second problem is related to the skeletal samples themselves. Most of the skeletal collections were poorly dated and as such the studies had little or no temporal control on the collections of individuals diagnosed with treponema. In many cases they had difficulty in determining whether the skeletal samples were pre-European or post-European contact. This is particularly the case with much of the Murray River collections, which were collected without detailed archaeological recording of their spatial or temporal integrity. The major study by Stephen Webb concluded that the 'extent and prevalence of Treponema in pre-contact Australia cannot be determined from skeletal material held in collections around Australia until some of it is dated'.[33]

Endemic or Non-endemic?

In order to establish which form of *Treponema* was affecting the Murray River groups Sturt encountered on his journey along the Murray consideration must now be given to yaws, non-venereal syphilis (endemic syphilis) and venereal syphilis. As discussed above, all can under certain conditions display clinical symptoms similar to those seen by Sturt.

Yaws certainly appears to have been common until recent times in some Aboriginal populations but its distribution is restricted to the tropical regions of central and northern Australia.[34] Long-standing endemicity of the disease has been noted in tropical Australia,[35] among the Arrernte of central Australia[36] and in the Kimberley region of Western Australia.[37] However, no trace of active yaws has ever been found among the Aboriginal groups of southern Australia.[38]

The temperate climate along the Murray River corridor does not favour yaws. The yaws bacterium (spirochaete) is a fragile organism outside its host and highly intolerant of seasonal changes, particularly seasonal cold and low humidity such as are characteristic of the Murray River and southern inland regions of Australia. The optimum environment for the organism and for the disease to become endemic in human populations is the humid, equatorial, lowland rainforests, where all months have a mean temperature exceeding 18 degrees centigrade and a rainfall exceeding 65mm per month.[39] The contemporary worldwide distribution of yaws in tropical and subtropical regions reflects this optimum environment. On this basis it is unlikely that yaws was the disease that Sturt saw.

Yaws can be excluded further. It is primarily a disease of children and adolescents, with males being more frequently affected than females.[40] It is usually contracted in infancy or early childhood through surface contact with infected children or adults. The condition may last for several years into adulthood, often in latent form.[41] The initial lesion commences as a large, rounded papule (mother yaw) at the point of inoculation, usually on the leg. It may also occur on the mouth of a suckling infant or on the breasts of a nursing mother. Within three to six weeks after initial infection, secondary eruptions occur and can extend over much of the body's surface. In many cases the disease is self-limiting and does not progress into the tertiary stage to involve skeletal structures, soft-tissue organs or the central nervous system. In later life all that may remain of an infection is scarcely perceptible scarring in the areas affected.

Bone lesions in yaws occur in about one per cent of cases and are commonly confined to the limbs. The most frequent bone is the tibia, followed by the fibula and the distal third of the femur. Cranial involvement in yaws is even less common and much less destructive than from syphilis. The main involvement in yaws is destruction around the nasal region. The frontal bone of the skull may be involved, but only in rare cases of tertiary yaws. When affected, the frontal bone usually displays shallow, pitted depressions that do not perforate the ectocranial surface and are not characteristic of the bone destruction (caries sicca) common in tertiary syphilis.[42]

With yaws then seeming unlikely, could the disease Sturt saw be an endemic form of syphilis that had flared up into an epidemic just as he was proceeding down the Murray River? This is possible but again unlikely. Endemic syphilis, like yaws, is a disease of childhood, usually contracted before the age of 15 years, with self-limiting symptoms and a low case fatality rate.[43] Several examinations of skeletal samples along the Murray River have shown that there is no definitive evidence of treponema dating before European contact.[44]

There are still problems with accepting endemic non-venereal syphilis as the disease Sturt observed. Was it just by chance that it was, for some reason, in a severe form of an epidemic phase, when Sturt passed through the region? How often an endemic disease flares up into a severe epidemic is dependent on the number of susceptible individuals in the community. In most cases of infectious endemic disease – endemic syphilis and yaws included – those susceptible are the young who have not been exposed to the pathogen and who have not developed immunity to the disease. Such a scenario does not sound plausible for the Murray River populations Sturt observed. The disease Sturt saw was affecting all ages, both young and old, and the symptoms were severe.

A further problem in accepting the existence of endemic syphilis along the Murray is that a considerable degree of cross-immunity to venereal syphilis would be expected in the Aboriginal groups if endemic, or non-venereal, syphilis was present. An example comes from the Pacific Islands. Until yaws was largely eradicated in many Pacific Island populations as a result of concentrated medical campaigns, venereal syphilis was virtually unknown, even after close contact between the indigenous populations and European colonists had been well established.[45] If endemic treponema had been present along the Murray River before European contact a low prevalence and attenuated clinical signs of venereal syphilis, when it was introduced, would be expected. Sturt's observation strongly indicates that this is not the case.

Venereal syphilis became a serious and common infection within Murray River groups after Sturt's return to Sydney. George Taplin, who spent from 1859 to 1879 among the Ngarrindjeri groups of the lower Murray and coastal regions as founder and superintendent of the Point McLeay mission settlement, writes:

> I have seen cases, even bad cases of syphilis amongst the natives. I am sure the disease was imported among them; they knew nothing of it before the advent of whites – this is the testimony of the natives. I have known fatal cases, also cases where the tibia was affected, and bony excrescences on the skin, with atrocious neuralgic pain.[46]

During his residency at Moorundie Aboriginal station from 1841 to 1843 as Aboriginal protector, Edward Eyre observed many inflicted with venereal syphilis. His account (originally written in Latin) reveals more about the disease:

> Of the diseases from which they suffer since the arrival of the Europeans by far the most frequent and the most deadly is the venereal strain … Among the natives this disease manifests itself in the same way as in many Europeans, yet for various causes it is even more hateful, especially

> because round pustules, commonly the size of an ounce weight, rise at the same time from the skin. The centre of these is gradually filled with flowing pus; then as they grow larger and larger and disperse, the surface of the whole body is affected with wasting and scab which cause horror and disgust to those near them. These ulcers sometimes may persist for six or eight months; but generally when irritants or caustics are applied locally they are cured within three weeks … After the first or second year the disease disappears, but sometimes causes death.[47]

Eyre appears to be in no doubt that the disease was venereal syphilis and that it followed a similar symptomatic course among the European population as it did among the Aboriginal population. His description of 'round pustules' rising from the skin and dispersing over the body corresponds to the secondary stage of untreated syphilis, with a maculopapular rash that disseminates in a variety of organs, most strikingly the skin over much of the body. Secondary symptoms of syphilis often spontaneously disappear within weeks and up to a year after formation, so it is doubtful whether Eyre's 'irritants or caustics' were effective. The disappearance of the disease symptoms after the first or second year, as noted by Eyre, would equate to the latent period between the secondary and tertiary stages of the disease. This observation is interesting because it suggests that Eyre was seeing only the primary and secondary stages of the disease and not the third and final stage. The pathological signs of tertiary syphilis, as seen by Sturt, would indicate that the disease had been present among them for some time and many would have been initially infected much earlier than when Eyre was seeing the disease.

The most parsimonious explanation for the disease Sturt observed is an epidemic of introduced venereal syphilis spreading along the Murray River corridor. This is supported by osteological evidence of treponema and by further historical documentation of venereal syphilis in the Murray River populations, elsewhere in South Australia and in the other eastern colonies.

An Early Introduction into South Australia

A final set of questions must now be addressed. If venereal syphilis was the disease seen by Sturt in 1830, it was present before the establishment of the colony of South Australia. When was it introduced, by whom and where?

Sexually transmitted diseases were among the first of the European pathogens introduced into Australia, almost certainly arriving with the First Fleet at Sydney Cove in 1788. Syphilis and its companion traveller, gonorrhoea, were firmly established as a health problem among Aboriginal groups within four years of the start of the settlement.[48] Lieutenant Governor David Collins was the first to comment on its presence. He recorded:

> The venereal disease also had got among them, but I fear our people have to answer for that; for though I believe none of our women had connection with them, yet there is no doubt but that several of the black women had not scrupled to connect themselves with white men.[49]

Within four years of the establishment of the Port Phillip (Melbourne) settlement in 1835 sexually transmitted diseases were being recorded in the Aboriginal groups surrounding the European settlement.[50] The source of the diseases may have been from the settlement itself or via sealing and whaling ships on the southern waters of south-eastern Australia since the early 1800s, preceding European settlement.[51] However, the inland timing and spread of these diseases is unknown.[52] Treponemal disease, along with gonorrhoea, may have reached the Murray River populations through Aboriginal individuals or groups moving inland from the European settlements but we have no evidence of the extent of the disease.

When observed by Sturt in the summer of 1830, the extent of syphilis among the middle and lower Murray populations suggests that it was introduced on the coast of South Australia and was even then spreading upstream towards the east. Sturt first recorded the symptoms of syphilis at a point upstream of the Darling River junction. He then continued to make similar observations among the Aboriginal people he met along the remainder of the river to its mouth. He makes no mention of the disease among the Aboriginal communities before this point. It would appear that the disease was not spreading from the established European settlements in the eastern colonial regions where it was already established.

A strong contender for its introduction is the sealing and whaling industry that began around the islands in Bass Strait and off the Victorian and South Australian coasts in 1803. Small base settlements were established on Kangaroo Island around this time[53] by the sealers, and ships often visited the mainland coast to kidnap Aboriginal women.[54] In 1819 Captain Sutherland of the brig *Governor Macquarie* recorded in his diary the activities of other ships' crew while at Kangaroo Island:

> They have carried their daring acts to extremes, venturing on the mainland in their boats, and seizing on the natives, particularly the women, and keeping them in a state of slavery, cruelly beating them on every trifling occasion, and when at last some of the marauders

> were taken off the island by an expedition from New South Wales, these women were landed on the main with their children and dogs, to procure a subsistence, not knowing how their own people would treat them after a long absence.[55]

An 1837 letter from John McFarlane, head of the South Australian Company's Rosetta Head fisheries, sheds further light on such an introduction of syphilis to the southern coastal regions of South Australia. He writes about the difficulties of keeping men employed and the inconvenience incurred by their absconding from his service.

> There are two more of my men which have run away, Mr Morgan and Richard Ralph, which I trust you will punish without any leniency as they have left me in a very disgraceful manner. Richard Ralph was ill with the venereal disease some considerable time and in fact gave the same to some of the poor natives about here which [*sic*] are now a spectacle of horrible misery to which Mr Cooper can testify. As for the lad Morgan which [*sic*] is only a boy I assure you brought the disgrace from Van Diemen land and gave the same to some of the poor creatures here. I used all of my medicines upon him, made him well after which he went again with them, which served him right for his own disorder given back to him. I do assure you the Blacks are quite enraged about it here.[56]

Although written several years after Sturt described the disease among the Aboriginal groups, the important point of this letter is the manner and means by which sexually transmitted disease could be introduced into Aboriginal populations ahead of the establishment of colonial settlements. In all probability, venereal syphilis was introduced to the coastal and lower Murray River populations several times over a period beginning in the first decade of the 1800s.[57] This is an acceptable timeframe for syphilis to have spread along the Murray River populations to a point where Sturt observed the severe and destructive manifestations of the disease among the Aboriginal populations.

* * *

The disease that Charles Sturt observed among the Aboriginal groups along the Murray River in 1830 was in all probability an epidemic of sexually transmitted syphilis. The introduction of the disease into the Aboriginal groups would have initially been through sexual contact between European males and Aboriginal females on the southern coastal regions following the arrival of sealing expeditions in the first decade of the 1800s. Infection readily spread within the Aboriginal communities by further sexual relationships. The severe nature of the disease described by Sturt, affecting males and females of all ages, is consistent with an introduced disease into an immunologically unprotected population with little or no herd immunity. A similar pattern of infectivity and severity of symptoms was documented in the early 16th century when syphilis reached epidemic proportions in Europe,[58] in the post-contact period in America[59] and the Pacific Islands.[60]

At the time Sturt observed the disease state among the Aborigines along the Murray River, syphilis, gonorrhoea and a suite of other sexually transmitted infections were becoming the foremost causes of serious chronic morbidity among populations throughout the continent. Either spreading far ahead of the settlements or following step by step the expansion of colonial settlements, these diseases were destructive and cruel among Aboriginal populations whose collective immune systems, isolated by thousands of years from the Old World civilisations, could not protect them.

Coda: Imagining the Consequences

What would it have been like to suffer from syphilis with no effective treatment? Consider an anonymous Aboriginal person living on the Murray River in the 1800s, either male or female, in their early 20s and sexually active. Following sexual intercourse this person is infected by the syphilis spirochete *Treponema pallidum*. After around three weeks this patient begins to notice an ulcer, or a group of ulcers, developing around the genital area. The ulcers are not painful but are accompanied by a fever, and the inguinal lymph nodes in the groin area begin to swell and feel uncomfortable. A rash may appear. The patient experiences periods of overwhelming malaise – restlessness, depression, anxiety, unhappiness, a general feeling of being ill and having no energy. The genital ulcers heal in a few weeks, but the malaise lingers. The rash spreads across the body and on the palms of the hands and soles of the feet. Warty growths begin to emerge around the genital areas. A severe headache develops, it comes and goes but is debilitating at times and the patient seeks rest. This is the beginning of meningitis, which will continue. The rash may settle but chances are that it will appear again. This cycle of symptoms may then disappear, and the patient begins to feel well again and can continue a normal daily life. The patient may experience weeks, months, even a few years of freedom from the disease, and may begin to think that the illness is over. But this period of apparent health will not last.

The syphilis spirochete remains in the body and is slowly spreading and reproducing throughout the internal organs. It begins to cause damage to the heart, blood vessels and liver. Severe arthritis begins to be experienced as the spirochetes invade the bones and joints. Around this time the spirochetes have established themselves in the central nervous system causing further debilitation and pain. The brain is invaded, and the patient begins to develop psychotic symptoms. They may experience episodes of joyous energy, creativity, heightened perception, dazzling insights leading into a sense of mystical knowledge. In between these episodes come those dreaded periods of malaise and depression, severe headaches and body pain. It is a continual cycle of euphoria and depression.

The spirochetes have now established themselves throughout much of the body and painful ulcers are developing on the surface of the nose and mouth and beneath the hair on the patient's head. The ulcers spread across the face and skull, eating through the skin and beginning to invade the underlying bone, and by now have most likely resulted in damage to the ears and eyes causing deafness and blindness. The end is now near for the patient.

The immune system is weakening, trying to cope with the spread of the disease, and secondary bacterial or viral lung infection occurs, causing lower respiratory damage and making it difficult to breathe and to exercise. By now the internal organs are shutting down and the patient is suffering insanity and speech impairment as the damage in the brain cells continues. The central nervous system begins to malfunction and the patient experiences periods of uncontrollable nervous spasms and lapses into a coma. Death from a cerebral infarction (stroke) is the outcome, and the patient is finally free of the terrible suffering.

This whole sequence of events and cycles may have taken a few months from initial infection by the spirochetes or may have taken several years. During the periods of symptom suppression the patient may have had further sexual interactions, either passing on the infection or receiving further infection. Whatever the case, like hundreds of other young and healthy individuals, the patient has suffered terribly from a frightening and painful disease.

If this anonymous patient was a female, then there may well have been further complications. The syphilis spirochete has a habit of crossing the placental barrier of infected pregnant females and invading the developing foetus, making the disease even more insidious. If she had become pregnant before or after being infected with syphilis, there would be a significant risk of losing the baby through a miscarriage. Intrauterine growth restriction, where the baby is infected and undernourished, stillbirth or preterm birth are other likely outcomes. If the child survives through the gestation period and is born with congenital syphilis the child may have anaemia, pneumonia, syphilitic sores and lesions within the body and damaged internal organs, all of which would restrict the infant's growth and development and lead to a premature death. If these circumstances are not bad enough, syphilis can be even more sinister. The baby may go full term and be delivered normally with no outward signs of the disease. But the spirochetes are still in the small body, inactive and causing no symptoms. But complications are likely to arise later, even some years into the child's young life. Major organ damage and the signs and symptoms that affect the adult in the tertiary stage of untreated syphilis would result, denying the young victim a fair chance of life.

Syphilis among the Aboriginal populations of the Murray River, as documented by Charles Sturt, would have had to be something well beyond their cultural perception and experience. It would have been terrifying beyond belief. The irony of it all was that those outsiders who brought the disease into the Aboriginal populations had very little understanding of the full complications and implications of the disease in its tertiary forms and its effect on a people who had had no experience of the disease.

Syphilis is a highly contagious disease, especially so in the first years of its progress. Even so, there would not be many clinicians in Australia today who have seen a case of untreated tertiary syphilis. It is now successfully treated with penicillin-derivative drugs. In Australia, benzathine penicillin and procaine penicillin are the preferred drugs used to treat the primary stage of the disease. But, before the development of penicillin in the 1940s, and particularly so in the 19th century, there were no effective treatments and the disease would run its course, often taking years, leading to a lifetime of pain and suffering.

In the European populations of Australia, a great deal of personal shame was attached to the disease, particularly due to its mode of transmission by sexual contact. Often the symptoms were concealed by those individuals who were unfortunate enough to be infected. Many did not want it known that they had engaged in sexual relations, particularly outside of marriage. If a sufferer sought treatment, the real cause of their symptoms was often concealed from their families and associates, and never spoken about. Doctor–patient privacy was inviolable in the case of syphilis. In all strata of Australian society, the disease was ever present, always feared, but not often mentioned or admitted. Because the symptoms of syphilis could be explained away by the sufferer or the physician to other more socially acceptable causes, syphilis, 'the venereal' or 'the pox' were often not mentioned or recorded.

These social inhibitions towards syphilis, however, were not so durable when it came to physicians or missionaries observing the disease in Aboriginal populations. In the historical literature there is an enormous number of references to the disease across Australia. For the unwary researcher today reading through the archival files it could seem that the disease was restricted mainly to the Aboriginal populations and certain unsavoury elements of European society. It just did not exist in the upper echelons of polite society – but it did.

Chapter 5

SEXUALLY TRANSMITTED DISEASE AFTER COLONIAL EXPANSION

Prior to the advent of modern drug therapies, sexually transmitted diseases were a dreaded affliction on humans. Ever present in many populations around the world, they caused misery, suffering and pain for centuries. Sexually transmitted syphilis, once introduced by European sailors to the south coast, spread along the Murray River populations far ahead of the colonial frontiers, as shown in the previous chapter. As the British colonial expansion spread from the shores of Sydney in 1788 to penetrate the whole continent, disrupting Aboriginal populations, so too did the scourge of syphilis and other sexually transmitted diseases.

Understanding Sexually Transmitted Disease

A common travelling companion of syphilis is another sexually transmitted disease, gonorrhoea. Gonorrhoea is caused by the gonococcal bacterium *Neisseria gonorrhoeae*. Infection is usually limited to the epithelial tissues of the urogenital tract, most commonly the urethra in males and the endocervix in females. In males, symptoms begin to appear two to seven days after infection and are characterised by a painful burning sensation when urinating (dysuria) and a purulent discharge. The infection may be self-limiting, in that it is temporary, or in some cases develops into a chronic carrier state. In such cases, acute prostatitis or epididymitis can result in male sterility. In females, infections can be asymptomatic or mild enough to pass almost unnoticed. In untreated cases or continual infection, pelvic inflammatory disease and blockage of the fallopian tubes can often occur. In such cases female sterility can result, making this disease a major factor in population decline.

While in most cases gonorrhoea is not life threatening for either males or females, secondary infections, most commonly gonococcal septicaemia, arthritis, meningitis and endocarditis can occur. Neonatal infection can arise from infected amniotic fluid or an infected birth canal. Symptoms usually arise a few days after birth. The major form of neonatal infection is gonococcal conjunctivitis, which may lead to permanent blindness. Other sites of gonococcal infection in neonates are the pharynx, respiratory tract, vagina, anus, joints and bloodstream.

Both syphilis and gonorrhoea often occurred simultaneously among the Aboriginal populations, causing severe pain and tissue destruction for the individuals infected. They also had a profound effect in terms of rapid population decline.

Syphilis and Gonorrhoea among the European Population

Sexually transmitted diseases were common among the crews of European ships exploring the Pacific in the 18th century. For example, James Cook's crew, together with other European voyagers, left a trail of sexually transmitted diseases, particularly syphilis and gonorrhoea, throughout the islands of the Pacific. Syphilis and/or gonorrhoea came with the First Fleet to Australia in 1788. Before sailing from Britain, Governor-designate Arthur Phillip had been concerned about the medical fitness of the future colony, realising that its success would largely depend on the health of all who sailed. He made a special request to the Home Office that convicts selected for transportation should be in a good state of health and free from sexually transmitted diseases. His request was not given due consideration. With the ever-increasing number of convicts in the already overcrowded prisons, the Home Office was under pressure to increase the number of convicts to be transported and their health was given little attention in the selection processes.[1]

Sexually transmitted disease became an unwelcome passenger to Australia, not only among the convicts but among the military contingent as well. By the time the fleet had reached the Canary Islands, their first port of call after just three weeks at sea, Surgeon White reported ten cases of 'venereal' – eight of them were convicts, the other two were marines.[2] Further cases were reported among both groups before the final destination of Botany Bay was reached.

Attempts to keep the sexes apart while at sea met with some success, but when landed their separation became impossible to ensure. Heterosexual liaisons began soon after the arrival ashore in Port Jackson, particularly among the convicts. Within three months of the settlement's establishment the presence of sexually transmitted disease among the convicts began to concern Governor Phillip and his medical staff. Not only was it becoming more prevalent, but it was common for the sufferers to conceal their condition in an attempt to escape punishment. In a vain effort to flush out those with the disease and prevent it spreading through the colony, Phillip ordered that any man or woman found to be concealing the disease should receive corporal punishment and be put on a reduced allowance of provisions for six months. Marriage was also encouraged by both the medical and religious authorities as a further attempt at inhibiting the spread of the diseases. Neither method was successful in stopping the spread of sexually transmitted disease throughout the colony. In a five-year period between November 1791 to September 1796 'lues venerea' (another name for syphilis) accounted for 5 of the recorded 137 deaths (3.6 per cent) among the civilian, military and convict contingents.[3]

It continued to be a major cause of morbidity among the colonial population throughout the 19th century. Annual reports from the Sydney Dispensary and Infirmary record that syphilis was the sixth most common disease in 1838–39, accounting for 4.8 per cent of all diseases treated. By 1859 it was the third most common disease, occurring at 7.0 per cent, and by 1874 it had reached second, at 6.5 per cent, with the leading cause of morbidity being accidents and violence.[4]

Syphilis and Gonorrhoea among Aboriginal Populations at the Frontiers

It is not known exactly when syphilis and gonorrhoea began infecting the Aboriginal populations of Australia. The diseases may have been introduced prior to the arrival of the First Fleet in 1788 during the seasonal arrivals of Malay fishing fleets on the north coast but there is no record of the diseases among the northern Aboriginal populations. However, there can be little doubt of an entry following the arrival of the First Fleet on the eastern coast, when physical relations developed between the Europeans and local Aboriginal women. Because of their mode of spreading through sexual contact, the diseases would have transferred through Aboriginal groups in the same manner, reaching epidemic levels ahead and beyond of the colonial borders. This was in fact the case, first throughout eastern and southern Australia and then into the west and north of the country.

New South Wales

The first indication that a sexually transmitted disease was affecting the Aboriginal population was when David Collins, the new colony's lieutenant-governor, reported in 1789.

> The venereal disease also had got among them; but I fear our people have to answer for that; for though I believe none of our women had connection with them, yet there is no doubt but that several of the black women had not scrupled to connect themselves with white men ...[5]

Which disease Collins is referring to, and at what time after the arrival of the First Fleet he saw it, remains unclear. Collins served in New South Wales from January 1788 until August 1796 and published his account of the colony in 1798, so he is most likely referring to the presence of one or more of the sexually transmitted diseases among Aboriginal people during that eight-year period. He then goes on to say:

> It was by no means ascertained whether the lues venerea had been among them before they knew us, or whether our people had to answer for having introduced that devouring plague. Thus far is certain, however, that they gave it a name, Goo-bah-rong; a circumstance that seems rather to imply a pre-knowledge of its dreadful effects.[6]

How quickly the diseases spread throughout the Aboriginal populations is unclear. It may not, however, have become a serious health problem among them until after at least the first six months of settlement at Port Jackson because of the infrequent contact between the two groups. Governor Phillip's objectives towards the Aboriginal people were twofold. On the one hand the function of the Port Jackson community was to establish a penal settlement in New South Wales. It was therefore necessary to control the movements of the convicts, who made up the bulk of the settlement's population, and to keep them from freely fraternising with the neighbouring Aboriginal groups. On the other, Phillip had also been instructed to foster a friendly relationship with the Aboriginal people, to establish a system of trade with them and to teach them the 'benefits' of his own civilisation. In order to do this, he had to meet with them. The first contacts between Aboriginal people and the colonists were, however, sporadic. When they did occur, misunderstanding and mistrust between the two often resulted in the angry use of weapons. The Aboriginal response was to avoid the settlement and its occupants.[7]

Keeping the convicts from meeting with Aboriginal people outside the confines of the settlement was, however, a problem for the colonial authorities. Collins recorded:

> In one of the adjoining coves resided a family of them, who were visited by large parties of the convicts of both sexes on those days in which they

> were not wanted for labour, where they danced and sung with apparent good humour, and received such presents as they could afford to make them; but none of them would venture back with the visitors.[8]

By the 1820s sexually transmitted disease was perceived by Europeans as a serious problem among Aboriginal people in the Sydney region. Peter Cunningham, a naval surgeon who made five trips to New South Wales aboard convict transport ships between 1819 and 1828, commented on disease among Aboriginal people. He made a distinction between gonorrhoea and syphilis, although attributing one disease to females and the other to males, and for the wrong reasons.

> From their natural filthiness, the women soon become diseased with gonorrhoea, and propagate this infectious malady among the convict-servants who cohabit with them. I have often observed the men too, labouring under eruptions of the skin resembling syphilis, and open tumours also in their groins apparently of the same nature; but time with them cures all disorders.[9]

In all likelihood gonorrhoea and syphilis were affecting both sexes.

Cunningham's view that 'time ... cures all disorders', while reflecting the state of medical knowledge of the era, was correct in one point but incorrect in another. It has already been established that gonorrhoea in males can be self-limiting, and if no further infection is acquired the individual may be entirely cured. However, mild clinical symptoms may appear in females for a short period but lead to the more serious pelvic inflammatory disease. Cunningham also appears to be referring to the primary chancres of syphilis, which can spontaneously heal within four to six weeks of infection even without effective treatment. The second and third stages of development of this disease often lead to more serious life-threatening complications if effective treatment is not provided.

Port Phillip

Sexually transmitted diseases among Aboriginal people soon began to be noticed by colonists after the settlement of Melbourne was established on the southern coast of south-eastern Australia in 1835.

Within four years of the establishment of this settlement, syphilis was recorded by several observers to be widespread among Aboriginal people. During the late spring and winter months of 1839, an increasing group had been living on the banks of the Yarra River, on the fringe of the new European settlement at Port Phillip (now Melbourne). Many of these people were in a poor state of health and were suffering from a variety of symptoms, including dysentery and fevers.[10] After six had died Dr Patrick Cussen, assistant surgeon for the Port Phillip settlement, was instructed by Chief Protector G. A. Robinson to visit the group and offer what assistance he could. Cussen reported back to the chief protector that most of those who were ill were suffering from syphilis:

Syphilis had been present among the Aboriginal people of the colony before this incident, according to Cussen – probably as early as 1837, two years after settlement. In his report back to the chief protector he noted:

> From an experience of more than a year and a half of the tribes which frequent this neighbourhood, I can assert that syphilis is (generally speaking) committing the most extensive ravages amongst them, and shall most shortly, if unchecked, render them extinct in a very few years. I have had several of them from time to time under my care and they appear to receive with avidity and gratitude any measures that are adopted for their advantage.[11]

In May 1839 Assistant Protector Sievwright wrote to the chief protector reporting that 'nine-tenths' of Aboriginal people under his administration around the present city of Geelong, on the western side of Port Phillip Bay, were victims of syphilis. The symptoms, he claimed, appeared in a more 'violent' form than even the most 'extraordinary' European cases. Sievwright went on to report that neither sex was exempt from the disease and those infected ranged from infants to the aged.[12] His observations were later supported by Foster Fyans, who had moved to the region as the police magistrate in 1837. He stated that 'large families of natives – husband, wife, boys, and girls – were eaten up with venereal disease' and estimated that 'two thirds of the natives' of the colony had died from this infection.[13]

The disease in this district could have two sources. It may have been carried along from the Melbourne settlement, 60km east, with the movement of colonists and Aboriginal people between the two settlements. Another potential source may have been from the sealing and whaling ships that had been frequenting the southern waters of south-eastern Australia since the early 1800s. If the latter, then syphilis and possibly gonorrhoea may have been present among the Aboriginal groups in this area for 30 years before the settlement of Victoria.

In 1840 syphilis was reported by Assistant Protector Edward Parker in the northern district of the Port Phillip colony. From early December of that year an increasing group of up to 170 had been gathering at the Loddon River Aboriginal Station. Parker reported that he had found '… five cases of syphilis of a very severe character'. The rest of the people appeared to be free from syphilis. Parker was concerned about the frequent sexual fraternisation between Aboriginal women and European men. He saw the Aboriginal people '… sinking to a lower degree of moral degradation by the pernicious intercourse which they have with the vitiated portion of the lower classes in the colony'. He was concerned enough to write to Chief Protector Robinson and request that it would be 'highly desirable' for a medical officer to visit the station as soon as possible to instruct him and his overseer on ways to administer to the disease. Medical help was not immediately forthcoming and his predictions about the increasing problem of syphilis were realised ten months later. In an urgent disposition he wrote again to Robinson:

> The call for medical assistance is however rendered especially urgent at the present time by the rapid and extensive spread of syphilitic affections among the aborigines … At the present time I fear more than half the women are infected, and the disease is rapidly spreading.[14]

Similar reports were made by a third assistant protector, James Dredge, on the Goulburn River. Dredge reported to the chief protector:

> … it is extremely difficult to convey a correct report of the awful amount of disease amongst both sexes of every age, resulting from illicit and promiscuous intercourse with the Whites, and with each other. This disease amongst the natives originating, in every instance – as my observation goes – in their intercourse with white men. For the cure of this loathsome and deadly disorder, no medicines adapted for their use have been placed at my disposal.[15]

While neither the assistant protectors nor the police magistrate were medically qualified, their reports of what would appear to have been an epidemic of syphilis can be taken with some confidence. All three assistant protectors had close contact with the Aboriginal people in their regions and were required to investigate and report any disease among them. Moreover, there is a strong similarity between all their reports and with the observations of Dr Cussen, who was convinced of a highly virulent epidemic of syphilis present among the Aboriginal people of the colony.

The reports of Cussen and the three assistant protectors reveal several features of the disease they observed, which was almost certainly syphilis.

All but Dredge reported that the symptoms they saw were due to syphilis and referred to it by that name. Dredge, while not specifically naming the disease as syphilis, states that he is certain that it was spread by sexual intercourse, particularly when Aboriginal females and European males were involved. By 1840 it was widespread throughout the colony. Cussen reports it among Aboriginal people at the main settlement of Melbourne, many of whom had come from areas further inland to camp on the fringe. The assistant protectors observed the symptoms in the vicinity of the European pastoral settlements in the south-east and the north of the colony. All report that there was a rapid dissemination of the disease among the Aboriginal groups, and morbidity and mortality were excessive. Both sexes and a wide spread of age groups were observed to be affected. While the claims of 90 per cent morbidity and two-thirds of the Aboriginal population dying from the epidemic may be exaggerations on the part of Sievwright and Fyans, they lend support to Cussen's observation that syphilis was at a high level among the Aboriginal people of the colony at the time. The actual mortality from the epidemic is, of course, unknown but the general tone of the reports demonstrates that it was severe.

Further evidence of the extent, persistence and severity of the epidemic is available from the papers of Chief Protector Robinson. Between April and October 1844 Robinson travelled throughout the eastern interior of the colony. His purpose was to examine firsthand the state and welfare of the Aboriginal people living near European settlements and those in the regions not settled by Europeans. Robinson continually saw men and women suffering from syphilis at Lake Omeo and Twofold Bay in the south-east, on the Snowy River and Monaro regions of the highlands and at Gundagai on the upper Murrumbidgee River. On his return Robinson reported that syphilis was 'almost general throughout the land' and had 'extended [its] baneful influences to the remotest parts of the interior'.[16]

In the same year concerned settlers on the Murray River in the northern region of the colony wrote to Robinson calling his attention to the state of the Aboriginal people in their region:

> At the present moment there are few stations in the District at which there are not from one to three Aborigines suffering under the various stages of Venereal; and besides the mortality it causes amongst the natives themselves it is also the means of propagating the disease among the labouring men of the District to a very great extent. There is, and we fear will be, until religion gradually works a change, a great deal of

> promiscuous intercourse between the Europeans and the Aboriginal native, the consequence of which is the rapid increase of the disease in the District.[17]

In 1848, while Robinson was visiting the Aboriginal Protectorate settlements of the colony, he reported that along the main road between Sydney and Melbourne there were 'as usual a great number suffering from Syphilis'.

By 1860 reports on the health of Aboriginal people living in the Murray River corridor began to indicate that the cases of sexually transmitted disease had decreased. Published in the first report of the Central Board for the Protection of the Aborigines, Thomas Goodwin wrote of the Yelta settlement near the junction of the Murray and Darling rivers in the north-west of the colony:

> Venereal is not so frequent amongst the men as is generally supposed, I have seen very few cases, but I believe many of the young women, and even girls are afflicted with it.[18]

In 1864 and again in 1866 the reports of the board indicate an improvement in the general health of the Aboriginal people along the Murray and a decrease in the number of sexually transmitted disease cases being observed. Dr Neil Campbell, who had been employed as a medical practitioner among the Aboriginal groups on the Loddon River, reported in 1867 that he had not seen sexually transmitted disease among those residing or visiting the station during the past four years.[19]

Medical descriptions of sexually transmitted disease among Aboriginal people in the 19th century are not well represented in the historical records. Probably the earliest surviving description of a sexually transmitted disease comes from Dr William Wilmot, medical officer and Melbourne's first coroner. In 1842 he attended the sick at Narre Narre Warren (Lake Tyers) Aboriginal Station, 40km south-east of Melbourne. His diagnosis of a 'syphilitic disease' he saw among Aboriginal people was based on his own observations of the clinical signs of the disease in what he took to be its various stages of development, from a few weeks through to six months after the suspected time of initial infection:

> It generally originates with a small cluster of irritable papulae on the inside of the thigh or scrotum and perineum, which rapidly coalesce, and degenerate into foul ulcers, terminating ultimately in a warty excrescence; in a few weeks it spreads very widely, and the skin becomes at length

> affected with a scaly eruption of a circular form, with a well-defined margin, giving it much the same appearance as lepra vulgare.
>
> The action of the virus [*sic*] is singularly modified by the habits and constitution of the native as it does not appear to pass through the ordinary channel of the lymphatic system into the constitution, but directly through the general circulation or capillary vessels as only in one instance and of a dubious kind did I meet with any appearance of specific glandular affection.
>
> In no case did I find any other than the inguinal glands affected; in no case was there any ulceration of the fauces [mouth and throat], nor did I meet with a single instance of a venereal node.[20]

The signs Wilmot describes are not compatible with the clinical signs of syphilis or gonorrhoea. Primary syphilis typically presents as a single painless ulcer or chancre at the site of inoculation, usually on the shaft of the penis, vulva, labia or cervix. The secondary stage of syphilis is characterised by a spreading maculopapular rash in a variety of organs, most commonly the skin of the palms and soles, mucosa, lymph nodes, stomach and liver. The rash is apparent in the moist genital surfaces, as well as the mouth, although in Wilmot's description the latter was not the case. Other secondary symptoms include the broad, flat plaques of lesions (condylomata lata) in warm, moist areas and lesions around hair follicles, neither of which can be reconciled to Wilmot's description. Gonorrhoea infections are commonly localised to the urogenital tract in both sexes, with males displaying the characteristic purulent discharge from the anterior urethra. No cutaneous lesions are associated with the infection.

The small clustering of 'irritable papulae on the inside of the thigh' is more suggestive of genital herpes. Herpes simplex virus type 2 produces a spectrum of vesicular and necrotising lesions localised to the genitalia and immediate surrounding regions. The principal sites of primary infection are the penis, cervix and vulva, with recurrent disease involving the perineal skin, legs and buttocks. The degeneration of the primary rash into 'foul ulcers', described by Wilmot, may represent localised secondary bacterial infection, particularly if those afflicted were living under unhygienic conditions, as was possibly the case. The 'warty excrescence' may represent genital warts (*Condylomata acuminatum*). They commence as small swellings in the perigenital and perianal regions, and rapidly grow into grouped pedunculated lesions. A number of lesions may fuse into a cauliflower-like mass.

A final possibility is that the pustular lesions may be due to chancroid infection (another sexually transmitted disease) caused by *Haemophilus ducreyi*. This bacillus is highly infectious and invades on contact through the skin or mucosa of the genitalia. A papule develops up to 14 days after inoculation, becomes pustular and ulcerates. The ulcers are usually small, but large mutilating ulcers can occur. Multiple ulcers are common. The lesions may spread locally to the perineum, anus, scrotum, thighs and/or lower abdomen.[21]

From examining Wilmot's description, it is not possible to come to any firm conclusion in identifying the disease, or indeed diseases, he saw. However, two of the most common sexually transmitted diseases of that time – syphilis and gonorrhoea – can be ruled out as contenders in this case, due to the incompatibility of the symptoms. This then leaves the other possibilities – herpes simplex, genital warts and chancroid. The latter is unlikely because the disease is mostly confined to the tropical and subtropical regions of the world, although introduction by infected sailors recently arrived via a tropical port is a possibility. An outbreak of herpes simplex, possibly accompanied by cases of genital warts, seems the most likely.

South Australia

The initial introduction and dissemination of sexually transmitted disease among the Aboriginal groups of South Australia differs somewhat from the two other colonies already discussed. A disease, most likely syphilis, had been introduced on the southern coast by the crew of sealing and whaling ships, and Captain Charles Sturt, on his exploration, had observed it spreading along the Murray River corridor with extreme morbid effect far ahead of European settlement. But, once settlement was established in Adelaide in 1836, sexually transmitted diseases, particularly syphilis, began to be recorded in Aboriginal populations.

There is little surviving evidence of syphilis among the Kaurna living around Adelaide and the surrounding coastal plains during the early years of the settlement. Dr William Wyatt was the third Aboriginal protector appointed in South Australia and held the post for two years from 1836. In an inquiry into the state of the Aboriginal people of the colony, Wyatt remarked that he first became aware of sexually transmitted disease, although 'manifested as very considerable difference in appearance and symptoms', after his first year as protector.[22] It is not clear, however, whether Wyatt was referring to syphilis, gonorrhoea or some other disease. Neither is it clear that he was referring specifically to Aboriginal people in the immediate vicinity of the settlement or along the coast and Murray River corridor with whom he also had contact.

Following Wyatt, Dr Matthew Moorhouse was appointed Aboriginal protector in June 1839. Moorhouse was an ardent supporter of Aboriginal rights but passionately believed in instilling a Christian education among those he administered. In a brief report on the health of the Aboriginal people, Moorhouse indicated that syphilis was present among those in Adelaide.[23] Again there is some doubt as to whether he was referring to the local Kaurna groups or groups from elsewhere. In 1843 Moorhouse estimated that 300 Aboriginal people in the Adelaide district were in regular contact with the settlers but many of these were Ngarrindjeri from the lower Murray and coast and Meru from the Murray River, who regularly visited the region following European settlement (which it is apparent that the Meru did not do prior to settlement).

The diffusion of sexually transmitted disease into the Adelaide area and its subsequent morbidity and mortality among Aboriginal people may have been lower than it had been among the other Aboriginal groups living near the settlements of Sydney and Melbourne. Summers has argued that the more liberal, humanitarian background of the first settlers to South Australia, and the more orderly nature of colonisation there, had the effect of creating amicable relations with the Kaurna.[24] The absence of convicts in the colony may also have had some effect in reducing sexual relations between the two groups and consequently the prevalence of sexually transmitted disease. Alternatively, it would seem highly unlikely that sexual relations between free European males and Aboriginal women did not regularly occur. It was a common practice for Aboriginal women to be prostituted in exchange for tobacco, alcohol and food from the early days of the settlement. The timing of sexually transmitted disease into the Kaurna population occupying the Adelaide Plains is unknown.

Its timing and distribution north and west of Adelaide is more readily substantiated. During the 1850s and 1860s European pastoral leases and settlements became established on Eyre Peninsula and in the recently surveyed regions north of Spencer Gulf. As early as 1852 sexually transmitted disease was being reported as a serious health problem among the Banggarla and Nawu people who had contact with the pastoralists. Moorhouse reported to the South Australian Government that there had been a 'considerable mortality' among the adults. Thirteen men and one woman had died chiefly of 'secondary symptoms of venereal'. Moorhouse wrote that he could do little about the problem other than send 20 blankets to be given to those suffering.[25]

The process of settlement and Aboriginal dispossession north and west of Adelaide continued into the final decades of the 19th century, with recurrent releases of pastoral land tracts at the head of Spencer Gulf and into the Flinders Ranges. Sexually transmitted disease spread among Aboriginal people at an equally comparable and disastrous pace. In 1867 newly appointed Sub-Protector E. B. Scott travelled 2000 miles (3200km) along the spine of the Flinders Ranges and between Lake Frome and Lake Torrens. He met with the Banggarla, Adnyamathanha and Kuyani groups and reported to Protector Buttfield, with some ambiguity, that their general health was good but there had been a great amount of 'sickness' among them.[26] Subsequent reports by Protector Buttfield to the Commissioner for Crown Lands (by now the body responsible for Aboriginal affairs in South Australia) allude to a satisfactory state of health and make no reference to any sexually transmitted disease present among them.

By the mid-1870s further pastoral development and an increase of the European population altered the Aboriginal health situation. In 1874 Buttfield now reported that there was 'a great deal of sickness' and syphilis was one of the principal diseases.[27] Once established, syphilis was maintained among Aboriginal people who had frequent contact with Europeans. In his annual report on the state of Aboriginal people in the northern district of the colony for 1887, Sub-Protector Beasley recounted that:

> … there are a great many suffering badly from venereal disease, caused principally by contact with Shearers and those from Town, this is a sad thing for these unfortunate creatures, but what can we do. The evil cannot be stopped, nor the disease cured in most cases, as they cannot be induced to use or submit to the necessary Medicinal remedies … Consequently this terrible disease is spreading.[28]

By 1879 the pastoral frontier had moved north of the Flinders Ranges and was now into the arid regions beyond Lake Eyre. Syphilis had spread with the northern movement and was infecting the Dieri, whose lands centred around Cooper Creek on the edge of the Strzelecki Desert. Missionary C. A. Meyer, at Kopperamana mission, reported to the sub-protector:

> The general health of the Aborigines has not been very good during the past year as they all – with only a few exceptions – suffer from Syphilis [emphasis in the original] it would therefore be very advisable to have medicines for them.[29]

Syphilis developed into a major health problem among the Dieri, with little or no treatment or help available to them. In some circumstances, help for the inflicted was actively denied. It was the policy of the Lutheran missionaries at the Killalpaninna mission settlement (of which Kopperamana was an outstation) to expel those suffering the disease because of their perceived 'immoral behaviour'.[30]

The effects of chronic sexually transmitted disease on the fertility of the Aboriginal groups cannot be assessed with any degree of precision from the historical records, as there is not enough quantitative demographic data. It is reasonable to assume, however, that where there was a high prevalence of sexually transmitted disease, particularly where it was likely to go untreated and the chances of reinfection were high, there is a strong likelihood of associated infertility. A hint of such a situation among Aboriginal people at Kopperamana was given by Meyer in 1885. Although Meyer kept no written record of births and deaths, he observed that there had been no increase among the 65 living on the mission settlement or among the 40 or 50 living nearby.[31] Meyer did not specify whether this was an effect of a reduction in the birth rate, mortality or migration. If it was due to reduced births, then gonorrhoea may have been involved. Tubal destruction from pelvic inflammatory disease in females and testicular inflammation (epididymo-orchitis) in males is a complication of untreated gonococcal infection leading to sterility.

Several years earlier George Taplin, in a report on the Ngarrindjeri living on the Point McLeay settlement (Raukkan), stated:

> I am well aware that the temptations held out by white men to the native girls are constant and attractive, especially to those who can earn so little money ... I notice that decent, chaste women among the natives almost invariably have large families. I know of three who have had three children in five years.[32]

Taplin is referring mainly to those who were living on the Point McLeay settlement and its outstation. Like most missionaries, Taplin strongly opposed premarital sexual relationships and encouraged monogamous marriages. Such a practice, if maintained, would reduce the incidence of sexually transmitted infection. The implication of 'decent and chaste' women having large families may then be an indicator of the reduction of sexually transmitted disease, particularly gonorrhoea, and a reduction of associated tubal infertility.

Bernier and Dorre Islands, Western Australia

In Western Australia, 'lock hospitals' were set up on Bernier and Dorre islands and operated from 1908 to 1918. The name dates back to the early leprosy hospitals established in London during the reign of Henry VIII. 'Lock' refers to the ragged bandages that were used to cover the leprosy lesions of the patients.[33] In later years lock hospitals were established during the peak period of the British Empire in the 1800s. They were originally built to confine women, in British garrison towns in the colonies and at home, who had contracted venereal disease (usually from British soldiers and sailors). Their aim was more towards protecting the military personnel from acquiring venereal disease than caring for and treating the local infected women. While they came under much criticism and opposition from the public in the homeland, they were continually established under acts of parliament in the colonies well into the 20th century. In Australia, lock hospitals were set up in Melbourne and Brisbane, specifically designed to treat and confine prostitutes who were deemed as showing the signs of a venereal infection, and on Fantome Island, in the Palm Island group in Queensland, from 1928 to 1945 for Aboriginal people.[34]

The Western Australian lock hospitals on Bernier and Dorre islands were located at the north-west extremity of Shark Bay, today a popular tourist destination, 45km from the mainland coast at Carnarvon. These islands, washed by the rolling waves of the Indian Ocean, are elongated and narrow fingers of land, remnants of former ice-age coastal dunes formed on a landscape that drowned as the sea rose, a consequence of melting ice sheets. Uninhabited by Aboriginal people in the past, they are lonely windswept places even today, guarding the entrance of Shark Bay. The islands are listed on the National Heritage Register and are part of a World Heritage-listed area significant for its scientific, flora and fauna values. But their Aboriginal history, albeit brief and forlorn, goes unrecognised on state and Commonwealth heritage lists.[35]

The lock hospital scheme was the first attempt by the Western Australian Government to systematically deal with Aboriginal health and particularly the long-standing problem of syphilis among Aboriginal and European populations. In 1905 a royal commission was held to investigate the administration of the pearling industry in the north of the state, particularly its employment and treatment of Aboriginal people. One of the commission's concerns was the spread of sexually transmitted diseases, particularly syphilis, emanating from the pearling industry. Among the advisers to the royal commission was Dr Richard Wace, resident magistrate and district medical officer at Derby. He informed the commission that the influx of foreign crew members from the pearling ships was:

> ... most thoroughly demoralising to the blacks. In the laying-up season of this year several pearling luggers laid up at Cygnet Bay. Several cases

> of supplying liquor to the blacks were brought down here. In every case I asked why the defendants had given the liquor, and in every case I was informed that the reason was that they wanted one of the women. I think that liquor is seldom given in these cases – in fact in any cases – to the aboriginals except for that specific purpose. It is the recognised payment. I have treated several cases this year of specific diseases amongst the pearling boats, and I know from my own knowledge that it is extremely prevalent amongst these crews and cannot but have an extremely bad effect amongst the blacks. It is readily communicable, and its worst point is that it is hereditary [*sic*]. It has a morally and physically deteriorating effect both on the one who contracts it and the one to whom it is communicated by descent. To my own knowledge, girls have been taken from a mission station in accordance with the tribal marriage customs – young girls of 14 or 15 years, who have only just arrived at maturity and in perfect health – taken away and prostituted amongst the crews of the luggers, returning after some time suffering from specific disease. One of the main reasons of the dying out of the black race is the fact that, through prostitution, the women become infertile. This, by the way, applies throughout the district.[36]

The role of the lock hospitals was to curb the sexual activities between Aboriginal women and European males in the townships and cattle stations, and the Asian crew members of the pearling luggers, by isolating the infected Aboriginal people. Aboriginal men and women who were diagnosed or suspected of suffering from a venereal infection were forcibly removed from their country on the mainland and transported to the isolation of the island lock hospitals. In many cases the decision that an Aboriginal male or female had a venereal disease was made solely by police troopers, who had no medical training and often little experience in determining one disease from another. Expeditions by the police and sanctioned by the government were sent into the inland areas to round up those they suspected of having a venereal disease and then forced them to walk, often restrained in neck chains, several hundred kilometres to the coast. There they were then taken by boats to the islands. Males were sent to Bernier Island and females to Dorre Island. In 1911 one police expedition collected 99 people. On these long journeys many of the sick and aged would never make it to the islands.[37]

Grant Watson, a young Cambridge biological science graduate who accompanied English anthropologist Radcliffe-Brown on research expeditions, observed these round-ups of men and women being taken to Bernier and Dorre islands. He wrote that the journey:

> ... often took weeks, and many prisoners died by the way. Flies in clouds buzzed about suppurating sores. The chains were never removed, for if they had been the natives would have been quick to escape. Men and women mingled, and it was not surprising that all the survivors were thoroughly infected by a variety of ailments by the time they arrived at their destination.[38]

This practice often meant removal to an unfamiliar land, along with other Aboriginal people whose culture was foreign and languages unintelligible. Such separation from family and kin groups caused additional trauma and psychological stress to the infected individuals. If they were fortunate to survive the disease while incarcerated at the lock hospitals and diagnosed as cured by the medical staff, the government policy enabled them to leave the islands and, if again fortunate enough, they might find themselves back in their homelands. Once released from the island, however, there was no organisation in place to take them back. Many would have faced the prospect of finding their own way and many would not have attempted to cross regions with which they had no traditional affiliation or knowledge. Torn from their country and kin by a colonial government policy, they were left to fend for themselves.[39]

Many, however, died on the islands from a combination of the disease and psychological stress caused by their removal from country. Cross-infection with other diseases, particularly tuberculosis, would also have added to the morbidity and mortality on the islands.

Table 5.1. Documented number of admissions, discharges and deaths on Bernier and Dorre islands lock hospitals during their years of operation.

Gender	Admissions	Discharges	Deaths
Male	209	151	45
Female	426	273	116
Unspecified	2	26	8
Total	637	450	169

Source: Mary Anne Jebb, 'The Lock Hospital Experiment: Europeans, Aborigines and Venereal Disease', in Bob Reece and Tom Stannage (eds), *European-Aboriginal Relations in Western Australian History* (Nedlands: University of Western Australia, 1984), p. 81.

Table 5.1 shows a disparity between the admissions and the combined discharges and deaths, which almost certainly is the result of inconsistency in the stations' record keeping. Neverethless, it reveals several indications of the prevalence, morbidity and social attitudes to venereal disease. Two-thirds of all admissions over the ten-year period of the lock hospitals were females (67 per cent) compared with males (33 per cent). This gender disparity strongly suggests that the rate of infection and resulting morbidity from venereal disease in Aboriginal groups throughout the settled, rural and mining areas of Western Australia was much higher in females than males. This may well have been the case as it was commonplace for European and Asian men on the outlying rural stations and the crews of pearling ships to engage in sexual activity, often forcibly, with Aboriginal women, thereby infecting them time and again with venereal diseases.

The gender disparity in admissions may also reflect the prevailing opinion by the European population, government and civil, that the prevalence of syphilis was the direct fault of Aboriginal women spreading it among the population. The fact that the disease did not exist in pre-contact Aboriginal populations and that it was repeatedly introduced by colonists and seafarers into the Aboriginal populations was an inconvenient issue that was to be officially placed firmly into the moral abjurations of all.

Of those unfortunate enough to be admitted to the lock hospitals, 27 per cent were never to leave the islands. Such a high mortality exposes another damning indictment on the efficacy of the lock hospital program – and this figure does not include those who died on the long journeys to the islands or those who were discharged, seemingly cured, who would never make it back to their country.

In 1909, Frederick Lovegrove, the superintendent medical officer on the islands, reported to the chief protector that on arrival the Aborigines were provided with 'clothes, blankets, and rations of flour, sugar, tea, and tobacco', and those well enough were allowed to hunt and fish and, during the summer months, collect turtle eggs and meat. In many cases the Aboriginal inmates lived in mia-mias they constructed themselves from brushwood. These traditional structures were preferred over the tarpaulin shelters that had been originally provided. They were later able to live in small sheds constructed of a timber frame, a corrugated-iron roof and covered on three sides by canvas, leaving the front section open for a fireplace.[40] A 20-bed hospital was erected on Dorre Island for the females and a 12-bed building for the males on Bernier island.

While such a lifestyle might sound ideal, particularly in an official government report, the reality of the conditions experienced was far from ideal. Daisy Bates, who had cared for the welfare of Aboriginal people, visited the islands in 1910 with Radcliffe-Brown and Watson, as part of their anthropological research. Bates, who had originally been in favour of the lock hospital policy, later described the situation on both islands:

> Dorre and Bernier Islands: there is not, in all my sad sojourn among the last sad people of the primitive Australian race, a memory of one-half so tragic or so harrowing or a name that conjures up such a deplorable picture of misery and horror unalleviated as these two grim and barren islands off the west Australian coast, that for a period, mercifully brief, were the tombs of the living dead.[41]

Watson came away with the same damning opinion of the conditions and the people forcibly incarcerated on the islands:

> ... broken and helpless pieces of humanity who lay still all day and looked out across the bleak expanse of sand dunes, under which they were destined to be buried, and thought regretfully of their beloved and far away bush.[42]

Radcliffe-Brown, a Cambridge-trained anthropologist with a scientific outlook, who was later to take the chair of anthropology at the University of Sydney, oddly did not comment on the conditions on the islands or the deprivations faced by the Aboriginal inmates, although he collected and documented genealogies as they died.[43]

Each morning, after breakfast, the Aboriginal people were assembled at the surgery, with the necessary dressings changed and medication given. Medication was usually in the form of regular mercury, arsenic compounds and iodine of potassium treatments, all of which were largely ineffective. In fact, mercury-based treatments conferred more harm than good when applied or taken regularly as a therapeutic.[44] It would not be specious to suggest that those with syphilitic lesions being treated with mercury were more likely to suffer prolonged morbidity and have a higher mortality than those whose condition was left largely untreated.

Was It Only Syphilis?

While syphilis was common throughout the Aboriginal groups in Western Australia, as it was elsewhere on the continent, many who were sent to the lock hospitals may not have been suffering from that disease. Dr Hickenbotham, a medical practitioner at Carnarvon on the shores of Shark Bay who was familiar with syphilis and who had examined the Aboriginal people at the lock hospitals, thought the cases he saw presented anomalies in their clinical presentation and history. He considered many were not suffering from 'true syphilis' but what he called 'ulcerative or infective granuloma'. Prior to the discovery of the treponeme causing syphilis in 1905, the disease was often confused by the medical fraternity with other skin and genital ulcerative diseases. Diseases such as leprosy, gonorrhoea, chancroid, cancer, lymphogranuloma inguinale (donovanosis) and lymphogranuloma venereum (LGV) could mimic the clinical signs and progression of venereal syphilis or exist as a coinfection. So there is a reasonable case that what Hickenbotham was seeing in the Aboriginal people he examined in the lock hospitals was not always or only syphilis. He had previously examined suspected cases of syphilis among European stockmen and Aboriginal women with whom they had cohabitated and noticed 'interesting discrepancies' between them and the syphilis patients he was familiar with.[45]

Hickenbotham, together with the government pathologist, Professor J. B. Cleland, described the clinical aetiology of the disease:

> In the male, the first signs of the disease are small round nodules on the glans penis, varying in number from one or two to a condition in which the glans is thickly studded with them, and presents as sort of tessalated [*sic*] cauliflower appearance. These nodules are prone to ulceration especially when covered by a tight foreskin, and great destruction of tissue may follow. It frequently happens that on removing a tight foreskin, half the glans has been eaten away, by ulceration, and the other half presents the characteristic nodules, coalescing with one another in parts and some them being ulcerated.[46]

In one of the worst cases Hickenbotham examined the ulcerations reached across the whole groin region. In the females he examined the infection showed a similar trend, beginning around the vaginal regions and spreading to adjoining skin areas. In some cases, they noted that the infection would mediate and appear to clear up, only to return again. Both Hickenbotham and Cleland found that the various local applications commonly used to treat syphilis had little effect and the ulcerations would eventually lead to permanent soft-tissue destruction and death of the individual.[47] The disease was becoming problematic at the two lock hospitals, incurring an increasing death rate preceded by long-standing suffering. The only treatment was to operate on the ulcerating tissue, removing, cleaning and scraping away the dead and infected areas, only to find the process reappearing. In other extreme cases, genital excision was resorted to. One can only imagine the physical and psychological trauma such a medical procedure would incur.

It is of course difficult to substantiate what the disease Hickenbotham was puzzling about on Bernier and Dorre islands during his examinations over a hundred years ago, but two suspects are donovanosis and LGV. Both diseases are transmitted by sexual contact and both can cause inflammation and ulcerations of the genitals and perigenital regions, leading to severe disfigurement and life-threatening situations if untreated.

LGV is caused by the bacterium *Chlamydia trachomatis*, which is more commonly known as the pathogen causing the eye disease, trachoma. Trachoma was in the past, and still is today, a problem mainly affecting Aboriginal populations living in the remote northern parts of Australia. *C. trachomatis* is more accurately classified as a serovar complex of strains of the same species of bacterium, each strain having slight differences in its DNA. *C. trachomatis* strains A, B and C cause the eye disease trachoma and strains L1, L2 and L3 cause LGV. Other strains of the bacteria can also cause inflammation of the urethra, cervicitis, pelvic inflammatory disease, particularly salpingitis (scarring of the fallopian tubes often rendering females infertile), and pneumonia.

Donovanosis is caused by a different bacterium, *Klebsiella* (formerly *Calymmatobacterium*) *granulomatis*. The disease is now rare in Australia but, until recently, it remained a problem with Aboriginal and Torres Strait Islander people in the remote tropical and subtropical areas of northern Western Australia, far-north Queensland and the Northern Territory, and often went misdiagnosed.[48]

Whatever the disease was that puzzled Hickenbotham, and it could have been both LGV and donovanitis occurring in the inmates, the treatments applied by the medical staff were not effective. Along with the ever-present venereal syphilis, it was causing serious distress among the Aboriginal inmates of the lock hospitals. Lovegrove, most likely at the end of his wits and skills, requested that an experienced bacteriologist familiar with venereal diseases might be required to join him on the islands to investigate the disease. In the early 1900s bacteriology was a developing branch of medicine in Australia, following on from the research on bacteria in Europe by Louis Pasteur in the 1860s and the germ theory of disease causation by Robert Koch in the 1870s. In an effort to avoid expense, however, Lovegrove suggested to the Western Australian Government that a junior pathologist from a university could be given the opportunity to do original research, using the infected Aboriginal inmates as case studies, to isolate the causative agent of the disease. Dr Steele, a newly appointed pathologist for Central Health Services in Western Australia, was sent to the islands in 1910 to investigate. He came with a new arsenic-based drug that had been used in Europe and had been purported to be the wonder-drug cure for venereal syphilis – compound 606.[49]

Compound 606 (later known as Salvarsan) had been developed by Paul Ehrlich, a German scientist (and 1908 Nobel Prize winner), and had quickly shown to be effective against syphilis in many cases. It came in a powder form and had to be mixed with pure, sterilised water and injected intravenously. But it was not the magic bullet that the medical profession thought it was to be, even though it remained a worldwide treatment for syphilis until penicillin became available in the late 1940s. Nor was it the blockbuster cure for Steele and the Aboriginal patients he treated at the lock hospitals. Steele stayed on the islands until June 1911, but could not find an effective treatment for the terrible diseases affecting the Aboriginal people. If the diseases were LGV or donovanosis, he would have had to wait at least another four decades before effective antibiotics became readily available to provide the cures he was looking for.

The two lock hospitals on Bernier and Dorre islands closed in 1918. The remaining 24 surviving inmates who were thought to be suffering from syphilis were transferred back to the mainland to another lock hospital in Port Hedland to see out their time. Known as the 'Depot for Diseased Natives', the Port Hedland facility was to eventually close in the early 1960s, ending an ineffectual and traumatic government policy in the treatment of Western Australia's Aboriginal people.

Coda: Examining Recent Outbreaks

In the first years of the 21st century the medical profession was beginning to believe they were close to eliminating syphilis from the remote Indigenous communities where it had been constantly simmering. But, like many past attempts to rid communities of infectious diseases, such speculation (hopes) can be premature. Moving towards the third decade of the 21st century syphilis is still a concern in remote Indigenous communities.

In January 2011 an outbreak of syphilis started in an Indigenous community located in far-north Queensland on the Gulf of Carpentaria. At that time sexual health services across Queensland were subjected to budget cuts by the state government, and surveillance and treatment services were affected. What started as a handful of cases in the community began to spread. Further cases were detected in the Northern Territory in July 2013, and then in the Western Australia's Kimberley region in June the following year. In 2016 and 2017 further cases were detected in the western, central and far-north regions of South Australia. The slow spread of the outbreak followed the movements of

Indigenous people throughout the regions as they travelled to visit other communities. By mid-2018 more than 2088 had been infected. In all the regions, the disease occurred mainly in the younger age groups and in females more than males.[50] Amid the outbreak six infants died from congenital syphilis.

In 2012, in response to the increasing notifications of active infectious syphilis, the state and territory governments responded by developing *Interim Guidelines for the Public Health Management of Syphilis in Remote Populations in Australia*.[51] As the disease spread and its incidence increased, the Multijurisdictional Syphilis Outbreak Group was formed, in 2015. During the outbreak a general Australia-wide health survey of Aboriginal and Torres Strait Islander people reported that there were 433 syphilis notifications for that year alone among Aboriginal and Torres Strait Islander people, accounting for 16 per cent of the notifications in Australia. The notification rate for this disease was over six times higher than for non-Indigenous people (61 per 100,000 and 10 per 100,000 respectively).

The disease was highest in the 20–29 years age group (164 per 100,000 in males and 166 per 100,000 for females), and for non-Indigenous people it was highest for the 30–39 years age group for males (39 per 100,000) and the 20–29 years age group for females (1.5 per 100,000). The percentage of infectious syphilis notifications for Aboriginal and Torres Strait Islander people was slightly higher for males (55%) than for females (45%).

For the same period there were 3518 notifications of gonorrhoea, which accounted for 19 per cent of total notifications in Australia. The notification rate was ten times higher for Aboriginal and Torres Strait Islander people than for non-Indigenous people. The majority of cases occurred in the 15–29 years age group. The diagnosed rate in Indigenous populations was slightly higher for females, whereas in the non-Indigenous populations it was four times higher in males. The survey report suggested that the transmission of syphilis and gonorrhoea occurred largely through heterosexual contact in the Aboriginal and Torres Strait Islander populations, whereas sex between males was the predominate mode of transmission among non-Indigenous people.[52]

Back to that outbreak of syphilis. In November 2017 (six years after the first notification) an action plan was put into place by the Australian Health Protection Principal Committee, a federal agency. The objectives were first to control the outbreak of syphilis in all the communities, then to undertake control efforts for other sexually transmitted diseases and finally to investigate 'long-term sustainable responses' to prevent further outbreaks with an 'ultimate goal of reducing rates' of sexually transmitted diseases to a 'sustainably low level'.[53]

This outbreak of syphilis, a disease that can today be successfully treated and controlled, serves as a warning that, even in this modern age of medical technology, fully functional and funded medical surveillance and disease management services must be maintained across the whole country for Indigenous and non-Indigenous communities alike, particularly for remote areas. As the old cliché goes, history has a way of repeating itself.

Part 3

Respiratory Diseases

Chapter 6

TUBERCULOSIS AMONG ABORIGINAL POPULATIONS 1788–1901

On Tuesday May 1st 1770, a gentle northerly breeze blew over Botany Bay in what was to be the colony of New South Wales. Lieutenant James Cook, commanding officer of Her Majesty's Barque *Endeavour*, anchored in the bay, wrote in his log:

> Last night Forby Sutherland, Seaman, departed this Life, and in the A.M. his body was buried ashore at the watering place, which occasioned my calling the south point of this bay after his name.

Sutherland had died 'of consumption with which he had been Afflicted ever since our departure from Streigtes le Maire'.[1]

Forby (Forbus) Sutherland became the first recorded European to be buried in Australia and his death was the first recorded mortality from tuberculosis in the country.

Tuberculosis is recognised as a disease of considerable antiquity among human Old World and New World populations.[2] Examinations of archaeological human skeletal collections dating back around 6000 years show osteomyelitis destruction of bone attributed to tuberculosis infection in European and North African populations and pre-Columbian populations in the Americas.[3] The disease may have a greater antiquity, possibly having an early progenitor present in East Africa as early as three million years ago, infecting early hominids at that time and evolving together with modern humans.[4]

Tuberculosis is an infectious disease caused by pathogenic responses of the genus *Mycobacterium* in human and non-human mammals. There are many species of the bacterium throughout the world, of which around 30 have been known to cause debilitating disease in humans.[5] The most common and regularly pathogenic to humans are *M. tuberculosis* and *M. bovis*. *M. tuberculosis* is usually acquired through human-to-human contact and is the more harmful of the two. *M. bovis* is acquired from cattle, often through drinking unpasteurised milk. An attack from the bovine type, often confined to children, can induce protection against a later infection by *M. tuberculosis*. Childhood infection by *M. bovis* can then act as a safeguard to adults exposed to the human bacterium. Other species of mycobacteria, *M. africanum*, *M. canettii* and *M. microti* can also induce a pathogenic response and, together with the human and bovine species, make up a complex of closely related bacterial infections in humans.[6] *M. leprae*, the causative agent of leprosy (Hansen's disease) is another closely related species but has a different pathogenic reaction to tuberculosis.

In England, towards the end of the 18th century, tuberculosis was well entrenched in the population, reaching a peak prevalence causing the death of 1–2 per cent of the population each year.[7] 'Consumption' was the most common term for tuberculosis used by 19th-century medical practitioners, including those in the Australian colonies. It refers to the most prevalent form of the disease, pulmonary tuberculosis. Other common terms were 'phthisis', referring to the slow wasting away of the body, and 'scrofula' (tuberculous cervical lymphadenitis), referring to the direct extension of tuberculosis into the skin from underlying lymph nodes (scrofuladerma). Tuberculosis has also been known under other names, such as 'tabes' or 'tabes mesenterica' (tuberculosis in the mesenteric glands), 'lupus' (scrofuladerma) and 'inflammation of the lungs' (again referring to pulmonary involvement). Many of these terms have largely been abandoned by Western medicine today. The actual name 'tuberculosis' was introduced during the first half of the 19th century to designate a group of symptoms characterised by the presence of tubercles in different body organs. More recently it has come to mean any infection caused by tubercle bacilli, whether or not tubercles could be found in the infected organs.[8]

Today, the World Health Organization (WHO) recognises tuberculosis as one of the top ten causes of death worldwide. In 2015 it was estimated that 10.4 million people fell ill with the disease and 1.4 million of those died. Over 95 per cent of deaths have occurred in low- to middle-income countries.[9]

Tuberculosis in Australia pre-1788?

Bearing in mind the long-standing association of the disease with humans, and the worldwide distribution of the *Mycobacterium* genera, there is no direct evidence of tuberculosis in or its effects on the Aboriginal populations of Australia prior to 1788.[10] The same scenario applies to New Zealand, where there is no evidence of tuberculosis as a human disease among the Maori people until the arrival of Europeans in the 18th century.[11] Yet in both countries the disease would become one of the major causes of sustained morbidity and mortality among Indigenous peoples during the colonial periods.

Human skeletal collections previously held by museums in Australia showing pathological changes have been examined to determine the presence of tuberculosis.[12] The osteological expression of the disease is mostly detected in the joint surfaces such as the lower thoracic and lumber spine, and the hip and knee joints, but other joints and the ribs can be involved.[13] The infection causes a septic arthritis with characteristic destruction of the joint surfaces and, if chronic, can extend to fusing (ankylosis) of the joints. This can be particularly severe and debilitating in the vertebrae joints (Pott's disease). However, none of the examinations on Australian skeletons found any definitive indication of characteristic bone lesions that can be attributed to tuberculosis. Nevertheless, invoking the well-known axiom, 'absence of evidence is not necessarily evidence of absence', could well be appropriate in this case. Ancient DNA examinations of archaeological skeletal collections outside Australia are now throwing light on the presence of tuberculosis infection in bones of individuals that do not show osteolytic changes, leading to the high possibility that infection and the clinical expression of the disease may be much higher in ancient populations than assessed by skeletal samples alone.[14] But the case for an Australian presence of the disease prior to European settlement must, for the moment at least, remain undetermined, as most of the former skeletal collections have been repatriated to Aboriginal organisations and are now out of reach of scientific examination.[15]

Tuberculosis among the European Population of South-eastern Australia

The Early Years

When the First Fleet left Portsmouth for Australia in 1787, tuberculosis was near its peak in the industrial cities and towns of Britain. Mycobacteria infecting humans also travelled well and was particularly suited to the conditions aboard the convict ships. Damp living conditions, poor diets, deteriorating health, lack of fresh air and enclosed living spaces in the crowded holds would have made ideal conditions in the ships that made their way to Australia.

Tuberculosis was also, along with other diseases such as smallpox and scurvy, a particular problem in the Royal Navy.[16] It is quite likely, therefore, that the pathogen was a common affliction among the First Fleet convicts, and survived the long trip to Australia particularly well.[17] It is also quite likely that the disease was brought in continually with subsequent fleets.

Although there are no surviving official medical statistics on tuberculosis, the first reports of death among European settlers that could be attributed to tuberculosis came several months after the arrival. John Easty, a marine private of the First Fleet, recorded several deaths in his personal diary, among which are cases that he considered to be tuberculosis. He recorded for October 10th 1788:

> This Day John Jones A marine Departed this Life of a concumtion [*sic*] and fever

And for February 2nd 1789:

> This Night att [*sic*] 10 oclock Captn John Shea of Marines Departed this Life after a Long illness of a Concumtion [*sic*] and was Buried the next Day in Miliantary [*sic*] form very Neat and handsome.[18]

Easty also recorded four other deaths from long illness and fevers between June 1788 and June 1791 that may have been from tuberculosis. Little is known of Easty, apart from his service in the marines, and he almost certainly had no medical education, so his descriptions must be taken as a lay opinion only. Nevertheless, he was probably recording the general opinions of the medical officers' diagnoses.

A sounder confirmation of tuberculosis in the new settlement comes from records of the newly established Sydney General Hospital, which listed in their 1803 returns of death, two males and two females dying of consumption during that year.[19] Tuberculosis, however, was stated as being responsible for just 4.2 per cent of deaths recorded in the hospital's register. The major cause of mortality in the settlement at this time was due to dysentery, which accounted for 52.1 per cent of recorded hospital deaths. Nevertheless, the limited diets, stringent rationing of food supplies, particularly to the convicts, the lack of sanitation and crowded living conditions would have increased individual susceptibility to tuberculosis infection and delayed recovery from the diseases.[20]

The first recorded non-European death from tuberculosis was a Tahitian who was visiting the new colony. Mowie, who had returned from a visit to

England on HMS *Glatton*, arrived in Port Jackson on March 11th 1803 and died on August 6th before there was a ship available for his return home. The cause of death given was 'inveterate Scrophuli and decay'.[21]

From the beginnings of European settlement in Australia, tuberculosis was constantly present among the first colonists. Governor Phillip considered that, up to February 1790 (two years after landing), about one-third of deceased convicts under his command 'died from disorders of long standing, and which it is more than probable would have carried them off much sooner in England'. Historians Gandevia and Cobley, outlining the mortality at Sydney Cove, consider this comment by Phillip to be based on the observations of his medical officers and most likely to be made in regard to chronic tuberculosis.[22]

The disease was maintained in the population of the colony, being supported by the new arrivals in the Second Fleet in June 1790 and in subsequent arrivals.[23] Of the 1026 Second Fleet complement, 267 died en route and 488 arrived at Port Jackson ill, many requiring medical treatment.[24] McLeod, writing in the fourth decade of settlement stated:

> Consumption of the lungs (phthisis pulmonalis) is much more frequent than from the mildness of the climate might be expected, and more in advanced life suffer from this disease than in England. It is remarked that in people who arrive in this Colony labouring under this complaint, it runs a much more rapid course than it is observed to do in colder climates.[25]

Tuberculosis among Aboriginal Populations

While the presence of tuberculosis in the First Nations people of Australia prior to the arrival of European colonisation must remain an open question, for the present at least, subject to further research, the disease was to find its way through the populations across the continent with devastating effect. Considering the excessive morbidity and mortality caused by other introduced infectious diseases, tuberculosis was possibly the most destructive. It was a disease that could kill in a matter of weeks or months after initial infection, or linger for years, slowly destroying the lungs and vital organs. A healthy immune system could hold the pathogen at bay but, when an infected individual's immune system was compromised by coinfection from other pathogens or was subjected to a low nutritional diet, the disease would erupt.

The First Decades of the 19th Century

When and where the first cases of tuberculosis occurred among Aboriginal populations are unknowns. Following the establishment of the first settlement at Sydney Cove, there was intermittent close contact with the local Aboriginal groups. Governor Phillip endeavoured to establish cordial and close relationships but was often unsuccessful. There is little doubt, though, that sexual relationships between the male convicts and Aboriginal women did occur in the early months of the settlement but there is no evidence of tuberculosis then being transferred to the Indigenous population.

The first reference to tuberculosis among Aboriginal people comes from a visiting French expedition. René Lesson, the second surgeon and naturalist on the French ship, *La Cocquille*, which visited the Sydney settlement from January 17th until March 20th 1824, noted:

> These natives are susceptible to a large number of illnesses, which their miserable state makes them bear more readily than would the more robust European. Most have chronic catarrh; some women are consumptive ...[26]

Although this observation cannot be accepted at face value, it is possible that some of the Aboriginal people (both male and female) seen by Lesson were suffering from tuberculosis. The disease appears to have accompanied the First Fleet colonists in 1788 and become established in the colony at that time, or soon thereafter. The observation by Lesson was then some 36 years later, which is ample time for the disease to have spread from the Europeans into the Aboriginal populations.

The first reliable records of tuberculosis becoming a major health problem among Aboriginal people is among those interned at Wybalenna settlement on Flinders Island in Bass Strait.[27] In November 1831 the Van Diemen's Land (later Tasmania) colonial government moved 150 Aboriginal people from the main island to temporary settlements on Flinders Island, and later, in 1833, the settlement of Wybalenna was established. The mortality of the Aboriginal people was high and by 1847, when the establishment was closed and the inmates were moved back to the main island, just 47 had survived.[28]

Before 1835 the causes of deaths on the main settlement and in the transit camps went largely unrecorded. From October 1835 to February 1839, however, when George Augustus Robinson was in charge of Wybalenna, causes of death were recorded and 32 autopsies were undertaken. After February 1839, the reporting of mortality again lapsed, although the sickness did not. During 1837 and 1838 autopsy reports show at least 13, or 35 per cent of all autopsies, involved extensive tuberculosis infection.[29] The post-mortem investigations commonly displayed lung adhesions, extensive external and internal tubercular lesions throughout the lungs and internal organs – liver, pancreas, spleen, gall bladder and heart – often extending to the small intestines and throughout the peritoneum and mesentery tissue of the abdominal cavity.[30] Three of the post-mortem cases were children ranging in age from two to seven years.

The number of deaths from tuberculosis in the settlement may have been higher. Surgeon Allen stated he had been informed that most of the old and infirm Aboriginal people had died of consumption and scrofula before he took up his position as medical officer of the station.[31] The records do not give the cause of these deaths but, in 1838 alone, the autopsy reports show that 9 deaths of the 14 recorded can be diagnosed as tuberculosis. After 1838 tuberculosis seemingly loses its prominence in the records and influenza, pneumonia, catarrh and 'pleuritis' were recorded as the most common causes of death on the station.[32] This does not, however, indicate that tuberculosis was becoming less of a problem. Mistaken diagnosis of the cause of death and the underlying immunosuppressant nature of chronic tuberculosis could well have predisposed many of the Aboriginal people to life-threatening influenza and pneumonia infections that were then recorded as causes of death.

On the Australian mainland, for the first 60 years of European colonisation, tuberculosis appears to have had little impact on Aboriginal populations as there are few references to it. With the instigation of Aboriginal Protectorates in Port Phillip (Melbourne) in 1835 and South Australia in 1836, reports on the health status of Aboriginal people were sent by the assistant protectors from their various stations in country and urban regions. In many cases these reports allude in general terms to severe and chronic diseases. Few, however, refer to consumption, phthisis, tabes or scrofula, the usual terms for tubercular infection.

The disease is not mentioned as a major health problem among the large groups who regularly left their homelands and congregated on the fringes of the major settlements of Sydney, Melbourne and Adelaide. One large group who met during April 1839 on the banks of the Yarra River in Melbourne was described as being in a state of 'wretchedness and disease' by the assistant protector for that area.[33] Dr Patrick Cussen, a leading Melbourne practitioner, was instructed by the chief protector to examine them and administer treatment. He reported that they were suffering from dysentery, typhus, syphilis, rheumatism, catarrh and starvation.[34] He made no direct mention of any tuberculosis infections.

The disease also appears to have been uncommon among Aboriginal people living among the pastoral settlements of Victoria. In 1840, Dr Watton, the medical officer of the Mount Rouse Aboriginal station, listed one case out of 142 presenting to him for treatment that could be ascribed to tubercular infection. This was 'a very old woman' who died while suffering from 'tabes'.[35] Of a further 87 Aboriginal people treated by Watton at Mount Rouse during the last four months of 1842, just 2 were diagnosed as suffering from tuberculosis. One young female, aged eight years, was diagnosed with 'tabes mesenterica' and another female six years of age was diagnosed with 'tabes'.[36] Doctors William Baylie and Neil Campbell regularly examined Aboriginal people in the north-east and north-west districts of Victoria between 1841 and 1845, while acting as medical officers for the Aboriginal Protectorate. Neither diagnosed any as suffering from consumption or phthisis, but Baylie described one case, a nine-year-old male, suffering from 'inflammation of the mesenteric glands', which could possibly allude to tubercular infection.[37]

Edward Curr, pastoralist and strong advocate for Aboriginal people, compiled one of the most extensive accounts on Aboriginal people in the 1800s. He recorded the absence of tuberculosis among the tribes of the Murray River in northern Victoria during the early period of European settlement:

> During the first eight years of my residence amongst several large tribes near Echuca, in 1841, I can recollect no instance of consumption; nor, though I have made inquiries on the subject of a few old residents who were good observers, have I heard of more than one death of that disease at that period.[38]

In South Australia the situation was similar. Edward Eyre spent a decade in close contact with Aboriginal people during his residence in Australia, initially as a traveller and explorer, but in particular during three years, from 1841 to 1844, as resident magistrate and Aboriginal protector at Moorundie, a police post and Aboriginal depot on the Murray River. During this time Eyre made regular journeys along the Murray as far as the Darling River junction and had frequent contact with many large groups living along the river corridor. In regard to tuberculosis he recorded:

> Phthisis occasionally occurs … Scrofula has been met with, but rarely.[39]

The Last Decades of the 19th Century

Tuberculosis reporting among Aboriginal populations began to increase in the second half of the 19th century, when it was to become a major cause of death. William Thomas, a Victorian medical practitioner, reported to the Victorian Parliament that 'eight-tenths' of the mortality he had observed among the Aboriginal people of the colony arose through pulmonary disorders, mainly pleurisy, pneumonia and consumption. Thomas, like most medical practitioners of that time, kept few or no health statistics on Aboriginal people he examined, so his statement must be seen as an impression based on his own recollection. Nevertheless, it suggests that tuberculosis was becoming a major cause of morbidity and mortality among Aboriginal people. He related the cause of these deaths to Aboriginal people's addiction to alcohol, which, when coupled with infection, led, he believed, to their deaths within days of showing the first symptoms.

> Although the aborigines of this colony are liable to the usual disease of Europeans, I invariably found years back that they seldom had the common diseases, as rheumatism, &c., to the extent Europeans have. Yet, I may state that eight-tenths of the mortality among the aborigines of Victoria arises through intemperance, bringing on pulmonary disorders, pleurisy, pneumonia, disorders of the chest, consumption, &c., which carries them off so speedily that the ablest medical treatment when available seldom save them. I may safely state, that when their respiratory organs are once affected, recovery becomes hopeless. I have witnessed this so invariably within the last ten years, as to look forward for death as soon as they are afflicted in the chest.
>
> The aborigines, however, were not so affected in their respiratory organs years back as at present; they have only been carried off so precipitately since they have become slaves to intoxicating liquors. I have known blacks years back to labour under diseases of the lungs for nine or more months, but now seldom so many weeks, and often not so many days.
>
> There is a peculiarity even in their pulmonary disorders to the European; there is not that straining distressing cough, which Europeans labour under, the phlegm comes free without much exertion and pain to the invalid, but accompanied with blood.[40]

Thomas then described a form of treatment (which he had presumably observed or been informed of) Aboriginal people took for those infected:

> The blacks study much the colour of the spittle in those affected in the lungs, and know well its stages. When the patient begins to expectorate blood, much attention is paid him; should this increase, which is generally the case, the doctors hold a consultation, and when once a consultation is held the doctors will not allow the patient to take any more medicine from the whites. The invalid is laid on his back and held firm by three or four blacks, whilst the native doctor keeps continually pressing with his feet, and even jumping on his belly. I need scarcely state that this cruel practice brings on premature death.[41]

Peter Beveridge, a Scottish-born grazier with property along the Murray River, had for 28 years closely observed Aboriginal culture among the Wadi Wadi people[42] wrote that the high prevalence and incidence of chronic venereal disease (primarily syphilis) was the chief reason for high morbidity and mortality from tuberculosis.

> Hence the numberless cases of consumption, or decline, together with almost countless disarrangements of a pulmonary character; whilst yet another phase of this fell disease is the wasting away of the tissues, until the frame becomes attenuation personified.[43]

This particular observation by Beveridge, who had no formal education in medicine but had been closely associated with the Aboriginal groups in the area and had written several ethnographic accounts,[44] is innovative for its time in that he is referring to the debilitating effects on the immune system of one disease, syphilis, causing an increase in the prevalence and severity of another totally different disease state, tuberculosis.[45]

The Ngarrindjeri, whose homelands extended along the lower reaches of the Murray River and coastal Coorong district of South Australia, also became victims of tuberculosis. This group had been in contact with Europeans since 1803, when sealing enterprises began to be established on Kangaroo Island and the southern mainland coast of South Australia[46] (as reported in Chapter 4). They were soon infected with syphilis and gonorrhoea spread by the sealers[47] but their early experience with tuberculosis is unknown.

George Taplin, a missionary and teacher, established the mission station, Raukkan (Ancient Way), at Point McLeay in 1859 and spent 18 years in close association with the Ngarrindjeri as well as other groups from further upstream on the Murray River. He noted the importance of tuberculosis among them:

> My observations have led me to the following views of the principal disease from which the natives suffer, which is evidently tuberculosis in its different forms. I think that a large number of deaths arise from this cause – of fifty deaths of adults which occurred here between 1859 and 1869 twenty-five were caused by tubercular consumption. In infancy the tuberculous diathesis shews itself frequently in the form of hydrocephalus, generally occurring at the time of dentition; it also very often manifests itself in the form of tabes mesenterica, about the third or fourth year or even later; I have even known of a very bad case occurring in a man of twenty-five. This constitutional tendency often appears in the form of induration and ulceration of the glands of the neck; where it comes out thus it is generally cured, and the person becomes healthy afterwards; but its most usual and fatal form is that of tubercular consumption. Any accident to the chest seems to lead to the deposition of tubercule. I knew a case of a previously healthy young woman who received a blow on the chest from her jealous drunken brute of a husband; she vomited blood immediately after, then her case gradually assumed the form of tubercular consumption. I had a case of a white woman on my hands at the same time as this one. I was struck with the exact similarity of the symptoms in each case – the two women died within an hour of each other though living miles apart.[48]

Tuberculosis on Mission Settlements

The extent of tuberculosis among Aboriginal people in the latter half of the 19th century is best seen on Aboriginal settlements from which reliable records are extant. For the purpose of this book, the registers of births, deaths and marriages compiled by settlements in south-eastern Australia in that period were examined. Causes of death recorded in the registers as consumption, phthisis, phthisis pulmonatis, tabes mesenterica, tubercular peritonitis and tuberculosis, have been extracted and recorded under 'TB' in Table 6.1.[49]

The table lists recorded deaths from tuberculosis, as extracted above, on eight Aboriginal settlements for varying periods and is compared with deaths from all other recorded causes. It should be noted, however, that tuberculosis was not confined to Aboriginal people living on established settlements but affected those who were able to live away from European settlements. In many instances migration of Aboriginal people to and from the settlements would have facilitated the spread of the disease to those who lived most of their life on their traditional homelands.

Table 6.1. Cause of death: the extent of tuberculosis as the recorded cause of death on Aboriginal settlements in the 19th century for which there are reliable data.

Station	Period	TB	Other	Unknown	Total	% TB
Framlingham	1876–1883	4	14		18	22.2
Lake Condah	1876–1900	30	66	1	97	30.9
Lake Wellington	1876–1900	20	68	1	89	22.5
Lake Tyers	1876–1900	8	85		93	8.6
Coranderrk	1878–1900	22	49		71	31.0
Lake Hindmarsh	1876–1900	18	64		82	22.0
Point McLeay	1859–1900	60	226	94	380	15.8
Point Pearce	1880–1900	12	25	5	42	28.6
Total	1859–1900	174	597	101	872	19.9

Source: P. Dowling, '"A Great Deal of Sickness": Introduced Diseases among the Aboriginal People of Colonial Southeast Australia 1788–1900' (Canberra: PhD thesis, Australian National University, 1997), https://digitalcollections.anu.edu.au/handle/1885/7529 (accessed July 2016).

Figure 6.1. Tuberculosis as a percentage of the recorded causes of death on Aboriginal settlements in Victoria and South Australia, 1859 to 1900.

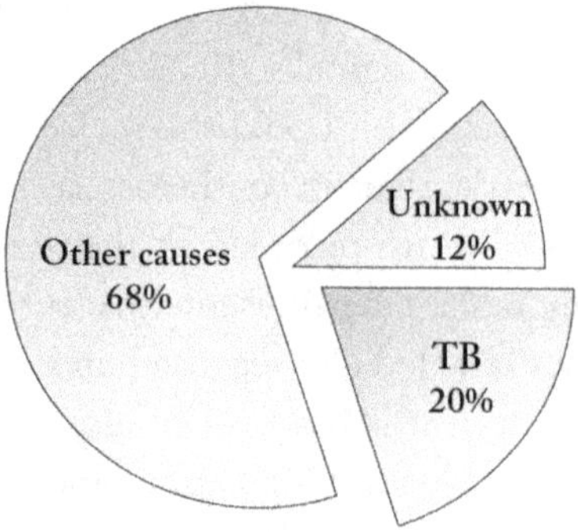

Source: P. Dowling, '"A Great Deal of Sickness": Introduced Diseases among the Aboriginal People of Colonial Southeast Australia 1788–1900' (Canberra: PhD thesis, Australian National University, 1997), https://digitalcollections.anu.edu.au/handle/1885/7529 (accessed July 2016).

It can be seen from Table 6.1 and Figure 6.1 that tuberculosis was a major cause of mortality among Aboriginal people living on the settlements, accounting for 20 per cent of all the recorded deaths. The records from Point McLeay, however, contain a substantial number of deaths (94 out of 380, or 24.7 per cent) for which no cause was given. This may have occurred because the cause was not known by the recorder or that it was simply a failure to record the cause at the time of death. This has most probably distorted the data for both tuberculosis as well as all other causes of death on this settlement and for the combined total. In such a case the extent of tuberculosis, as a cause of death at 20 per cent of all recorded deaths, should be seen as an approximate figure only. However, it may be an underestimation because of the chronic nature of the disease, making the sufferer more susceptible to secondary infections, particularly respiratory, whose symptoms would be more readily recognised by the recorders at time of death. In such cases tuberculosis would most likely have been the underlying cause of death. An indication that this figure may indeed be an underestimation comes from George Taplin, who estimated that 50 per cent of the deaths he observed among the Ngarrindjeri of the lower Murray River between 1859 and 1869 were of those suffering from tuberculosis.[50] While this estimate should, of course, be taken with caution, Taplin's observations do intimate that tuberculosis was inflicting an excessive level of mortality and by implication a high morbidity.

The Increase in Tuberculosis among Aboriginal Populations: Component Causes

The causes leading to the occurrence and establishment of an infectious disease are usually multiple and interactive. In the case of tuberculosis, a person's susceptibility is first determined by exposure to the tubercle bacillus (a necessary cause) and a host of other component causes, leading to morbidity and mortality, including environmental and social conditions to which a population or community is exposed.[51]

The historical literature indicates that tuberculosis infection was not a major problem among Aboriginal communities in the first half of the 19th century but then became one of the major causes of morbidity and mortality among them during the second half of the century. The reason for this rise in the prevalence of tuberculosis is multifaceted.

A major component cause of the increased prevalence of tuberculosis began with colonial government-sanctioned institutionalisation of Aboriginal people. The processes of 19th-century institutionalisation centred on the development of settlements controlled by missionary bodies and colonial governments through Aboriginal protection boards. These practices, aimed at control of the Aboriginal communities, ultimately led to their subsequent displacement and dispersal from traditional lands, eroding of culture and language, crowded living conditions and low nutritional diets often leading to long-term individual distress and increased susceptibility to infection.

In May 1879 two members of the Aboriginal Protection Board, Edward Curr and A. C. Le Souef, visited the Ramahyuck and Lake Tyers Aboriginal settlements in Victoria's Gippsland region. They reported back to their board:

> We observed, however, with deep regret, that consumption, or lung disease, here as elsewhere, was very prevalent, and the natives are rapidly decreasing in numbers; few of those born on the stations seem likely to attain the age of thirty years. The disease is always, sooner or later, fatal, and it has been for many years a terrible scourge among the blacks, thousands having no doubt died from its effects in the last thirty years. The complaint was most likely engendered in the first instance by an entire change of life, consequent on coming into contact with the whites.[52]

In the second half of the 19th century there was a sharp increase in the population of Australia due mainly to the discovery of gold in the 1850s. In 1852 alone, 370,000 immigrants arrived, many heading for the goldfields. The 'rush' continued at varying rates for the next 30 years. The total population of Australia trebled from 430,000 in 1851 to 1.7 million in 1871.[53] The newcomers comprised people from all strata of life and all economic circumstances. They often became wanderers, crowding on to the goldfields while there were payable seams, then moving on to the next after each worked out. Most of the immigrants were in the 25–35 years age group.

While it may have been a 'golden decade' for the economies of Victoria and New South Wales, it was a bleak period for those on the goldfields in regard to infectious diseases. In the period from July 1st 1855 to June 30th 1856 phthisis and scrofula were recorded as accounting for 8 per cent of all deaths in the European population; by the end of 1856, the proportion had more than doubled, accounting for 18 per cent of total deaths in Victoria.[54] Dr W. L. Richardson was a physician practising at the Ballarat District Hospital near to the largest goldfields in Australia during the gold rush period. He commented:

> Tubercular pulmonary consumption presents frequently; it certainly has become more frequent within the memory of the writer.[55]

With the increase of the population and tuberculosis cases came the increase in contact by the Aboriginal people with the mycobacteria and the subsequent increase in prevalence of tuberculosis among them.[56]

It was not just the gold seekers who came to Australia in the latter decades of the 19th century. Following the gold rushes came the arrival of convalescent tuberculosis sufferers to Australia. During the first half of the century it was generally, but falsely, believed by the English medical profession that a long sea voyage in the clear air of the ocean to a place with a mild and unchanging climate was of great therapeutic value to sufferers of pulmonary tuberculosis.[57] There was also little or no suspicion that tuberculosis was communicable and quite often the tubercular emigrants were not separated from healthy passengers.[58] Many, therefore, would have passed on their infection to others within the crowded confines of below-deck accommodation. Shipping companies catered for those sufferers of tuberculosis wishing to migrate to Australia, offering them special facilities on ships fitted out for convalescents. Many 'consumptives' fled England, choosing to immigrate to Australia to affect a last-resort cure. By the 1860s a growing number were making the trip. No doubt the decision was made more enticing after 1851 by the prospect of finding gold.[59] In a period of five and a half years from 1865 to 1870, within the city of Melbourne and its environs over two thousand deaths from phthisis were recorded; just over 86 per cent of these deaths were those of immigrants. Not only did the influx of tuberculosis immigrants increase the population; they also added substantially to the increased mortality from the disease in the colonies and were the vectors for the disease that then enabled it to become more firmly established in Australia.[60] As a result, the reported mortality rate from pulmonary tuberculosis in Victoria alone increased to 138 per 100,000 in 1880 from a rate of 115 per 100,000 population for the period between 1864 and 1871.[61] In New South Wales, Queensland, South Australia and Tasmania the trend was similar, with a steady rise in the rate of tuberculosis mortality peaking around the mid-1880s followed by a slow but steady decline as a major factor in the overall decline of deaths from infectious diseases.[62]

A fourth component cause in the increase of tuberculosis among the Aboriginal communities was the lack of an effective cure for the disease and effective medical care for the sufferers. It should be noted, however, that this also applied to the non-Aboriginal population. It could be argued that the application of medicines had little or no efficacy whatsoever in the treatment of any of the introduced infectious diseases suffered by Aboriginal people at this time. Conversely it could be argued that some of the treatments favoured by medical practitioners, particularly the widespread use of mercury-based prophylactics, had a deleterious effect on the patient rather than a curative.[63]

* * *

The human history of tuberculosis in Australia prior to 1788 is unknown. Paleopathological examinations of skeletal collections have not detected definitive evidence for the disease prior to the arrival of European settlement. Tuberculosis probably arrived in Australia in 1788 with the members of the First Fleet, as deaths from the disease were recorded among the colonists before the subsequent arrival of further fleets. It is uncertain, however, how soon after the arrival of Europeans the disease spread to the Aboriginal population.

Little is known about tuberculosis among Aboriginal people in the early years following the colonisation process in Australia. The first medically identified cases of the disease were diagnosed as a result of autopsies on Aboriginal people interned at Wybalenna settlement on Flinders Island in 1837 and 1838. The post-mortem investigations commonly displayed lung adhesions, extensive external and internal tubercular lesions throughout the lungs and internal organs, often extending to the small intestines and throughout the peritoneum and mesentery tissue of the abdominal cavity, and were most likely the primary cause of death.

In the second half of the 19th century tuberculosis became well established and was a major cause of mortality among the Aboriginal communities of south-eastern Australia. The causes for the increase in mortality from the disease can be related to the internment of Aboriginal people in defined settlements as a result of government and mission society policies; an influx of migrants during the gold rushes; an influx of tuberculosis sufferers from Europe seeking a cure; the persistence of other diseases, such as influenza, emphysema, syphilis and gonorrhoea, impacting on, and compromising, immune systems and leading to reduced resistance to tuberculosis infection; and the lack of effective European medical treatment, which in some cases further added to the stress on individual immune systems.

Coda: Tuberculosis in Indigenous Communities Today

While today tuberculosis is considered to be well under control in Australia, with one of the lowest rates of notification in the world, the disease incidence is much higher in the Indigenous population than in the non-Indigenous.

The most recent information about tuberculosis among Indigenous people is for 2009–13, when 158 (21 per cent) of the 761 notifications of the disease among Australian-born people in Australia were identified as Indigenous. Around one-third (35 per cent) of the new cases among Indigenous people were reported in the Northern Territory (56 cases) and around another one-third (32 per cent) in Queensland.

Australia-wide, the crude notification rate of tuberculosis in 2009–13 was 5.5 cases per 100,000 population for Indigenous people, with the highest crude notification rate being for the Northern Territory (16 cases per 1000,000 population). After age adjustment, the notification rate for Indigenous people was 11.3 times that for Australian-born non-Indigenous people. The notification rate of tuberculosis was higher for Indigenous people than for Australian-born non-Indigenous people across all age groups, with rate ratios being highest for the 45–54 years age group.[64]

Today in Australia, tuberculosis is rarely seen as a cause of sickness or death other than in some Aboriginal communities. But there is a lurking devil in this perception. Multi-drug-resistant tuberculosis is becoming more prevalent in developing countries in Africa and is causing high mortality and serious health issues in India. The modern medicines now used to treat and to cure the disease are becoming less effective as the drug-resistant strains of bacteria emerge and spread throughout communities. High and consistent surveillance methods are needed to control the spread of these resistant bacteria in those countries already affected, and also to prevent it from entering Australia – particularly Indigenous communities – and other countries that these strains haven't yet touched. Tuberculosis was a major cause of death and lingering illness for centuries past. It can be the same in this or later centuries. Tuberculosis has not gone away.

Chapter 7

INFLUENZA

As air-breathing mammals, humans are continually susceptible to the many airborne bacteria and viruses taken into the lungs with each breath. In most cases the immune system quickly destroys a potential pathogen before it can cause a disease response. In order to do this the immune system must be able to first recognise the invader as a health threat. This ability of the immune system comes about and develops during the early years when infants and children are exposed to mild doses of the pathogens and often suffer from coughs and runny noses. Once recognised, and neutralised, in most cases the immune system retains a memory of the pathogens it has encountered and when infected again will quickly be able to mount an attack before the pathogen can multiply and cause a disease. People may be completely unaware of their immune system's activity and have no symptoms when exposed to a potential pathogen. In other cases, when they may have breathed in a large number of pathogens and the immune system is in action, they may feel a little ill or off-colour or develop mild symptoms that last just a few days. In other cases, where the immune system is unable to deal with the pathogen and/or the pathogen has itself developed a defence against the immune system they begin to suffer from a disease. It is a two-way battle between the infecting pathogens and the immune system, with the stakes being survival and replication for the invading virus or bacteria and a continued state of good health for the human host. It is a battle that is fought within people every day.

One airborne pathogen that has developed a means to counter the human immune system is the influenza virus. This very familiar virus has been causing reoccurring periods of morbidity and mortality around the world for centuries. Influenza epidemics (local or regional outbreaks) and pandemics (global outbreaks) affecting human populations can be traced back with some accuracy for the past three hundred years and with somewhat less certainty into the distant past. Annual epidemics of the disease are common today, particularly in the cooler, moister months of the year, which suit the survival and transmission of the virus.

The virus causing influenza is a cunning and complicated creature. It is able to change its genetic appearance regularly to enable it to first survive the resistance of the human immune responses, then replicate and spread. The virus is roughly spheroid in shape, made up of an outer lipid membrane beneath, which is a rigid protein layer that protects the genes (the RNA) of the virus. Just think of what the now-familiar COVID-19 virus (or its designated World Health Organization name, SARS-CoV-2) looks like to get an idea of the surface morphology of the influenza virus.

Poking up from the outer surface of the influenza virus, like small spikes, is an array of glycoproteins (proteins linked with sugars) two of which are haemagglutinin and neuraminidase. Or, to give them their abbreviated names, H and N. The H protein, shaped somewhat like a lollypop on a stick, penetrates the outer surface of the human cells and allows the virus to enter. The N protein has the task of breaking back out of the infected cells to release the replicated viruses.

The genes that produce these two proteins, referred to as antigens, determine the subtypes of the influenza virus and are important to the effectiveness of the human host's immune system. Over time, sometimes as little as one or two years, the structure of the spiky antigens on the surface of the virus are altered by the interchange of RNA segments between the human host and the virus during reproduction within the human cells. For example, if a cell is invaded by two or more viruses with slightly different RNA subtypes (viruses can be very promiscuous), these can be intermixed during the viral replication process within the invaded cell, resulting in yet another subtype of influenza virus emerging. It is like human sexual reproduction, where the resulting offspring share their genes with each parent but usually (if not twins) have a different genetic profile from each other.

The bad news for humans, with all this viral genetic recombination, is that when this happens the immune system is 'tricked' by the virus and does not immediately recognise the invader as a pathogen, allowing it to reproduce and reek its havoc, sometimes with life-threatening results.

If these abilities were not bad enough for humans, the virus has another trick up its sleeve. Approximately every 10 to 50 years the virus in its various genetic cloaks infects other non-human species, such as birds and pigs, mixing its genetic identity even more. This reassortment of genes results in a larger change to its surface protein structure and a new subtype of the virus emerges. These subtypes are not immediately immunologically recognised by humans and animals, and the destructive spread of influenza occurs again. The influenza virus is a master of disguises, a real shapeshifter able to continually change its form to outwit the human immune system. Pandemics occur when these new forms of the virus spread across continents and around the world. In recent years new forms of influenza pandemics have spread across the globe causing excessive morbidity and, in many cases, excessive mortality.

Influenza epidemics usually occur without warning, quickly infecting a large percentage of people and spreading throughout communities, and then disappear after a few weeks or months. At first they can be highly destructive and cause high mortality, but many of those people infected recover and acquire an immunity to the particular form of the virus. If reinfected, their immune systems now recognise the virus as a pathogen and quickly eliminate it with little or no illness incurred. The virus then steadily loses its ability to replicate in its human hosts and the initial pandemic dies out.[1] However, many of the various genetic forms of the virus remain 'hidden', unobtrusively infecting humans and animals that are yet to be infected and have developed no immunity.

It was not until 1945, with the advent of the electron microscope, that the influenza virus was identified as the cause of influenza. Prior to that, several theories (or to be more precise several beliefs) surrounded the cause of this well-known and very destructive disease. In medieval times the suggested causes included acts of God, or a false god or the devil, who regularly sent the disease. In later times the causes suggested were related to comets that have on occasions coincided with outbreaks of influenza or poisoned air emanating from volcanoes. Electrical conditions in the atmosphere, excess ozone in the air and high and low air pressure have also been blamed, as well as miasmas (bad air) arising from swamps and spread by high winds or following wet weather. Plagues of flies, caterpillars and locusts have been blamed. In fact, many frequently occurring natural (or supernatural) phenomena were associated with the cause of influenza outbreaks.[2]

Even into the early 20th century, natural phenomena were given as the cause of outbreaks of influenza. William Ramsay Smith, physician, naturalist, anthropologist and principal medical officer in South Australia, commented on the common and long-held view of the cause:

> For many hundred years past a strange disease has from time to time appeared in various places on the habitable globe, has spread widely and unusually rapidly, has devastated whole countries, killing multitudes, and

> causing much permanent ill-health among the survivors, and then has seemed to die out, only to re-appear, perhaps several times in the course of the next century. No other disease has ever been so widely diffused. So strange was it in its mode, or modes, of origin, so unaccountable in its methods of spread, and so often associated with strange meteorological or other phenomena, that its cause was suspected to be some peculiar stellar or telluric [atmospheric] 'influence'. Hence it was named 'Influenza'.[3]

But, by the turn of the 20th century, the development of microbiology was leading scientists and medical practitioners towards realising that infection by a microorganism was the cause of influenza. Initially it was thought that a bacterium, *Haemophilus influenzae*, was the cause, because it had been isolated in some influenza patients. Following a series of trials that did not produce influenza symptoms in test subjects, this cause was abandoned.

Today much more is known about the identification of the causative virus. Further investigation has revealed three major types of influenza virus infecting humans, based on their genetic differences: Type A is the major cause of severe epidemic outbreaks in humans; Type B also causes influenza epidemics but less frequently and less severe; and Type C, a rare form of the virus that can cause a mild cold-like illness in humans. (A fourth variant, Type D, primarily infects cattle and is not known to cause illness in humans.) To make the virus more complicated, it has the ability to change and exchange its genes, resulting in different strains within the main A and B types. Today the US Centers for Disease Control recognises at least 29 subtypes of Type A influenza alone.[4]

During the later decades of the 20th century, microbiologists studying the influenza virus determined that the deadly human type, influenza A, has as a natural reservoir of many species of migratory aquatic birds throughout the world.[5] In Australia, the short-tailed shearwater, or mutton bird (*Ardenna tenuirostris*; formerly *Puffinus tenuirostris*), was a carrier and could in cases, when the virus mutated, become a victim to the disease. These birds, along with other aquatic birds that had been a common source of food for Indigenous populations for centuries, could be the vectors for influenza A epidemics in Australia long before the arrival of European colonists. In Tasmania, for example, mutton birds were captured by reaching into their nesting burrows, grabbing the birds, pulling them out and then gutting them prior to cooking and eating. Close handling of the birds and their internal organs could well facilitate cross-species infection of the virus, with humans as the recipients of influenza. We may never know if the disease had broken out as an epidemic across Australia some time in the past, causing high mortality and morbidity among Indigenous people, but current knowledge of the biology and behaviour of the virus suggests that could well have occurred. Whatever the case, the introduction of the influenza A virus of European origin, genetically different from the Australian type, was to cause havoc among the Indigenous populations of Australia.

While the virus itself can cause disruption and damage to the respiratory system, quite commonly its association with another common human pathogen, *Staphylococcus aurens*, a bacterium that causes pneumonia, can have a devastating effect. While the immune system of a person infected with an influenza virus busily combats the invading virus using much of its energy sources, the ever-present staphylococcus bacteria, now no longer kept in close check by the immune system, begins to replicate and causes respiratory distress and destruction, which in turn can lead to the death of the victim. Throughout history the two pathogens have, in association, caused excessive deaths, particularly in the elderly or those suffering from other chronic diseases of the heart and lungs and whose immune systems have already been compromised.

Influenza is a highly contagious disease that can, if untreated, cause severe illness and lead to death. In its mildest form, infection by the virus may result in an asymptomatic condition or may produce mild symptoms like the common cold, such as a low fever, sinus blockage and excessive nasal secretion. More serious forms, often occurring among the very young and the aged, may cause an acute, prostrating febrile illness with the sudden onset of a range of symptoms, including fever, malaise, headache, muscle pain (particularly in the back and legs) coughing, nasal and sinus congestion, shivering and a sore throat. Infection may be accompanied by undifferentiated acute respiratory complications such as viral pneumonia, bronchitis and the common cold. Gastrointestinal manifestations presenting as nausea, vomiting and diarrhoea, and prolonged fever and convulsions may occur in children.[6]

During epidemics, the disease is often severe in young and elderly victims, and in victims with pre-existing underlying conditions. The latter include victims with compromised immune systems caused by underlying chronic diseases such as tuberculosis, cardiovascular disorders, other respiratory disorders such as chronic bronchitis, asthma, emphysema, renal or metabolic disorders, anaemia, nutritional deficiencies (starvation and alcoholism), advanced age, a history of inflammation and inadequate therapy and medicinal treatment. Many of these medical states were common among post-contact Aboriginal populations in various degrees of chronicity last century.

Spreading Far and Wide

The influenza virus has been a great sea traveller, spreading itself around the world with the help of its human hosts. From the end of the 15th century to the late 18th century sailing ships have traversed the globe. Led first by the Spanish and Portuguese voyages of discovery and colonisation of the Americas and followed by Dutch, French and English ships, the influenza virus has been carried around the world. The introduction of the European virus in its various forms has resulted in excessive mortality among the native populations of the New World and the Pacific, including Australia. The virus found an excellent host in these ships, enabling it to survive the long sea passages by infecting the crew members and most likely altering its genetic makeup on the way. (Today, with air travel and ever-increasing passengers travelling across global hemispheres within hours, the virus in all its present forms regularly and continually circumnavigates the globe.)

Entering the New World populations, the virus found virgin soil in the native populations and spread rapidly and repeatedly, causing untold morbidity and mortality. An outbreak of what was probably swine influenza emanating from the Spanish settlement of La Isabela in Santo Domingo in 1493–94 has been blamed for the disappearance of the indigenous populations of the Antilles. Accounts of the outbreak describe an acute infectious disease that was extremely contagious, with a noticeably short incubation period, affecting much of the population and having the signs of a high fever and prostration, and inflicting excessive mortality. A Spanish observer recorded that 'so many Indians died that they could not be counted ... all through the land the Indians lay dead everywhere'. Following the first epidemic, a second outbreak of what was possibly influenza, in 1539, spread among the northern Andes and into populations further inland. Further epidemics of influenza and other introduced maladies caused severe population loss among the Inca (estimated to be around nine million) in the 16th century.[7]

Influenza epidemics and associated respiratory complications among American Indians became common during New World colonial expansion. Such outbreaks were responsible for many deaths in the south-west of North America, the north-east, the Saint Lawrence Valley and New Spain during the 17th century; among the Aleut of Alaska from the early days of contact in the late 18th century; on the north-west coast in the early 19th century; and among the Chumash on the mid-west coast in the 18th and 19th centuries.

Europeans began venturing into the Pacific Islands early in the 16th century. Ferdinand Magellan crossed the Pacific from the Americas, making initial contact with the Marianas Islanders. A few decades later a Spanish trade route was established between Mexico and the Philippines. Dutch trading ships followed, establishing commercial enterprises in the Indonesian archipelago and exploring the northern, western and southern coastlines of Australia, looking (unsuccessfully in Australia) to extend their commercial opportunities. British, French, German and American merchants, whalers and missionaries were to follow, bringing the once-remote islands of the Pacific into the world sphere. Influenza came with them. The first reported major outbreak of the disease was among the indigenous populations of Tahiti in 1772. This was followed by outbreaks in Fiji in 1791–92, Samoa in 1830, Cook Islands in 1832 and Papua New Guinea in 1889.[8]

Influenza in Australia

There is a reasonable chance that influenza arrived with the First Fleet to Australia but its effect among the first colonists and on the Aboriginal groups around Botany Bay and the Sydney settlement is unknown. The first recorded epidemic of the disease occurred in 1820, 32 years after European settlement. Since then influenza has been a constant companion and traveller to Australia, ever present among the European colonists and the Aboriginal populations, as shown in Table 7.1.

Apart from localised epidemics in New South Wales in 1820 and 1826, in Victoria and South Australia in 1844–45 and the non-appearance of the disease during the pandemics of 1800–02 and 1830–33, the epidemics of influenza in Australia have paralleled the pandemics of the northern hemisphere.[9] However, it is interesting to note the substantial historical evidence for an influenza epidemic sweeping through the Maori of New Zealand around 1804–08, before any recorded in Australian Aboriginal populations.[10] This epidemic, not associated with the known pandemics, appears to have entered the Maori populations from a source in the Bay of Islands that, since the early 19th century, was a favoured port of call for European shipping. The epidemic among the Maori was reported to spread through both main islands and was particularly severe. Mortality rates of up to 50 per cent of settlements were estimated. Although this figure appears high, it is feasible in a virgin-soil population exposed to a pathogen for the first time.

Just a handful of extant references document the first recorded influenza epidemic in Australia, in New South Wales in 1820, and these were written at various times after the event. Deputy Inspector of Military Hospitals Dr D. McLeod referred to the epidemic when he replied to a set of questions posed by the Royal College of Physicians:

> In July and August, 1820, an Epidemic Catarrh prevailed throughout the Colony; occasional cases of it had been appearing from the beginning of the Year, but most Families began at this time to suffer severely, there being hardly a House that had not cases of more or less danger. It proved chiefly fatal to infancy and old age; the symptoms of this Complaint were common Cold, Cough, pains in the forehead, sneezing, Soreness and Spasms in the Chest, copious discharge of mucous [*sic*] of various Colours from consistencies from the Lungs.[11]

Table 7.1. Pandemics and periods of epidemic and unusually high morbidity from influenza in Australia in the 19th and early 20th centuries.

World Pandemics	Australian Epidemics					
	NSW	Vic	SA	Tas	Qld	WA
1800–02						
	1820					
	1826					
1830–33						
1836–39	1836–38	1837–38	1838	1838		
		1844–45	1844–45			
1847–48	1847–48	1847–48	1847–48	1847–48		
1850–52	1852	1852		1852		
1857–60	1860	1860	1860	1860	1860	1860
1873–76	1875	1875	1875			
	1885–90	188–905	1885–90	1885–90	1885–90	1885–90
1889–91	1890–91	1890–91	1890–91	1890–91		
	1894–95	1894–95	1894–95	1894–95	1895–95	1894–95
	1898–99	1898–99	1898–99	1898–99		
1918–1919	1918–19	1918–19	1918–19	1918–19	1918–19	1918–19

Epidemic dates derived from multiple sources.[12]

The epidemic was considered serious enough to be recorded in the 'Chronological Table of Remarkable Events' of the *Australian Almanac of Sydney*:

> An epidemical catarrh prevailed throughout the Colony about this period. Many families suffered severely from this strange complaint. The symptoms of this disease were unaccountably varied. In many instances it appeared in a hectic cough, accompanied by violent spasms. In others, it produced, independent of the violent cough, a severe affection in the ear, with pus occasioned by internal inflammation. Some cases were visited with external eruptions, accompanied with extreme debility, and intense pain. The complaint was general. Many of the inhabitants were consigned to the grave in a few days, from the violence and fury of the attack; and some few, to this day, have the remains of this visitation still as a painful companion. Great numbers of the poor Aborigines fell victims to this novel and severe distemper.[13]

Peter Cunningham, surgeon superintendent on convict transport ships, made five trips to New South Wales between 1819 and 1828. Writing some six or seven years after the event, he made a brief reference to the epidemic and listed some of the more prominent symptoms:

> An epidemic influenza carried off a number of the old Europeans some years ago [1820], and also not a few of the aborigines, while many of our younger individuals occasionally feel the effects of it to this day. It appeared at the time, or immediately in the rear, of a hot northern wind, the symptoms being violent headaches, cough, sneezing, and inflamed eyes; with a quick pulse, and other general febrile concomitants.[14]

After the first epidemic subsided, the infection may have persisted in the colony at a low level of morbidity. Although there is little evidence for this in the records of the colonists, the second surgeon aboard the French ship *La Coquille*, which visited Port Jackson between January and March 1824, recorded:

> The sailors of our crew, during this long stay presented only a numerous series of catarrhal complaints, ephemeral inflammatory fevers, colds in the head, illnesses neither interesting nor serious.[15]

A second epidemic of influenza struck the colony in November 1825 and lasted into the next year. There is little evidence of the morbidity and mortality levels in the European populations from subsequent epidemics up to 1890, other than to say that they were substantially higher than normal. The 1860 and 1885 epidemics were general throughout the south-eastern Australian colonies and beyond (Table 7.2). The 1860 epidemic was called 'Fog Fever' in Victoria, where 'the cases were very numerous, some very severe in nature – whole families being affected'.[16]

The epidemic for which there are reliable estimates of mortality is the 1890–91 event.

Table 7.2 shows the mortality rate per 100,000 population in the south-eastern colonies from influenza and pneumonia in 1890–91.

Table 7.2. Mortality rates from 1890–91 influenza epidemic (deaths from pneumonia included).

Colony	Mortality Rate (per 100,000)
New South Wales	87
Victoria	98
South Australia	84
Tasmania	80

Source: J. H. L. Cumpston, in M. J. Lewis (ed.), *Health and Disease in Australia: A History* (Canberra: Australian Government Printing Service, 1989), pp. 313–317

This epidemic was severe in terms of the mortality and morbidity it inflicted on the European population. It has been estimated that in Sydney there were 100,000 cases of influenza, infecting approximately 25 to 26 per cent of the city's population. The mortality rate from influenza alone was 61 per 100,000 population for 1891.[17]

Influenza and Pneumonia among Aboriginal Populations

Evidence on influenza among Aboriginal people begins with the first epidemic of 1820 in New South Wales. This epidemic was a local event in New South Wales and was not connected with a pandemic. Observations made by a 'Medical Gentleman' in a letter to the Sydney Gazette describe the effects of the epidemic. Brief as it is, this description of the 1820 epidemic among Aboriginal people reveals the severity of the symptoms affecting the young and healthy, and the Aboriginal response to flee from a disease that was new to them. It is worth quoting at length. After giving an account of his own experience with the disease and that of his family he goes on to state that Aboriginal populations of the interior of the colony suffered excessively from the same infection

> … which had produced a great mortality; and the many young stout and robust people among them had become its victims, during the winter. In one severe instance a father, a very stout man, not exceeding forty years of age, with the mother and two daughters, and the infant of one of them, had all been carried off within the space of a month, leaving but one alive, a male about three years old, very distressed, until taken into protection by a European inhabitant of the settlement.

Some cases, this gentleman observed, appeared to him to have 'terminated in inflammation of the lungs' and that the people had

> … for the most part quitted the thinly wooded and more open tracts of the interior, and be taken themselves to the sea-coast, and brush and broken country, where were quantities of honey, and where they would undoubtedly remain until the return of summer. That these people should suffer intensely under every such contagion is not to be wondered at, when their state of privation from all comforts of life is considered; and that when prevented by bodily ailment from seeking their precarious means of sustenance, they are likely to become victims to famine, as unhappily from distemper.[18]

There are no further records of this epidemic among the Aboriginal communities of New South Wales so the severity of the diseases and its demographic and social effects on them remains unknown.

The second epidemic of influenza spread through the European populations of the colony in 1826.[19] There is little known of its effects on the European population and it went largely unrecorded among the Aboriginal population. However, the German missionary, Reverend Threlkeld, at Lake Macquarie reported incidences of whooping cough associated with an outbreak of measles among Aboriginal populations in the Port Macquarie region in 1835.[20]

After these early reports, the records on subsequent influenza epidemics and accounts of acute respiratory disease allow a better insight into the effects influenza and pneumonia had among Aboriginal people.

Tasmania, 1831–67

In May 1831, an epidemic of influenza, or a disease resembling influenza, broke out among Aboriginal people who were taken from the mainland of Tasmania to the small settlement established on Gun Carriage Island, part of the Furneaux Group in Bass Strait. This was the last temporary settlement before the establishment of the major Aboriginal settlement on Flinders

Island.[21] On March 20th of that year, prior to their arrival on the island, a young female died. Archibald MacLauchlan, a convict surgeon, submitted the following report on her death:

> Died at eleven o'clock am, Mary, a native child aged six years, having been afflicted with catarrh for some length of time, and from these last few days past, from fresh exposure to cold, she was seized with acute inflammation of the lungs which terminated her existence.[22]

By the end of March, the epidemic had spread. Several were reported to be ill and by late April two more had died, an adult male and adult female. On May 2nd Protector George Augustus Robinson reported that 15 Aboriginal people at the settlement were in 'a sickly state' and that the disease persisted and was taking its course among all the Aboriginal people.[23] The population on Gun Carriage Island at this time was about 50, including several women who had been living with European sealers until the settlement was established.

It is quite likely that this outbreak was associated with the 1830–33 world pandemic (Table 7.1), although there are no records of major outbreaks among the European population.[24] If so, the virus may have been introduced by one of the sealing ships that frequented Bass Strait, although by then large-scale commercial sealing had ceased and only local sealers remained.[25] The epidemic ran its course among the Aboriginal people and by November, when the settlement was eventually moved to Wybalenna on Flinders Island, eight had died.[26]

Wybalenna functioned as a place of incarceration of Tasmanian Aboriginal people from 1833 to 1847. The colonial government sought to solve the problem it had with the Aboriginal population by removing them from the main island of Tasmania, isolating them on Flinders Island. From the beginning of the settlement on Flinders Island Commandant Darling impressed on the Aboriginal people the need to eat European food in the European manner. The change from their traditional diet was drastic. Their daily diet consisted largely of the colonial rations of salt meat and flour supplemented by local food sources collected from the land or obtained by hunting. They had to learn new methods of cooking – boiling and baking – the new food with unfamiliar European utensils. Dampers made from the flour, stews made from the salted meat with cabbage and turnips, and tea were the staple diet. Arrangements for supplying the settlement were often unsatisfactory, with food running short, largely due to the irregular arrival of shipping at the island. The Aboriginal people often had to leave the settlement and live on whatever they could obtain in the bush. Game animals quickly became scarce and, on several occasions, the annual migration of mutton birds (*Puffinus tenuirostris*) to the island averted a more serious food crisis.[27]

Water for Wybalenna had to be obtained from brackish lagoons and brought to the settlement in containers. A freshwater creek near to the settlement ran only in the rainy season. No attempts were made by Robinson or the other commandants of the settlement to dam the creek to create a permanent source of fresh water.[28] In 1835 the combined European and Aboriginal population was more than 150, putting a serious strain on water resources.[29]

Prior to Robinson's arrival at Wybalenna in 1835, the houses or huts offered to the Aboriginal people were neither warm nor comfortable. In the early period of the settlements on Flinders Island, huts were made from bush materials collected by the Aboriginal people. They were simple A-frame constructions expected to house six persons but were unsuitable as a permanent structure against the prevailing cold westerly winds of Bass Strait. Robinson attempted to improve the living conditions first by repositioning the doorways, so the wind did not blow directly into the huts. Later he built brick houses with grass-thatched roofs in an L-shaped block of 20 dwellings, which were to be the permanent accommodation for the Aboriginal residents until their removal from Flinders Island in 1884. Each dwelling had one room, with two beds for four people. The dwellings later became infested by vermin. In the last years of the settlement the living conditions experienced by the Aboriginal residents had seriously deteriorated, largely due to neglect by Dr Jeanneret, commandant of the settlement from June 1842 to early 1844 and again in 1846, and a severe reduction in financial commitment by the colonial government.[30]

An indication of the poor conditions at Wybalenna comes from a petition written in February 1846. Signed by eight Aboriginal residents, it was forwarded to Queen Victoria through the secretary of state for the colonies.

> Dr Jeanneret kept plenty of pigs in our village which used to run into our houses and eat up our bread from the fires and take away our flour bags in their mouths also to break into our gardens and destroy our potatoes and cabbage … Our houses were let fall down and they were never cleaned but were covered with vermin and not white-washed. We were often without clothes except a very little one and Dr Jeanneret did not care to mind us when we were sick until we were very bad. Eleven of us died when he was here. He put many of us into jail for talking to him because we would not be his slaves. He kept from us our rations when he pleased and sometimes gave us bad rations of tea and tobacco.[31]

In 1847 Wybalenna was finally closed and the Aboriginal survivors moved to Oyster Cove on the main island of Tasmania.

Although the medical and mortality records at Wybalenna are inconsistent, they do reveal a high level of acute respiratory diseases among the residents.[32] Table 7.3 displays the number of deaths at Wybalenna and their recorded causes, with special attention to acute respiratory diseases.

Table 7.3. Causes of death and total deaths recorded at Wybalenna Aboriginal settlement 1833 to 1847.

Year	Pneumonia	Influenza	Other ARD	Other Causes	No Cause Recorded	Total Deaths
1833	-	-	-	-	31	31
1834	-	-	-	-	9	9
1835	11	-	-	3	-	14
1836	-	-	-	1	3	4
1837	3	-	-	8	18	29
1838	4	-	-	10	-	14
1839	-	8	-	-	-	8
1840	-	-	1	1	1	3
1841	-	-	1	-	2	3
1842	-	-	-	3	-	3
1843	-	-	-	1	-	1
1844	-	-	-	1	-	1
1845	-	-	-	2	-	2
1846	-	-	1	-	-	1
1847	-	-	4	-	-	4
Total	18	8	7	30	64	127

Source: N. J. B. Plomley, *Weep in Silence: A History of the Flinders Island Aboriginal Settlement* (Hobart: Blubber Head Press, 1987, pp. 939–944.

Respiratory diseases (n = 33) accounted for 26 per cent of the total recorded deaths. This figure should, however, be seen as a minimum because of the high number of deaths for which no cause was given (n = 64). The 18 deaths recorded as pneumonia all occurred within the first six years of the settlement. This may indicate the decline of this disease as a major cause of morbidity and mortality. Within the first seven years of the settlement 111 deaths, or 87.4 per cent, occurred, causing a severe population loss from an estimated original population of 150 in 1833. (Although just three years later the population was given as 140 yet 40 deaths were recorded in that period, this is assumed to be the result of movement on and off the settlement and poor record keeping.)

A number of individual cases of acute pneumonia leading to death were documented by Dr Allen in 1837.[33] Two have been selected here in order to indicate the severity of symptoms suffered. Both show severe inflammation, adhesion and destruction of lung tissue, oedema in the alveolar spaces, and hepatisation. A diagnosis of severe pneumococcal pneumonia is consistent with the recorded signs for both cases and possibly additional tuberculosis infection with the second.

Case one was a three-year-old child seen by Allen and described as 'of spare habit of body with a large abdomen large joints small unshapely limbs head disproportionably large, with a pustular eruption over the scalp. It [*sic*] was asleep or dozing when I saw it, skin hot and dry, tongue furred, pulse full and quick, respiration rather difficult'.

> 2nd day – Febrile symptoms increased with hurried respiration, and small quick pulse.
>
> 3rd day – Pulse small and quick, dry hot skin, tongue furred, cough accompanied with a glary [*sic*] expectoration which formed thick dark crusts on the lips, a wheezing noise in the chest as if the breath was passing through a fluid, a peculiar motion in the abdomen on inspiration and expiration as if respiration was carried on in and not in the chest in which latter [*sic*] there was very little motion. Comatose.
>
> 4th Day – Pulse small and quick. Thirst will take nothing but water. Skin dry and shrivelled, difficult respiration, troublesome cough.
>
> 5th Day – Great difficulty of breathing; towards evening convulsions set in accompanied with dilation of the pupils; greatly emaciated; lingered until the morning of the seventh day when the respiration having become very laborious died.
>
> Post mortem examination. The lungs and pleura were highly inflamed, extensive adhesions had formed between them in several places, the parts were joined together by thick layers of coagulable lymph, there was a considerable quantity of a serous fluid in the cavity of the thorax. The air cells [*sic*] were filled with a glary serum. The diaphragm was also inflamed. The abdominal viscera were healthy.

Case 2 described by Allen was a 'short stout native man about 26 years of age, short thick neck and flat chest, complained of a pain behind the ear which prevented his hearing on that side. Pulse full but a little accelerated, disinclination to move about, tendency to sleep, lounge clean, skin rather dry and hot'.

> 2nd day – Skin cool but dry, pulse not so full but rather quicker than yesterday, inclination to sleep continues, the pain has shifted half way down his neck, loss of appetite, tongue furred.
>
> 3rd day – Skin dry and hot, pulse small and quick, dry cough, difficult respiration; the pain has shifted from his neck, it is now down in his chest.
>
> 4th day – Much the same as yesterday, cough increased with expectoration of blood and mucus. Skin hot and rough, continually drinking cold water.
>
> 5th day – He seems very much relieved, skin moist, cough much easier, no blood expectorated, the tendency to sleep has gone off, pulse soft and nearly natural.
>
> 6th day – Improving fast. Pulses soft, skin moist, has been smoking this morning which is a sign of favourable termination.
>
> 7th day – Improving rapidly.
>
> 8th day – Still improving.
>
> 9th day – He got up this morning and walked about and during the course of the day he eat [sic] a large quantity of kangaroo meat and in the night was taken ill again.
>
> 10th day – Complains of a pain in his left side, cough. Pulse small and quick, skin dry and hot, considerable difficulty of breathing, prostration of strength.
>
> 11th day – The pain in his side still continues, febrile symptoms rather increased, cough accompanied with a glary expectoration, difficult respiration.
>
> 12th day – The difficulty of breathing much increased, he is now very much emaciated, feeble quick pulse, dilation of the pupils, coma.
>
> 13th day – Greatly agitated, extreme difficulty of breathing, hot dry shrivelled skin, lips and mouth thickly coated with the expectoration which flows from his mouth and nose, in the evening he became convulsed and towards morning he expired.

> *Post mortem examination* – On cutting into the peritoneum a quantity of serum escaped, the diaphragm and liver were inflamed and adhering firmly together, on attempting to remove the latter which was indurated and of a dark colour, it was easily torn. The spleen was indurated and thickly studded with strumous tubercles. In the thorax – the pleura and pericardium contained a large quantity of serum, the lungs and pleura were highly inflamed, and several extensive adhesions had formed, a layer of coagulable lymph of considerable thickness in some places united the pleura which covers the lungs to the pleura that lines the chest. The lungs were of a dark colour quite inelastic and very much resembled indurated liver. The air cells were filled with lymph and pus – there was several small tubercles interspersed through the substance of the lungs, which contained a clot of hard dark blood, these tumours were surrounded with a number of small blood vessels containing dark blood, the heart was healthy.

Acute respiratory diseases were not confined to the epidemic events of influenza at Wybalenna. Prior to the first recorded pandemic or epidemic event of influenza in 1836–37, Allen reported that between 1834 and 1837, he had treated 230 cases of new, or aggravated, pneumonia at the settlement in a population that averaged 140 individuals.[34] Out of the 140 estimated on the settlement, 40 of them had not displayed symptoms of pneumonia. That leaves, according to Allen, 100 individuals who presented 230 times with cases of pneumonia during the three-year period leading up to the first influenza epidemic. A further indication of the prevalence of severe pneumonia comes from the records of death in 1835,[35] with 14 deaths recorded in that year (Table 7.3), 11 of which (79 per cent) were recorded as due to pneumonia. Of the remaining three deaths, two were recorded as 'anasurea' (nephritis) and one as 'phthisis' (tuberculosis). All this strongly suggests that pneumonia became an acute and chronic disease among the Aboriginal inhabitants of Wybalenna soon after its establishment in 1831 and prior to the first recorded epidemic of influenza in the main Tasmanian colony.

Influenza caused serious morbidity and mortality at the Flinders Island settlement in 1837 during the course of the 1836–37 pandemic. On January 16th Robinson reported to the colonial secretary that a 'direful epidemic the influenza' had swept through the settlement. The Europeans were attacked by the virus, but it was the Aboriginal inhabitants who, according to Robinson, were the most severely affected. For that year 29 deaths were recorded in the settlement, an unusually high number. For most, no details of death were given, but for three adult females pneumonia was listed as the cause of death and four more died of the same cause in the following year.[36]

Surgeon Walsh performed an autopsy on one, an adult female, who died in October 1837. The right lung revealed considerable empyema (pus in the pleural cavity) and the characteristic consolidation of pneumonia.

> On opening up the thorax the pleura was found considerably thickened and highly vascular ... a large quantity of thick brownish fluid spurted out, which appeared to have occupied the greater part of the cavity ... The right lung not only adhered firmly to the ribs but also to all the neighbouring parts; it was of a firm and solid consistency its cellular texture being quite obliterated ... The adhesions of the left lung were not extensive, and it was on the whole healthy in appearance.[37]

A second wave occurred in 1839, when influenza again inflicted a severe morbidity and mortality among the Wybalenna Aboriginal population. A week before his final departure from the settlement, Superintendent Robinson wrote of the epidemic:

> I regret exceedingly to state that the influenza has already commenced its ravages among the aborigines supposed to have been communicated by the government vessels recently at this station. More than two-thirds of the natives are now affected, several of whom are not expected to recover. The aged and infants it is thought will suffer most although the worst cases at present are among those who are the most hale and robust. This epidemic has not confined its attacks to the natives, many of the whites being seriously indisposed, though I do not anticipate any fatal results as regards them.[38]

The two government vessels referred to by Robinson were the *Vansittart* and the *Eliza*. Both vessels had previously been to Hobart, where an epidemic of influenza had been spreading among the European population for some months.[39] A second source of introduction may have been Robinson himself. He had returned from Sydney in January 1839, immediately prior to the Wybalenna influenza epidemic.[40]

George Robinson Jnr, the son of the commandant of the Flinders Island settlement, began to record the epidemic among the Aboriginal people on the day his father left to take up the position of chief protector on the mainland at Port Phillip. The following are extracts from his journal. The first entry begins on February 24th 1839:

The Commandant left the settlement about mid-day to proceed to Port Phillip with several of the Aborigines, and as he proposed walking down to the Old Settlement Mr Clark with myself accompanied him part of the way thither. During our walk we met with several of the natives belonging to the settlement proceeding to some of the others who were staying in the 'bush' with provision as we were informed they were in a bad state of health from the influenza which had not long visited the settlement.

25 February
The influenza today [has] shown itself to be very general amongst the natives who had all or most of them encamped themselves in the 'bushes' environing the settlement … Several of them were violently attacked with the epidemic.

27 February
The influenza was spreading itself to a still more alarming extent among them. The boat arrived near mid-night during a heavy gale of wind with the sick people from Long Point.

28 February
The native woman Semiramis died about break o'day. The rest of the natives returned home from their 'breakwinds' [small brush shelters] this morning, those most affected with the influenza being brought in the truck by the others.

1 March
On proceeding as usual to the square early in the morning I was greatly surprised to hear that two of the natives, Phillip and George Robinson, had died both about one time during the night … A native child belonging to Sarah died this afternoon. One of the native men 'Billy' died in the early part of the night.

2 March
The natives still dangerously ill.

3 March
About midday 'Sabina' died and in the evening 'Jane'. Both the females had been for several days in great suffering from the disease.

> 4 March
> Interred at the usual hour, viz four o'clock pm, two of the deceased natives Sabina and 'little Billy', and as rather a remarkable occurrence one of the sick natives Queen Adelaide breathed her last as we were placing the corpses in the coffins.[41]

By March 6th Robinson Jnr was infected with influenza and soon after he records the disease striking several members of his family, the staff and convict labourers of the settlement. The last reference to the disease in his journal is on March 14th, when Robinson Jnr records that he was still suffering. How long it lingered among the Aboriginal population is unrecorded but by March 9th Robinson Jnr states that some of the males had begun to recover. According to his journal and the register of births and deaths for the settlement, eight of the Aboriginal people (three males, four females and a child) died of influenza during the epidemic.[42] The real total is almost certainly much higher, as many of the Aboriginal people had no faith in the efficacy of European medicines and, to escape the sickness, left the major settlement to live in the surrounding bush during the period of the epidemic. Their suffering was probably made greater by Robinson Jnr and his staff withdrawing rations, in particular freshly killed mutton, from the Aboriginal people during their illness:

> In consequence of the general prevalence of the present epidemic among the natives it becomes necessary to restrict them from the use of animal food for some time. I have therefore to direct that there be no issue of fresh meat made to them till further notice, but in lieu of which let them have an additional ration of the tea and sugar for dinner.[43]

In August 1847 Wybalenna was abandoned. Two weeks before they left the settlement the influenza pandemic of 1847–48 reached them. It lasted 10 or 12 days on the settlement and there was one more death reported because of the disease.[44] The remaining Aboriginal people, now numbering 47 (of the original population in 1831 of 150) were transported back to the Tasmanian mainland to the Oyster Cove settlement.

Living conditions were worse at Oyster Cove than at Wybalenna. The settlement was built on the drainage plains of the Great Oyster Bay and Little Oyster Bay rivers. The buildings were made of wood, which offered little protection from the cold southerly winds. The floors were mostly damp and often flooded by excess water draining from the rivers. Oyster Cove had originally been built as a probation station and in 1843 used as a penal settlement but by 1847 it had been abandoned because it did not meet convict health standards.[45] James Bonwick, teacher and local historian, described the station in 1859 as

> … a miserable collection of huts and outbuildings … profoundly dirty and swarming with fleas … in a ruinous condition, roofs not waterproof, windows broken and furniture gone.[46]

While it was considered to be below the accepted health standards for European convicts, Oyster Cove was deemed by the colonial government to be suitable for the few remaining Tasmanian Aboriginal people from the Flinders Island settlement.

At the Oyster Cove settlement, the Aboriginal population continued to suffer a high level of morbidity, principally from acute and chronic respiratory infections. Mortality persistently reduced their number until, by the end of 1861, just two men and six women remained. There was scant concern shown by the colonial government towards the Aboriginal people and little commitment was given to basic healthcare.[47] While the Flinders Island settlement was functioning, a medical practitioner had always been on staff to provide for the needs of the Aboriginal people, although in most cases he would have been of little use to them. At Oyster Cove there was no resident doctor despite the well-known poor state of health of the Aboriginal residents.[48] William Smith, a surgeon from Kingston, made periodic visits to the settlement between 1858 and 1869, summoned by the superintendent when emergency cases occurred, and more regular visits were made when outbreaks of influenza occurred on the settlement, particularly during the winter months.

During these visits Smith recorded his diagnoses and recommended treatments of the patients he examined in the settlement's visiting officers' book.[49] They appear in a chronological sequence according to the date of each of his visits to the settlement but, when separated and rearranged into a sequence for each of the Aboriginal patients, they reveal a progression of symptoms for each of the individuals Smith examined.

Influenza and pneumonia were common diseases throughout the period of Smith's visits. In the winter of 1860 Smith reported an epidemic of influenza on the settlement with at least 8 of the 15 Aboriginal residents affected, as well as the European superintendent and his family. During the period of the epidemic, from July to September, two females and two males died from symptoms suggestive of an infection of influenza.[50] This epidemic was most likely part of the 1857–60 world pandemic, which was recorded during 1860 in all the colonies of south-eastern Australia (Table 7.1).

Two individual cases depict the recurring morbidity of these diseases at Oyster Cove. Both cases are adult Aboriginal women whose symptoms were recorded by Smith over a period of three years in the first case and seven years in the second. The previous medical histories of both cases are unknown but both women had come to the Oyster Cove settlement from Flinders Island in 1847, where influenza, pneumonia, bronchitis and tuberculosis were major health problems. It is quite likely that both women had a long history of tobacco smoking and alcohol consumption. Pre-existing chronic bronchitis and emphysema may also have been present in both cases.

The first case is an elderly female, Sophie (Dray), around 60 to 70 years of age. In 1829–30 she was living on Bruny Island, approximately 50km east of Hobart. She accompanied George Robinson on his first expedition around the island, locating Aboriginal clans, and was later sent to Flinders Island in September 1833.[51]

Smith records:

> 23 Sep 1858
> Suffering from flu with swelling of the glands of the neck.
>
> 25 Sep 1858
> Still some swelling of the glands of the neck but in other respects better.
>
> 27 Sep 1858
> Appears much better.
>
> 27 Aug 1860
> … affected by the influenza. [She] appears to me to be in a depressed state and the physical powers lower than natural under the circumstances. I have recommended beer daily with beef tea and mutton broth and linseed tea as often as [she] can be induced to take it.
>
> 29 Aug 1860
> Sophie not so well, her cough is very troublesome and like many others, the phlegm appears to accumulate in the air passages. The bowels are much constipated. I have recommended Croton oil liniment to rub into the chest.
>
> 1 Sep 1860
> Sophie is still complaining of her cough and has some pain in the

epigastrium [upper central region of the abdomen]. The conjunctiva of the eyes have a very yellow tinge.

5 Sep 1860
Sophie appeared somewhat better but still complained of cough, the Croton Oil liniment has produced rather more eruption on the chest.

21 Aug 1861
… Sophie suffering from debility – she is supposed to be 70 years of age …

25 Aug 1861
Sophie has been poorly for several days and is apparently suffering from Bronchitis and general disability being upwards of seventy years old. I have recommended Brandy and Beer to be given at frequent intervals with as much Beef Tea as she can be induced to take.

27 Aug 1861
Sophie is sitting out having an Airing in the sun which she seems to enjoy much. Her breathing is still bad and there appears to be much mucus accumulated in the air passage. She does not take too much nourishment as she aught.

29 Aug 1861
Sophie died early this morning. Probably from exhaustion and the accumulation of mucus on the air passages.

The second case is an adult woman, Wapperty (or Wobberrertee). She was probably of the Pyemmairrener people, born on the north-east coast of Tasmania. Little is known of her early life. As an adult she was abducted by sealers and lived on the Bass Strait islands before being moved to the Flinders Island settlement in 1844 and thence to Oyster Cove in 1847.[52]

16 July 1860
Wapperty not so well. Complaining of pain in the chest with cold chills.

18 July 1860
Wapperty somewhat better and is apparently free from pain.

21 July 1860
Wapperty more lively.

14 July 1863
Wapperty is suffering from influenza with pain on the left side attended with some cough. I ordered a mustard plaister [*sic*] and mixture with taitan emetic and compound camphor mixture.

17 July 1863
Wapperty is complaining of pain in the right side with difficult breathing and symptoms of Bronchitis, to continue the mixture and have the taitan emetic ointment rubbed into her chest and a blister on her right side.

19 July 1863
… the pain in the right side has left her, the cough somewhat better but the tongue coated with thick brown fur. Pulse not so strong, her appetite is not ample. To take Gin in linseed tea or milk if it be procured.

21 July 1863
suffering symptoms of Bronchitis, in other respects better, the brown fur has left the tongue the bowels are acted upon, she does not sleep very well. To have Dovers Powder at bedtime in place of Gin, to have bottled porter with egg and nutmeg.

23 July 1863
Wapperty is still suffering from Bronchitis. The bowels are regular, appetite pretty good, breathing somewhat difficult. To continue the mixture and let her have rum in linseed tea.

25 July 1865
Wapperty is in many respects better but the cough is still troublesome. The Tartar Emilie has brought out a slight eruption on the chest, her appetite is pretty good.

27 July 1865
Wapperty appears greatly improved and the breathing seems natural. Her

appetite is very good. She is allowed beer daily which is recommended to continue.

22 July 1865
Wapperty is complaining of pain in the stomach.

29 July 1865
… complains of cough.

24 June 1867
[Wapperty was sent to hospital suffering from dysentery.]

29 July 1867
[Wapperty recovered from dysentery and returned to Oyster Cove.]

8 August 1867
Wapperty suffering from Catarrh and debility, respiration difficult.

9 August 1867
[Wapperty appears to have improved.]

11 August 1867
Wapperty does not appear well, pulse weak and pain.

12 August 1867
[Wapperty died.]

During the periods leading up to their deaths, both women suffered repeatedly from acute respiratory tract infections. No post-mortem examinations were recorded for these women but the cause of death given for Sophie in the settlement's records was 'congestion of the lungs' and for Wapperty 'catarrh debility'.[53] While the official records giving causes of death among Aboriginal residents on settlements can be vague, there appears little doubt that the deaths of these two individuals are closely related to the respiratory disorders they had.

Port Phillip, 1839

The 1836–39 influenza world pandemic reached mainland Aboriginal populations in 1839. In that year, the disease caused serious morbidity and mortality among the European and Aboriginal populations of Victoria. The first signs of the disease began to be noted early in the year and by July and August it reached a peak, prevailing throughout the European population of the colony. In a report to the Royal College of Physicians, the deputy inspector of hospitals stated that hardly a household had escaped the disease.

Sub-Protector William Thomas had just arrived in Melbourne and one of his first encounters with Australian Aboriginal people was with the Boonwurrung and Woiworung on January 17th and 18th. He noted in his journal:

> Saw several blacks. The inhabitants of Melbourne say that they are about returning to the settlement, having left it on account of the influenza that prevailed. The natives considered that the whites brought the disorder.[54]

Some four weeks later Thomas noted in his journal that a family group of four, all suffering from influenza, were the first to come into the settlement for aid.

During February and March 1839 larger numbers began to arrive in Melbourne. They came from the outlying regions to the north, south-east and south-west. The reason for their going to the European settlement was seemingly to meet newly appointed Aboriginal Chief Protector George Robinson.[55] Robinson arrived in Melbourne by the government cutter *Vansittart* on February 27th, which had also visited Wybalenna and Hobart the previous month. By this time four hundred Aboriginal people had gathered in a large encampment on the Yarra River opposite the main European settlement. On the very day of his arrival Robinson reported he was suddenly attacked with influenza symptoms and was so severely incapacitated that he was unable to perform his duties for several days.[56]

By the last week in March 1839, five hundred Aboriginal people had gathered in Melbourne to meet Chief Protector Robinson and his assistants.[57] It soon became apparent that many were suffering from influenza. Sub-Protector Thomas reported in his journal that he, in company with Chief Protector Robinson, visited the Aboriginal encampment on May 5th and found a scene 'truly appalling'.[58] There was little that Robinson could do. The Protectorate had limited financial reserves and no medicinal resources of its own to dispense among the Aboriginal communities. Repeated requests by Robinson for extra financial support were more often than not denied by Governor Gipps. The protectors could do no more than distribute just four blankets, which they took from their own beds, among the Aboriginal people who were sick.

On his return to the European settlement Robinson immediately instructed Dr P. Cussen, the assistant surgeon for the colony, to go to the encampment and give what aid he could. Cussen visited the encampment the next day and witnessed what he called 'a most distressing scene of disease, destitution and misery'. According to his report he found the Aboriginal people displaying the symptoms of 'dysentery', accompanied with 'typhus fever of the worst description', 'rheumatism' and, in many, the symptoms of chronic syphilis. The prevailing influenza epidemic, which Cussen referred to as 'acute catarrh', had already had a serious effect on the group gathered on the banks of the Yarra River, with six of them having died within the four days preceding Cussen's visit and many more expected to die within the next days.[59]

The *Port Phillip Gazette* expressed its serious concern, not particularly about the wellbeing of Aboriginal people, but of the threat of influenza being further disseminated into the European population. It warned its readers that it was well known that influenza was epidemic, and the Aboriginal people should be removed as quickly as possible. It further advised

> ... all mothers to be careful of allowing their children to be taken in the direction of the native camps, the slightest attack of the influenza is sufficient to carry off an infant in a few hours.[60]

Across Port Phillip Bay the situation was similar among the Wathaurong.[61] In August Assistant Protector Sievwright requested the assistant colonial surgeon for the Geelong district, Dr J. Clerk, to attend an individual who was suffering severely from influenza with secondary lung complications. Clerk's response succinctly reveals the plight of the Wathaurong in particular, and the Aboriginal population of the Port Phillip colony in general, as well as the inadequacies of the Protectorate and helplessness of the medical establishment to render assistance:

> In compliance with your [Sievwright's] request of yesterday, I visited the native black man and found him dangerously ill with inflammation of the pleura occasioned by exposure to the cold.
>
> I bled and prescribed for him accordingly but fear that medicine can produce little effect on him or any of the Aborigines whilst they are suffered to continue in their present exposed, helpless, and miserable state, destitute (when sickness attacks them) both of shelter and clothing and other necessaries for their comforts. It cannot under these circumstances be supposed that medicine can do much good ... Several

to my knowledge this season have been carried off by inflammation of the chest.[62]

By September, the epidemic had begun to subside among the European population of Melbourne but was still prevailing among the Aboriginal communities. Assistant Protector Thomas reported to his superior in September that many Aboriginal people living along the Yarra River were 'labouring under affections of the chest'. The number of Aboriginal people at Melbourne began to fall at the end of April, when groups started returning to their homelands. By October 1839 most of the visitors had left Melbourne, with fewer than 50 remaining, the majority of these reported to be from the local region.[63]

Elsewhere in Victoria, 1845–90

An epidemic of influenza, restricted to the colonies of Victoria (Port Phillip) and South Australia, occurred between 1844 and 1845. Although its origin is unclear, it was likely to have been introduced by ship and begun as an infection among the European populations of the two colonies, reaching a level of excessive morbidity towards the end of 1845.[64] Chief Protector Robinson reported that few families living in Melbourne escaped infection and out of a population of 12,000 at least two-thirds had suffered attacks of influenza.[65]

Aboriginal people, according to Robinson, were the greatest sufferers, especially those living in the interior of the colony. At the Goulburn River Aboriginal station morbidity was high among the Taungurong with 'upwards of one hundred' reported to be affected and at least one death occurring in 1845. A similar situation occurred among the Gunditjmara at the Mount Rouse Aboriginal station in the west of the colony. During the last three months of 1845, 65 individuals were treated, most of whom presented with 'influenza and diarrhoea with occasional dysenteric symptoms'. No deaths were recorded among those living on the station.[66]

Dr John Cumpston documents the next pandemic or epidemic of influenza beginning in November 1851. It prevailed extensively throughout Victoria during the following three months and continued to exist in other settlements of the continent throughout 1852 and into 1853.[67] The epidemic coincided with the beginning of the gold rush period, which attracted thousands of seekers from Europe, Asia and America. Few records of the effects of this epidemic on the Aboriginal population have survived. The source of much of the early information on the Aboriginal people of Victoria had ceased when the Aboriginal Protectorate was abolished at the end of 1849. It can, however, be assumed with reasonable confidence that the morbidity was severe among Aboriginal people. The great influx of gold seekers to the newly established goldfields and, with it, the pervasion of legal and illegal liquor outlets made it easier for Aboriginal people to obtain alcohol, much of which was of dubious quality.

In a letter to the lieutenant governor, Assistant Protector Thomas, wrote:

> The present condition of the Aborigines have no way improved but lamentably deteriorated, the discovery of Gold has greatly affected their moral condition, at all events those who locate these colonies or make transient visits to them ... the consequence is that their frames are enervated in the absence of regular exercise and their blood corrupted through continued dissipation, so much so, that when seized with a violent cold inflammation follows so rapid [*sic*] that it is impossible in most cases to save them; the old and middle aged do not die in any proportion to the young, who, do not live out half of their days.[68]

In 1861, following another pandemic or epidemic of influenza, Thomas reported to the Aboriginal Protection Board on the mortality from respiratory disorders:

> I may state that eight-tenths of the mortality among the aborigines of Victoria arises through intemperance, bringing on pulmonary disorders, pleurisy, pneumonia, disorders of the chest, consumption, & c., which carries them off so speedily that the ablest medical treatment when available seldom save them. I may safely state, that when their respiratory organs are once affected, recovery becomes hopeless.[69]

The second half of the 19th century saw many of the Aboriginal people of south-eastern Australia centralised on mission and government settlements. Acute respiratory disorders were regularly reported on all these settlements. Medical reports from the Aboriginal settlements of Coranderrk and Lake Condah in rural Victoria reveal respiratory disorders as recurring causes of morbidity. Dr J. Gibson made regular and special visits to the government settlement of Coranderrk between 1865 and 1875, and reported his diagnoses and treatments to the Aboriginal Protection Board. Over the 11-year period of his visits, Gibson's medical reports record periods of excessive morbidity from a possible outbreak of influenza in 1867; whooping cough (pertussis) in 1868; and influenza in 1873.[70] The periods of high influenza morbidity were most likely localised outbreaks as they do not parallel the sequence of pandemics or epidemics of south-eastern Australia (Table 7.4).

Table 7.4. Periods of excessive morbidity from respiratory and possible respiratory disease on Coranderrk Aboriginal settlement between 1865 and 1875.

Date of Visit	No. of Inmates	No. with Respiratory Disorders	%	Remarks
21 Apr. 1867	105	7	6.7	'Intermittent fever' Several others recovering
14 May 1867	-	16	-	Many leaving due to epidemic
8 Aug. 1867	78	5	6.4	'Influenza'
5 Dec. 1868	74	-	-	Whooping-cough attacking all children & most adults
29 Dec. 1868	65	-	-	Whooping-cough still present but incidence abating
16 Jun. 1873	125	11	8.8	'Influenza'
26 Jun. 1873	129	13	10.1	Nine children & four adults infected

Source: J. Gibson, Reports, in 'Annual Report of the Board for the Protection of the Aborigines', Papers Presented to Parliament, Legislative Assembly, *Victorian Parliamentary Papers*, Vol. 4, 1869; Vol. 3, 1871; Vol. 3, Part 2, 1872; Vol. 3, Part 1, 1873; Vol. 3, Part 1, 1874; Vol. 3, 1875–1876.

Gibson diagnosed the epidemic in April and May 1867 as 'intermittent fever', a common medical term of the day often given to the febrile symptoms of malaria.[71] It is unlikely, however, that this was the disease causing the symptoms. Cases of malaria among Aboriginal populations in the 19th century were restricted to the north coast of Australia and there is no evidence for appearance of the disease in south-eastern Australia.[72]

The term 'intermittent fever', together with 'fog fever', were occasionally used as euphemisms for the various 19th-century epidemics of influenza.[73] By his November 1867 visit the symptoms had ceased and Gibson described the general state of health of the settlement as 'good', with just three cases of illness out of a population of 76. The symptoms presented in both Aboriginal males and females between two years of age to adults, as well as the superintendent of the settlement and his children. In May of that year Gibson administered treatment to 16 (12 per cent) of the residents but many others had left the settlement to escape the epidemic. Against these periods of high morbidity was a backdrop of periodic influenza cases of lower incidence and severity occurring mainly in the colder months of the year.

Morbidity from respiratory diseases at Lake Condah settlement during the years 1886 to 1890 was higher than in previous years. The superintendent of the settlement, J. H. Stahle reported in 1886 an epidemic of whooping cough, followed two years later by a severe attack of influenza in the spring and autumn. Initially the epidemic caused only the confinement of people to their homes but in 1889–90 it became a serious health problem:

> We had several deaths during the first half of the year, and the latter half was not better as regards the health of the people, for influenza visited the station and was very severe on the poor blacks, all of whom were attacked and will probably not feel much better until the warm weather sets in again.[74]

The records of mortality from the settlement reveal 9 deaths of a total of 25 during the period 1886 to 1890 that could be attributed to infectious respiratory disease.

South Australia, 1850–93?

The first reliable records of influenza or acute respiratory diseases among Aboriginal people in South Australia do not appear until 1850, 14 years after the colony of South Australia was established. There is no evidence regarding the effect of the pandemics of 1838 and 1845–47, or of the local epidemic of 1845. Little knowledge of the health of the populations closest to the European settlements is available in this period. In 1844 Dr Matthew Moorhouse, Aboriginal protector, reported to the governor of the colony on the state of the Aboriginal population. He included a brief account of the diseases suffered by them, in the main, venereal diseases and tuberculosis, and concluded that they were

> subject to those [diseases] common to the human race, as inflammation and its consequences ...[75]

Moorhouse's reference to diseases was vague and whether or not he made any reference to influenza epidemics is uncertain.

By 1850 acute respiratory diseases were becoming a serious source of morbidity and mortality. In a quarterly report to the governor, Moorhouse reported on an epidemic that was most likely influenza with cases of secondary pneumonia:

> I regret to have to remark, that the epidemic characterised by inflammation of the lungs, continues to afflict the natives ... The deaths of

> three children and three adults have been recorded by me … I have little doubt that many more have died in the scrub, whose deaths will remain unknown to me for months, if not altogether. The aborigines … appear to have an instinctive knowledge of the approach of death, and a desire to let the breath of life depart at or about the place where it was first inhaled.[76]

In this instance Moorhouse may be referring to a local remnant of the major epidemic of 1847–48 in the eastern colonies.

Beginning in 1843 and continuing into the next decade, a regular migration trend developed when the Ngarrindjeri from the lower Murray River and Coorong and the Meru from the eastern river region of the colony began to gather in Adelaide.[77] They displaced the remnants of the local Kaurna and established encampments on the banks of the Torrens River with numbers often exceeding 70 or 80 individuals.[78] They became a common sight to the residents of Adelaide, staying each year for most of the winter months. Exposure to the cold, poor nutrition, inadequate sanitary conditions and alcohol abuse made them extremely susceptible to infectious disease. In 1855 a concerned citizen wrote to the *South Australian Register*:

> It is painful to every one who comes into contact with the natives to witness the dreadful colds with which they are nearly all afflicted in such a winter as the present. The severity of such complaints among them is no doubt chiefly owing to the want of shelter from the inclemency of the weather. Would it be too much for our Government to provide them, out of our abundance, with a building which would afford them some more substantial shelter than their wretched 'wurlies'? Their rude wants would require nothing elegant or costly.[79]

In 1852 the gold rush in the eastern colonies created a shortage of European labour on rural properties and the settlers wanted Aboriginal people to assist with their crops. As a consequence, many of the Ngarrindjeri and Meru moved to the agricultural districts, where good wages and ample food supplies were offered for their labour. A much larger number than usual came to the city late in the year. Moorhouse reported:

> In November, the City of Adelaide was visited by upwards of three hundred natives; Encounter Bay, Lake Alexandrina, and Murray River tribes, all met by appointment. The Lake Alexandrina tribe undertook to reap about ninety acres of crop … They would have done more, but the influenza was raging at the time, and the whole becoming more

> or less affected by it, ceased their reaping, and returned to their own district.[80]

The influenza epidemic had already reached the Ngarrindjeri before their arrival in Adelaide. Sub-Protector Mason reported to Moorhouse in July 1852 from Wellington on the lower Murray:

> I am sorry to report that a great amount of sickness prevails among the natives at the present time, many are suffering from complaints of the chest, and rheumatism. In such cases of sickness amongst them, they are generally treated with kindness by the settlers.[81]

West of Adelaide, on Eyre Peninsula, the Nawu, who occupied most of the south and west of the peninsula, were suffering the effects of the epidemic in 1852 and 1853. Archdeacon Hale informed Moorhouse:

> In reporting upon the state of this Institution for the past four months, the subject which, on account of its importance first demands our attention, is the great extent to which sickness and mortality have prevailed amongst the inmates during this period.[82]

The cause of the mortality is not clear from Hale's report but a later report by him, which includes a brief autopsy report, alludes to an epidemic of acute respiratory disease:

> I am again under the necessity of referring … to the frequent instances of mortality amongst our inmates. We had no less than three deaths since the date of my last report. In the last case a post mortem examination was made by our medical attendant, Dr. Lawson. He found the lungs to be extensively diseased; one lobe having a very large ulcer upon it and the other lobe being in a highly inflamed state.[83]

The pandemic of 1850–52 affected the colonies of New South Wales and Victoria but appears not to have influenced the morbidity or mortality of the South Australian colonists. The origin of the outbreak of influenza among the Ngarrindjeri and Meru living in Adelaide is then somewhat of a mystery. The best way to account for it is to assume that there was a low prevalence of the disease among the colonial population of Adelaide and it was transferred to the Aboriginal people, who suffered a more serious morbidity.

Between the pandemic or epidemic events of 1852–53 and 1885 localised epidemics of influenza and other respiratory disease recurred among the Aboriginal communities of South Australia. Acute respiratory disease continued to be a cause of high morbidity and mortality among the Nawu living both on and off the Poonindie settlement. In 1857, Octavius Hammond, a qualified medical practitioner who succeeded Hale as superintendent, reported that 'bronchitis' and 'pleurisy' were among the most commonly developed diseases. He observed the severe effects of the disease in the rapid onset of symptoms and little resistance offered by the patients. He further stated:

> While speaking on this subject, however, it should be borne in mind, that there has existed a similar state of disease and death among the natives in the bush, in this neighbourhood, in a proportion, probably equal to that experienced at Poonindie.[84]

The 1860 pandemic saw the return of influenza universally across south-eastern Australia. It was reported to be causing excessive morbidity and mortality, this time mainly among the Ngarrindjeri. George Taplin, from the Point McLeay settlement, informed the Aborigines' Friends' Association:

> The suffering of the natives from cold have been very great. The country from which they used to get their opossum-skins for rugs being nearly taken up, they are dependent on blankets for protection from cold. But it unfortunately happens that the blankets supplied by Government are not distributed when winter sets in. Had this been done, many who have this winter fallen victims to influenza might have survived.[85]

By the mid-1860s respiratory disease among the Aboriginal people of South Australia was common and widespread. Morbidity and mortality from respiratory infections in between the influenza epidemics of 1860 and 1885 was a constant factor of Aboriginal health. Sub-Protector Buttfield noticed 'catarrhal affection' among Narangga on northern Yorke Peninsula in July 1866. The elderly suffering from acute respiratory disease would regularly go to the Point Pearce settlement to obtain treatment and, after many deaths from 'inflammation of the lungs' on the mission, several children were taken by their parents to live away from the settlement and avoid the continuing infection.[86] And George Taplin noted among the inmates of Point McLeay in 1868, 'We have lost that very troublesome visitor the hooping [*sic*] cough which only carried off three or four children altho [*sic*] so many suffered with it.'[87]

In 1878 Inspector Hamilton reported that the Aboriginal people throughout the colony were 'exceedingly susceptible to colds, which often settle on their lungs'.[88] The *South Australian Government Gazette* listed respiratory diseases (influenza, whooping cough and 'inflammation of the lungs') as the highest cause of mortality after tuberculosis in the official returns of the causes of death in 1875 and 1879. The returns of sick Aboriginal people under treatment in Adelaide Hospital and among the Buandig in the south-east of the colony during 1874–76 show recurring cases of bronchitis, pneumonia, influenza, catarrh and 'pleuritis'.[89]

In 1874–76 acute respiratory diseases inflicted excessive morbidity and mortality. The respiratory infections accompanied a major epidemic of measles that spread throughout south-eastern Australia (see Chapter 3). Sub-Protector Hamilton reported a 'great deal of sickness' among the Ngarrindjeri on the south coast in February 1874, chiefly influenza accompanied by scarlet fever and rheumatism, and in the north of the colony Sub-Protector Buttfield reported high morbidity, though few deaths, from influenza.[90]

While acute respiratory diseases were becoming established in the settled southern and western regions of the colony, a localised epidemic began among the Aboriginal populations in the north. A boom in colonial expansion in South Australia began in 1869 into areas specially selected for their suitability to cultivation.[91] The spread of settlement north along the Flinders Ranges brought the Europeans into closer contact with the Banggarla, Kuyani and Adnyamathanha people. In May and June of 1870 unusually heavy rainfall was experienced along the Flinders Ranges. In a six-week period the rainfall was measured at ten inches (250mm), almost the average annual amount. Sub-Protector Buttfield, responsible to the commissioner of Crown lands for the welfare of Aboriginal people in the northern districts, recorded an epidemic of what was most likely influenza among the Kuyani and Adnyamathanha around Blinman in June:

> Owing to the heavy rainfall ... travelling has been quite impracticable during the month of May. My time has, however, been fully occupied for the cold and wet has increased the number of patients. Coughs, colds, sore throats have been very prevalent. I have three cases under treatment of a more serious nature – haemoorhage [*sic*] of the lungs.[92]

The three 'haemoorhage' cases may have been pulmonary tuberculosis.

Buttfield had been confined to the settlement and ration station at Blinman during the rains and had little or no contact with people living away from Blinman so was unable to report on their condition. Two months later, however, another report by Buttfield reveals that the morbidity from respiratory diseases had increased:

> Owing to the extreme inclemency of the weather my sick list was considerably augmented during June. The Aborigines suffering from

> Catarrh and other disorders. Scarcely a day passed without bringing some poor creature seeking for relief.[93]

By the end of the year the epidemic had waned and Buttfield reported in May 1871 that 'there has been less sickness during the past three months than at any similar period during my residence here'. During the remainder of 1871 Buttfield visited an area of the Flinders Ranges to the north and east of Blinman and had found the people in a satisfactory condition, with only a few cases of sickness. The continuing trend of improving health and the drop-in morbidity from respiratory diseases reflected in Buttfield's reports was attributed to the high rainfall in 1870. He reported that the rain had promoted growth of plant and animal food sources, which had enabled the people to move away from the European settlements and ration depots into the countryside. This in turn might have helped them to throw off some of the less serious infections and, while being dispersed and not living in crowded damp conditions near colonial settlements, enabled them to avoid further infection.[94]

However, in 1885 the disease was again reported in the northern regions of the South Australian colony, this time among the Dieri people. It claimed several living on the Killalpaninna mission settlement and an unknown number living in the Lake Eyre and Cooper Creek region.[95]

Of the remaining influenza epidemics of the 19th century, the most serious was the one that appeared in the last decade. It was reported to have come from Melbourne in March 1890 and spread rapidly in all directions, reaching Adelaide shortly thereafter. Of the 320,000 European population of the South Australian colony, 48 deaths from influenza were registered during the epidemic. It may have lingered among the Aboriginal populations in the north of the colony until 1893.[96] Sub-Protector Beasley reported influenza spreading among the populations following along the Trans-Australian Railway line to the Cooper Creek region, and among the Banggarla and Nukunu north-west of Port Augusta. The extent of morbidity and mortality from the disease is unknown as most cases were not seen by the sub-protector and most deaths went unreported.[97]

Western Australia, 1883

Rottnest Island (or Wadjemup, as it is known by the local Noongar people) is a low-lying island 18km off the coast of Fremantle on Australia's south-western coast. Originally formed from shore-bordering sand dunes in the Pleistocene, Rottnest became an island during the period of sea-level rise around 7000 years ago. Today it is a popular tourist destination drawing a stream of visitors to engage with the native quokkas (*Setonix brachyurus*) a small macropod the size of a cat, whose habitat is mainly restricted to the island. Rottnest acquired its name in 1695, when Dutch mariner and explorer Willem de Vlamingh observed the quokkas. Thinking the island was overrun with rats, he gave it the name *'t Eylandt 't Rottenest* (Rats' Nest Island). The island is on the Western Australian heritage register principally for its environmental significance (including the quokkas), and its settlement and military history. But it has a more insidious past. From 1839 to 1903 it was used as a penal settlement and prison, primarily for Aboriginal offenders sent there by the colonial courts. Some 3700 Aboriginal men and boys from all over Western Australia were sent to the island, with 369 (10 per cent) recorded deaths. The actual death toll was probably higher. The Aboriginal burial ground is one of several Department of Aboriginal Affairs registered sites on the island. Many of the deaths were from respiratory disease.

Following reports of the influenza outbreak and the deaths of 37 of the prisoners in 1883 the governor of Western Australia, F. Napier Broome, visited the island. He stayed a day, inspecting the prison and the inmates. Concerned about the situation he ordered the colonial surgeon of the colony, Dr Alfred Waylen, to the island to investigate and report back. Waylen arrived at the island shortly before noon on August 2nd and quickly submitted his findings to the governor:

> I arrived at the island shortly before noon of yesterday, the 2nd instant, and proceeded at once to inspect the native prisoners. As many as were sufficiently well were paraded in the prison yard. There were 79 men. And all, with the exception of 14, came from the country north of the Murchison River; of these 65 there were sick who exhibited symptoms of influenza; but all were generally well conditioned and sufficiently clothed. I then visited a large cell used as a hospital, and 8 smaller cells each containing from 2 to 3 sick men; also the two kitchens or associated wards – in one there were 21, in the other 13 men, all suffering from the epidemic, though some but slightly. The cases in the hospital and cells were the worst, and they numbered 25. Of these and several others I made a careful examination; the symptoms were all alike, those of general influenza, intensified in this instance by overcrowding and the cold wet weather which has been and is now prevailing. The object being, impossible, to remedy these evils, I directed that one of the large rooms in the Reformatory should be devoted to the purpose of a

> temporary hospital. A fire having been made and the room warmed, in company with Dr. Holmes (who has been in attendance since the 30th ultimo), I selected 14 of the worst cases for removal thither, and instructed that the warmth of the room should be kept up all night. The selection was an easy matter, from the judicious classification of the sick by Dr. Holmes. His treatment is in my opinion most appropriate, but I have recommended a more extensive use of mustard and linseed meal cataplasms, also a supply of broth and gruel in addition to the ordinary ration. The medicine, which the natives take pretty readily, is given to them at the proper intervals, and the exertions of Mr. Oliver and the other warders are most praiseworthy under the circumstances, and I may say that everything that can be done is being done for the sick natives.[98]

Waylen continued in his report that 23 deaths had taken place since the outbreak began and, in the absence of fine weather, he predicted there would doubtless be others. The deaths were to increase to 60. The prison had held 170 inmates at the commencement of the outbreak and over one-third had died.

Waylen took the opportunity of his visit to comment on the living conditions he observed during his brief stay on the island:

> The prison is, I consider, far too small for the number of men at present confined in it. There is accommodation for 106 at the most. At the outbreak of the epidemic there were 170, and in May last 179. With this crowded state, the cold wet weather, and the very infectious character of the malady, added to the nature of these aboriginals to despond and rapidly fail in vitality, the number of deaths which have taken place can hardly be wondered at. There is an ample supply of all necessary medicines and nourishment, and I have made arrangements for additional supplies being sent over in the course of to-morrow.[99]

Doctor Waylen departed the island and recommended that further visits, as deemed necessary, should be undertaken by local medical practitioners until the crisis was over. When he received Waylen's report, a concerned Governor Broome initiated a commission to inquire into the Rottnest prison and the condition and treatment of the Aboriginal prisoners. But the detention of Aboriginal people continued into the next century.

The 1918–19 Pandemic

The 1918–19 influenza pandemic was one of the greatest human disasters of all times. Hard on the heels of the terrible losses incurred by the First World War, the disease swept around the world in waves, affecting millions of people. The mortality varied from country to country and continent to continent, but estimates have ranged between 50 and 100 million worldwide in the space of little over a year. The first wave of the pandemic in 1918 appeared to have missed Australia. The Commonwealth and state authorities were aware of the disease in 1918 as it spread through Europe, South Africa and Asia, and in October introduced quarantine procedures at all Australian ports. This had the effect of blocking to a large extent the first wave of the pandemic. But the quarantine measures could not cope with the steady influx of service personnel coming home from the war zones of Europe. The disease reached Australia in 1919, causing more than 12,000 deaths out of as many as 2 million people infected. It was a social and demographic disaster for a population of just over 5 million (then about the population of the city of New York). But that estimate, as harsh as it was, did not include many of the Aboriginal communities throughout the country.

We do not know the morbidity and mortality rates of the pandemic among Aboriginal people because they were not effectively enumerated in the official statistics, but there can be little doubt that they were high. In New Zealand, the Maori population was seven times more likely to die from the influenza pandemic than European New Zealanders. The Maori death rate exceeded 42.3 per thousand.[100]

In Queensland, 1030 deaths were recorded, of which 315 (30.6 per cent) were Aboriginal. The real figure is almost certainly much higher than this because many Aboriginal deaths, particularly in isolated regions, went unnoticed and unrecorded. Because few records of Aboriginal deaths were taken, little is known of the impact of the pandemic on Aboriginal populations elsewhere, although high morbidity and mortality would be expected.[101] However, in some places an indication of the morbidity and mortality of the pandemic can be extrapolated.

At Taroom, Queensland, a government-operated Aboriginal settlement on the Dawson River had a population of approximately 400 people. Within 24 hours of the epidemic striking, more than half had contracted the pneumonic form of influenza. The superintendent of the settlement also contracted influenza and was among those who died. By the end of 1919, the chief protector reported that just in the southern camps an estimated 298 Aboriginal people had died.

It was the practice of Australian authorities to round up sick Aboriginal people and take them directly to disease compounds, government depots, mission stations and hospitals for treatment. In several cases, fringe camps developed in or near hospitals for those showing signs of illness. Many suffered from physical exhaustion and lack of nutrition while trying to escape and hide from the police conducting the round-ups or travelling the distances to medical care.

Indigenous historian Dr Gordon Briscoe, writing of the pandemic among the Aboriginal people in Queensland, has described the disease compounds:

> The specially constructed disease-compounds on the government depots consisted of fenced areas. Built with a 10-foot high cyclone fence and topped by barbed wire to prevent entry and escape, they resembled huge wire cages. There were no structures inside them where the sick people could shelter from the cold and rain. Patients were sometimes allowed to leave the compound during daylight. An Aboriginal attendant saw to it that those leaving by day returned before the gates were locked at nightfall. The huts in the general grounds of the relief depots were made of weatherboard and cooking fireplaces were erected outside. The disease-compounds, originally constructed as punishment for people infected with venereal disease, became hospital camps as the number of influenza cases swelled the populations of the relief depots.[102]

At the Barambah (later Cherbourg) Aboriginal settlement in southern Queensland, the visiting medical officer, Dr Junk, reported that 596 'natives' were affected by influenza and only 10 in the settlement remained unaffected. Of the 69 deaths on the station, 45 were female and 24 male, with 29 being aged or infirm. The settlement was in 'a state of panic' because of the 'dire effects' of the epidemic. Many panic-stricken Aboriginal people fled the station into the surrounding bush hoping to escape. Up to 300 became ill, many of whom died officially unaccounted for. The staff of the settlement, of whom half were also suffering from influenza, had great difficulty in rounding up the surviving runaways to bring them back into confinement.[103] It would seem that there was just nowhere safe to go.

Another policy widely implemented was to remove 'mixed-race' Aboriginal children from their parents and place them in the care of European families. The common thinking of that time was still that the 'pure' Aboriginal people were doomed to extinction, but those that had some European parentage ('blood') could be saved by removing them and placing them in the care of a more civilised white society. This was at the time when Aboriginal people were still dying in large numbers from other introduced diseases. These children, whether they survived or died, were to become part of the Stolen Generations of Australia.

In tropical northern Queensland, Jane Bardsley spent much of her life living on cattle stations. She wrote many letters to her cousin, telling of her life in remote areas. While living on a station near Bowen during the pandemic, she observed firsthand the effects of the disease on the Aborigines she was familiar with:

> The blacks arrived home in a frightful state, too ill even to make a fire for themselves. I being the only one over the flu, went over to help them and was grieved to see poor old Maggie dying. She had a temperature of one hundred and six, and when she saw me she could just whisper 'whisky'. I thought that there was no hope of her to recover so decided to let her die happy and gave her a good dose of whisky. Next morning I crept over to the humpies, afraid of looking at death, when to my amazement she peeped at me over the blankets and said quite cheerfully, 'More whisky please'. So from then on I gave whisky freely to the patients and am glad to say that we never lost a case. At Strathmore station they kept strictly to regulation treatment and lost many blacks. In fact, some of them were in such bad state that their limbs fell from their bodies before there was time to bury them.[104]

It is doubtful that whisky had such a curative effect on those suffering from influenza as Jane Bardsley claims. They were more likely to have recovered from rather than have been cured by taking alcohol. Nevertheless, Jane's care would have helped those suffering.

Some settlements, however, offered protection from the pandemic. Dr Parker, an Aboriginal protector in Victoria, referring to the Coranderrk Aboriginal settlement near Healesville, stated that the 60 or 70 inmates escaped with only minor symptoms and no deaths occurred throughout the pandemic. The accuracy of all these morbidity and mortality figures will always be open to question, with the caveat that they are most likely understated. The 'real' numbers will remain unknown.

The pandemic disappeared from the general Australian public by the end of 1919. But, for the Aboriginal communities, whether confined in the compounds, fringe camps or settlements, the morbidity and mortality continued for another year. It was the same situation across the country.

More than 60 years after the pandemic it was still remembered by some Aboriginal groups. In 1982 Professor Isabel McBryde from the Australian

National University was conducting archaeological surveys and excavations around Lake Eyre in South Australia's arid north. She worked closely with the local Arabana people. During the survey she was shown an area of sand dunes south of the lake by an Arabana Elder who knew it as a place where many of his people who had died 'of the 'flu' in 1919 were buried. The disease had swept through the communities living in and around the lake system, causing high morbidity and mortality. The burial site bore testimony to the destruction the disease had caused. Most of these deaths went unrecorded.

The Experience of Influenza throughout Australia

The introduction into colonial Australia of pathogens causing acute respiratory diseases had a long-lasting and severe effect on Aboriginal populations of the continent. The first recorded cases of influenza reaching Aboriginal people in south-eastern Australia are in 1820, during the period of the first pandemic to reach Australia. Was this then the first appearance of transcontinental respiratory disease to involve Australian Aboriginal people?

Although it cannot be said with certainty that there were no outbreaks of influenza in Australia prior to 1820 (for example there is no record of the 1800 world pandemic reaching Australia), its apparent absence during the initial years of colonial settlement can be accounted for epidemiologically. The colony of New South Wales was isolated geographically and temporally from the major Old World sources of infection. Outbreaks of influenza, which were common enough aboard ships leaving England, often flared up in the initial days following departure but in most cases were self-limiting, failing to survive the long sea journey to Australia. Even after calling in to ports where influenza was endemic en route to the colony, the disease often burned out before arrival at Sydney.[105] If the disease did persist on board and was to reach the colony, its progress would then have been impeded by the small and dispersed nature of the settlements in New South Wales, and the low proportion of susceptible children in the colony's population.[106] Nevertheless, infections of influenza may have resulted prior to 1820, but if they did they were most likely to have been localised and self-limiting, and so of minor impact on the colony in general.

A similar set of epidemiological circumstances applies to the Aboriginal people. Prior to 1820 many Aboriginal populations living along the south-eastern and southern coasts had had contact with the sealing and whaling fleets as early as 1798. Large-scale commercial sealing operations quickly developed, particularly among the Bass Strait islands and the southern coastline.

Kidnapping of women by the sealers for sexual purposes and to assist in the capturing of seals was a common practice that lasted into the 1840s, when the industry declined.[107] There are no records from this period of influenza, or any other respiratory diseases, affecting the Aboriginal people who came into contact with the sealers (and perhaps little reason to expect such documentary evidence, as many of the sealers were illiterate and those who did leave diaries were more concerned with the commercial aspects of the industry, with had little concern about the health of Aboriginal people). Nevertheless, the means and opportunity of passing on influenza did exist with contact between the Ngarrindjeri and the sealing ships (such as the previously discussed likelihood of venereal disease being introduced to the Ngarrindjeri this way).

The pandemics and epidemics of influenza occurring among the European colonies of south-eastern Australia were largely paralleled among Aboriginal communities. Table 7.5 shows the temporal relationship of periods of excessive morbidity and mortality from influenza and secondary respiratory infections among Aboriginal communities, and their relationship with world pandemics and localised epidemics among the European population. The six influenza pandemics of the 19th century that reached Australia all had an effect on the Aboriginal communities of south-eastern Australia. Preceding the first pandemic and following the second and fifth were four localised epidemics that spread through the European communities and into the Aboriginal communities. This table does not, however, detail the full extent of influenza throughout the Aboriginal communities in each of the colonies. There can be few doubts that many of the outbreaks either went unrecorded or those recorded events have not survived or are not included in historical archives. Nevertheless, what evidence is available shows a strong correlation between pandemics of influenza and outbreaks among Aboriginal communities.

The morbidity pattern of respiratory disease changed, from the initial epidemics of influenza and pneumonia, with few infections between epidemic periods, to a background of infection, particularly in sedentary populations, interspersed with epidemics affecting both the Aboriginal and European populations.

The history and pattern of epidemics of influenza in Australia has paralleled that of the northern hemisphere for both the European and Aboriginal populations. However, documentation of the severity of influenza among Aboriginal populations for most of the pandemics that reached Australia in the 19th century is missing, and little more can be said about them other than that the morbidity and mortality was severe in each case, and probably equal to, or more than, that among the non-Aboriginal population. The epidemics of 1839 and 1847 were notably severe, particularly in 1839 among the Tasmanians incarcerated on Flinders Island and among the populations in southern and central Victoria.

Table 7.5. Evidence of influenza epidemics among Aboriginal populations in south-eastern Australia showing their relationship to pandemics and localised epidemics.

Year	Pandemic or Epidemic	Colony or Region	Remarks
1820	Localised epidemic	New South Wales	Probable high morbidity and mortality
1826	Localised epidemic	New South Wales	Effect unknown
1831	Pandemic	Gun Carriage Is., Tasmania	
1836–38	Pandemic	Victoria; Flinders Is., Tasmania	High morbidity and mortality; acute respiratory diseases common on Flinders Is.
1845	Localised epidemic	Victoria; South Australia?	High morbidity and mortality; acute respiratory diseases becoming established
1847	Pandemic	Flinders Is., Oyster Cove, Tasmania	High morbidity and mortality
1852	Pandemic	Victoria; South Australia	High morbidity and mortality
1860	Pandemic	Oyster Cove, Tasmania; South Australia	High morbidity and mortality
1870	Localised epidemic	Northern South Australia	High morbidity and mortality
1874–76	Pandemic	Northern South Australia	High morbidity and mortality
1890–91	Pandemic	Northern South Australia	High morbidity and mortality

Source: Peter J. Dowling, '"A Great Deal of Sickness". Introduced Diseases Among the Aboriginal People of Colonial Southeast Australia 1788-1900', PhD thesis, Australian National University, 1997, p. 217, https://openresearch-repository.anu.edu.au/handle/1885/7529 (accessed 16 December 2020).

The documentary evidence reveals that Aboriginal populations suffered excessive morbidity and mortality when initially exposed to the influenza virus. The changing style of life in residential communities, such as the large gatherings in Melbourne and Adelaide, and the incarceration of Tasmanians on Flinders Island and at Oyster Cove, favoured the spread of respiratory diseases. Infection rates by the influenza virus increased and facilitated a rapid build-up of case-to-case transmission, which resulted in explosive epidemics and a persistence of the virus between major outbreaks.

By the 1850s the pattern of acute respiratory disease, particularly influenza and pneumonia as endemic diseases, had become established in the Aboriginal populations of south-eastern Australia. The diseases were regularly reported by medical and non-medical observers between the pandemic periods. While there were epidemic years with excessive morbidity and mortality, influenza and secondary respiratory complications became ever present. It would probably be correct to state that every year, since its first introduction into Aboriginal populations, could be termed an influenza year.

Compared with the south-east of Australia, knowledge of the course of influenza and respiratory disease in other areas is less well known. For example, knowledge of the disease in Queensland and the far north of the continent during much of the 19th century is sparse. This is not a consequence of its absence but simply that there were few European observers to record its presence. Queensland was first settled in the 1820s, with the establishment of the Moreton Bay colony and subsequently Brisbane, but it was not until the 1840s and into the 1860s that European pastoral settlements expanded further north and into the interior. Further north, on Cape York Peninsula, rugged terrain and Aboriginal resistance discouraged settlement into the 1860s.[108] In the west of the country, the whaling port of Albany was established in 1826 but the first significant establishment was the Swan River settlement (Perth) in 1829. The harsh and arid conditions of the interior to the east and north hampered pastoral expansion and population growth until the discoveries of gold in the 1880s.

The highly contagious nature of the disease and a period of communicability ranging from three to seven days makes influenza an efficient traveller among humans moving from one place to another. There is then a high chance that it accompanied the many Aboriginal people moving around their country and through the extensive trade routes that criss-crossed the continent. In 1915 two medical specialists, Dr A. Breinl, from the Australian Institute of Tropical Medicine, and Dr M. J. Holmes, the chief health officer from Darwin, embarked on a medical survey of Aboriginal groups in northern

Australia. They began south of Darwin at Daly River, on to Anson Bay, further westward as far as Cape Ford, then to Melville and Bathurst islands, and finally back to the mainland to the Alligator River and the Aboriginal community at Oenpelli (Gunbalanya) in West Arnhem Land. The two doctors recorded the health and disease states of the Aboriginal groups they met and conducted clinics in each place. The Aboriginal groups they saw were largely still living in their traditional lands and practising their cultural economy but had contact with European settlements. In summing up the health of the Aboriginal communities, they reported:

> Of cosmopolitan diseases, bronchitis, influenza and colds are common, causing a great deal of sickness.[109]

Daisy Bates, a welfare worker and anthropologist, spent many years among the Aboriginal communities in the north-west and south-west of Western Australia and on the edge of the arid Nullarbor Plain in South Australia's Great Australian Bight. In 1918 she set up a residence at Ooldea, a permanent waterhole on the route of the Trans-Australian Railway and encouraged the Aboriginal desert tribes to gather there. She recorded:

> News travels quickly by smoke signal, and soon my old Bight and Eucla and Fowler's Bay natives were arriving to sit down with me again. An epidemic of influenza broke out …[110]

The 1918–19 influenza pandemic was the worst the world had experienced, its tentacles reaching into the sparsely populated desert regions of southern Australia, infecting even the small groups of Aboriginal people gathered at Ooldea. It marked a final phase of the great world traveller, together with its partner pneumonia, into the Aboriginal communities across the continent. It remains firmly entrenched today.

Coda: A Reading from 1861

In March 1861, an anonymous person, signing off as 'CKH', wrote to the editor of the *South Australian Weekly Chronicle*, concerned about the poor state of health among Aboriginal people living along the Coorong on the southern coast of South Australia:

> Sir– May I, through the medium of your Open Column, draw the attention of the public to the condition of the aborigines in the neighbourhood of the Coorong? During last winter a great many died

> from the influenza, generally brought on from being warmly clad one day and being in a state of nudity the next; in many cases gambling being the somewhat uncertain medium which regulates their supply of clothing. As a remedy I would suggest that warm woollen shirts and trousers should be dealt out to the men, and gowns of the same stuff to the women, at the beginning of every winter, of course due care being taken that each one kept his own, and during the coldest parts of the winter some properly qualified person should be sent round with a supply of medicine and other necessaries. This should be the duty of the Protector, and the name is a perfect anomaly unless he does so. When we are sick we go to bed and send for the doctor, but we never think that the blacks want one sometimes also. Of course, a blackfellow will get proper care taken of him if he goes to Wellington, but as it is impossible for a sick man to go there, why [are they] allowed to perish like so many dogs.[111]

Concerned this person was, and with good cause, but unaware also of the cause of influenza. But so too was everyone in the 19th century, including the medical profession. It was not until the next century that the virus responsible for influenza (and other viruses responsible for influenza-like symptoms) was detected. Yet this letter effectively sums up the feelings and concerns of many of the colonists who had the opportunity to observe firsthand the Aboriginal people living on the fringes of the new settlements. It is typical of many across the colonies at that time who witnessed the poor state of health of Aboriginal people. They revealed compassion for their fellow human beings but a frustration, or guilt, at what they perceived. Often the perception was a pessimistic hopelessness for the future of the Aboriginal people, believing that they would eventually all die out.

But within this letter, as in others written by concerned citizens across the country, is a touch of realism in the treatment of the sick. There was no effective medicinal cure for the influenza sufferer back then and the same can be said today. Because of the very nature of the influenza virus and its ability to genetically change, there is still no drug that can effectively attack and eliminate the pathogen in the long term. Instead, medical laboratories around the world produce drugs that are specific to particular strains of the influenza virus and are at best incompletely effective. 'CKH' advocates warm clothing in winter, each person having their own and not sharing (presumably to stop the spread of the disease), personal care and bed rest. All would assist in surviving an influenza attack. Even today, this is what patients are advised by doctors when presenting with symptoms consistent with influenza (an antibiotic may also be prescribed to protect against bacterial pneumonia). But it would be bed rest, warmth and fluids (and of course the human immune system) that would most often do the trick. If these simple measures had been available to the Aboriginal people of the Coorong and elsewhere across the country, then perhaps the mortality from influenza and respiratory infections would not have been so severe.

Part 4

The Lived Experience: Communities Then and Now

Chapter 8

DISEASE IN ABORIGINAL SETTLEMENTS, VICTORIA AND SOUTH AUSTRALIA

The focus of the previous chapters has been the major epidemics that swept through the Aboriginal populations following the arrival of European colonisation. Much of that examined occurred either well beyond the established colonial boundaries, such as the smallpox epidemics and the state of disease observed by Charles Sturt along the Murray River in 1830, or on the fringes of established colonial settlements and influence, such as tuberculosis and to some extent influenza and measles. It is now time to look more closely at the diseases that caused high mortality after the initial periods of contact, by examining those causes for a group of Aboriginal settlements in Victoria and South Australia. To this end, I use the records of births and deaths kept by each of the settlements, but with an appreciation of the historical context of the Aboriginal settlements as they were in the 19th century.

Beginning around the mid-19th century and extending well into the next, colonial governments across Australia developed legislative processes that were aimed at the institutionalisation and management (or 'protection' as it was often termed) of the declining Aboriginal populations in their jurisdictions. Following Federation of the Australian colonies under the Commonwealth Government, the former colonies, now states, largely carried on with their Aboriginal policies of control but slowly gave way, step by step, to self-management by Aboriginal bodies as the century progressed. But it was a slow process and is, in some cases, still a work in progress.

Settlements were established across the continent with Aboriginal people (often from differing socio-cultural groups) encouraged or enforced to join and to live in semi-isolation from the Europeans. Settlements were established by governments or by religious and missionary groups. Officially, containment on the settlements was a means of protecting Aboriginal people from elements of the European population, educating them in a more European way of life and, for the religious organisations, converting them to Christianity and its values. For many Aboriginal people it meant loss of their traditional land, their country and their cultural being. For others it meant survival. I do not wish to analyse the political good and bad of these policies; they have been minutely discussed and examined by observers and historians almost since they commenced and are still the subject of many a research thesis by emerging historians. The subject of this chapter is still the main diseases that caused exceptional morbidity and mortality for Aboriginal people living in European-controlled settlements.

To achieve this I use the results of research I undertook in a previous study of disease mortality in Aboriginal settlements in the 19th century.[1] Specifically I look at the Victorian settlements of Coranderrk, Framlingham, Lake Condah, Lake Wellington (Ramahyuck), Lake Tyers and Lake Hindmarsh, and the South Australian settlements of Point McLeay (Raukkan) and Point Pearce. It is these settlements for which records of births, deaths and, in many cases, causes of death were recorded by the authorities responsible. Although in no way complete, and often with uncertain and ambiguous causes of death recorded, these settlement records can give an insight into the morbidity and the diseases most responsible for deaths in the settlements.

I have selected a period of 25 years between 1876 and 1900 to examine these records. This period saw a high proportion of the surviving Aboriginal populations of south-eastern Australia institutionalised in the settlements. In 1876, 46 per cent of the Victorian Aboriginal people enumerated in that year's census data lived on the six settlements selected for examination. By 1901, at the end of the period, the figure had increased to 65 per cent. It is from the beginning of the period of concern that the most accurate official records of Aboriginal births and deaths were kept. Each of the settlements were required by the colonial governments to keep a register of all births, deaths and marriages, together with resident numbers, and to furnish quarterly and annual reports. While there were most likely inaccuracies in the record keeping over the 25 years, they are the best available and deserve to be taken with a degree of rigor.

The proportion of the South Australian Aboriginal population institutionalised during the period is difficult to quantify from the official census records, mainly due to the complications encountered by census officials in reaching and counting Aboriginal populations, particularly in the northern and western arid regions away from the main European towns. In 1875–76 George Taplin, the superintendent of the large Point McLeay settlement, completed a census of Ngarrindjeri people, showing 511 living on the lower Murray River, Lake Alexandrina and Lake Albert and along the Coorong coast. The Point McLeay settlement on Lake Alexandrina had a population of 135, 20 per cent of the Ngarrindjeri people. By 1896, the average population of the settlement and its nearby outstation, 'The Needles', was 234, with few of the Ngarrindjeri living continuously on traditional lands, some returning to the settlement when food from traditional sources became scarce. The Point Pearce settlement on Yorke Peninsula averaged 52 residents, mainly Narangga and Kaurna people. The Aboriginal population on the peninsula was not enumerated in the 1876 census, but a figure of 439 was given for the Western District Pastoral Region. Many of these lived far from the influence of the Point Pearce settlement. By 1890, despite severe depopulation of the Western District, the population of the settlement was still roughly the same, at 56 residents. The number of Aboriginal people living in the colony's northern and eastern pastoral regions was calculated in the 1876 census to be approximately 3500. Distance would have precluded all but a few of these people having contact with the two settlements of Point McLeay and Point Pearce.

Throughout the remainder of the 19th century the colonial governments of Victoria and South Australia maintained their policies of moving Aboriginal people (sometimes by force) onto the settlements and the number living traditional lifestyles was steadily reduced.[2]

The settlements were often established on land not immediately required or wanted by Europeans and out of the way of established European settlements. Although in many cases the land was unsuitable for agriculture, the managing authorities and the colonial governments expected the settlements to become largely self-supporting, efficient in growing crops and grazing sheep and cattle for their own consumption to supplement the government rations, thereby reducing the government's financial commitment.[3] The result was that food shortages were common.

Historian Diane Barwick, researching the missionary-established settlements in Victoria, states that before the food ration was doubled in 1875 the men who were able to work subsisted on five pounds of flour, one pound of sugar and two ounces of tea per week, while others who were unable to work had to do with even less. By the last quarter of the 19th century, traditional game species had become scarce around the settlements and could no longer be relied on as a satisfactory supplement for the inadequate rations. The able-bodied men often had to disperse seasonally to find paid work in order to buy food, as well as providing capital for the development of their settlement. Barwick described the meat ration provided to the Aboriginal people in the government settlement of Coranderrk as meagre, often of poor quality and always causing discontent among the residents.

> … from 1871 'regular workers' were allotted one pound of meat per day and other men half that amount. From 1875 to 1877 all adults were entitled to six pounds per week with half rations for children, but for the next five years the Board expected residents to purchase meat, increasing wages on a sliding scale according to numbers of dependents, and gave rations only to the aged and ill.[4]

This economic measure imposed by the settlement supervisors was the cause of real hardship for the residents, reducing their ability to purchase other necessities.

Although living conditions varied between the settlements and, over the time of their operation, funding by the responsible missionary bodies and government agencies was almost always inadequate, failing to maintain long-term satisfactory housing and conditions. Some Aboriginal families had huts or cottages. They were often of one or two rooms and, while adequate for a childless couple, they were often inadequate when family size increased with surviving children or when needed for accommodation of extended family groups. The Aboriginal occupants were frequently required to meet the costs of maintenance themselves and, with limited financial resources, maintenance was often neglected. Not all those who lived on settlements had huts or cottages. Children often slept and ate communally in classrooms and dormitories. Single males and females were often required to sleep in segregated dormitories. Even by 1876, despite the passing of several years after their establishment, some settlements could only offer bark shelters that the Aboriginal people constructed themselves.

In 1876, towards the end of his 25 years as the chief medical officer of Victoria, William McCrea paid a visit to the Coranderrk settlement. He was far from impressed by what he saw of the living conditions.

> The huts of the natives are built on a street which runs nearly north and south across the face of the slope, instead of up and down it, the natural advantage of the fall of the ground for drainage being thus lost … The construction of the huts is, in a sanitary point of view, the worst possible; the walls are of slab, paling, or bark, mostly the latter, with openings in them so numerous that they may fitly be compared to bird cages. The roofs are almost always bark, with openings nearly as numerous as in the walls; some of the natives have endeavoured by paper and bags to

> cover the chinks and openings in the walls and roofs, but in most cases with little effect. The floors are of clay, and are damp even at this the driest season of the year, whilst in the winter the natives complain that the water rises to the surface of the floors after every shower of rain. In wretched hovels like these it is no wonder the mortality is excessive.[5]

The sanitary and human waste disposal facilities on the settlement were reported to be little better:

> There are few closets of a common description, covering mere holes in the ground, scattered about irregularly over the establishment, insufficient in number for the wants and decency of the population [approximately 150]. Even these are not always used, the Superintendent stating that at night the children and some of the adults pass their excrement in the water channels in the street opposite their huts.[6]

Few, if any, of the settlements had a resident doctor and medical needs were met by either the superintendent or local medical practitioners who were called on to attend ill Aboriginal people. Lack of money often severely reduced the number of times doctors were called to the settlements. Phillip Pepper, a descendant of one resident, Nathaniel Pepper, writing his family's history, centred on the Lake Wellington and Lake Tyers settlements:

> Once the reserves were established it became obvious that doctors would have to be called in and the managers were authorised to seek medical assistance if required. Over the years their accounts were often questioned, and the managers were told to find out from the doctors exactly what services they had rendered. As a result, some doctors reduced their fees and many did not charge for visits.[7]

Despite the willingness of some doctors to forego full fees for their attendance, the Aboriginal Protection Board of Victoria saw the cost of medical assistance as too high. In 1886 they advised settlement managers that they could not call a doctor without due authority, unless the patient, in their opinion, was going to die.[8] The result was that the limited medical care made available to Aboriginal inhabitants could not meet their increasing health needs. Alcohol and tobacco consumption was high throughout the settlements, adding further to the health hazards faced by the Aboriginal people.

While these conditions may be considered extreme, they were common throughout the settlements in various degrees of severity for much of the last quarter of the 19th century. The Aboriginal settlements across south-eastern

Australia during the 19th century can be summed up as being small (except for Point McLeay in South Australia), and located on infertile and often badly drained land. The houses or living quarters were generally poorly constructed, often cold and damp in winter and hot and dusty in summer. Few services were provided, resulting in no or inadequate fresh water availability to the houses and poor sanitation throughout. The people living in the settlements had poor diets and little access to professional or even basic medical care. In attempts to convert the Aboriginal people to Christianity on the settlements traditional cultural practices were actively discouraged by settlement superintendents. The erosion of long-existing social structures by frequent deaths and the mixing of different socio-linguistic groups within the confines of the settlements caused further anxiety to many residents.[9] Against this backdrop were infectious diseases, ever present and persistent in the mortality they caused.

In this study I began looking for the major causes of morbidity from infectious diseases and the major causes of death from the records of the Aboriginal settlements. I extracted the sex, age at death and the recorded cause of death during the period 1876–1900 for each of the eight settlements. This was not as straightforward as it might seem. It was often the case that the sex of the individual was unrecorded. When this occurred, gender could sometimes be determined by the European name given. (In order to maintain the sensitivity of the individuals, no names were extracted with the data.) If no name or an Aboriginal name only was recorded, the sex of the individual had to remain undetermined. In the entries where age at death was not recorded, attempts were made to trace the individual back through the register of births. This proved difficult for several reasons. Many deaths with no recorded age also had no recorded names, making a check of birth impossible. European names were sometime untraceable because the same name was given to more than one child. Finally, many of those who had their deaths recorded did not have their births recorded. This happened when an individual was born out of the settlement system but later came to live in one of the settlements. Despite these inherent problems in the registers, they did reveal a substantial amount of useful information. During the period of concern, a total of 714 deaths was recorded across the eight establishments. Of those, sex, age at death and cause of death could be determined for 634 (88.5 per cent).

A further problem arose for the cause of death. While many of the deaths could be ascribed to a particular disease state given in the records, others were ambiguous due to the use of vague terminology, common at the time for all, not just Aboriginal people. In order to overcome this added problem and to determine (as best as could be done) the cause of death I used a contemporary index of disease names (nosological index), which was in common use at that time.[10] For example, when coming across the term 'phthisis' or 'consumption', the cause of death using the nosological index was ascribed to tuberculosis infection. In other cases, however, the recorded cause of death was given as 'senility', 'general decay' and 'old age' and could therefore not be ascribed to a particular infectious disease. Likewise, causes of death such as 'weakly child', 'general debility' and 'decline' could not be determined. But, rather than throw out these ambiguities (after all they relate to people and their personal suffering), an 'ill-defined' category was created. In all, 121 (19 per cent) of all causes of death had to be ascribed to the ill-defined category, making it statistically the third highest cause of death. Having sieved my way through all the causes of death and putting the ill-defined group aside, I used a modern category of disease nomenclature, the *International Statistical Classification of Diseases and Related Health Problems* (or ICD for short) to broadly classify the causes of death into groups (respiratory, infectious, diseases of the circulatory system, diseases of digestive system, neoplastic diseases etc). The ICD is used as the international standard diagnostic tool for epidemiology.

A word of caution. These are historical death statistics here, relying on the recorded identification of causes made more than one hundred years ago. Formal diagnosis using modern medical technology and microbiology cannot be applied to definitively ascribe a particular disease as the cause of death. That is often the nature of historical data. But, by being cautious and willing to sacrifice data to an 'ill-defined' category, an acceptable degree of confidence can be achieved, doing what can be done with the data available – weeding out the obvious uncertainties and going with the most certain.

Now that the required information – sex, age, cause of death – had been extracted from the settlements' records, I wanted to know if there were any differences in the causes of death between the settlements before I began to examine them as a whole set. The reason for this was that not all the settlements had complete records for the 1876–1900 period. For example, Framlingham had records from 1876 to 1883, Point McLeay from 1876 to 1883, then from 1888 to 1900, and Point Pearce from 1880 to 1900. The other settlements had a continuous record between 1876 and 1900.

But by now there clearly needed to be some balance in the data sets. To achieve some comparative sense with this seemingly hotchpotch of information I turned to a multivariate statistical technique called 'correspondence analysis', sometimes referred to as reciprocal averaging. Correspondence analysis is particularly suited to the analysis of tables expressed in raw counts (in this case the number of times each disease group was reported as a cause of death) where some of the objects (settlements) have a greater abundance than others. For the non-mathematician (yours truly) it is a detailed yet elegant means of comparing data coming from such variable origins like the Aboriginal settlement records. Lucky for me it came in the form of a digital package. I just entered all the data into a table on my computer and pressed the go button.

The result was somewhat as I expected. Six of the ICD groups actuating to cause of death – respiratory diseases, infectious diseases, neoplasms, nervous disorders, circulatory disorders and injuries were the common causes of death across the settlements. Of these, respiratory diseases and infectious diseases were the most common. Less common across the settlements were digestive, endocrine, perinatal, pregnancy and genitourinary system disorders. I suspect that one of the reasons this latter group of reported mortality causes was less common was because of the problems with diagnosis of cause of death by the recorders. This is an inherent problem when analysing causes of death from historic records. In many cases who determined the cause of death is unknown – whether it was a medical practitioner familiar with the signs and symptoms or a non-medically trained recorder. I also suspect that many of the causes ascribed to the 'ill-defined' category would include this less common group. Having cleared that up, I now look more closely at the common causes of death.

Tuberculosis, in all its forms, was the main cause of death throughout the eight settlements examined. It accounted for 20 per cent of all deaths recorded. It was particularly severe in children up to the age of 15 years, much more so in young females. This high mortality in young females may be a result of their suspected increased susceptibility to the development of life-threatening symptoms of the disease during the onset of menarche and/or an increased period of exposure to other sufferers. There was no gender difference in mortality from tuberculosis in the adults throughout the settlements but alarmingly most of the deaths occurred before the age of 35 years. Given that tuberculosis infection can lead to either an early onset of severe symptoms and death or linger for several years causing frequent disability and a lifetime of ill health, the suffering among the Aboriginal people cannot be understated. While the statistical evidence shows a seriously high cause of mortality, the number of sufferers would have been much higher. A burden of chronic tuberculosis would have weakened the immune system and in many cases led to serious secondary infections that were then recorded as a cause of death. There can be little doubt that tuberculosis was indeed a killer.

Diarrhoea and dysentery were major causes of death in infants up to four years of age, with most under two years of age. These two causes of death were often recorded synonymously, referring to the symptoms observed. Diarrhoea is a condition that involves the frequent passing of loose or watery stools, while dysentery is an intestinal inflammation, especially in the colon, that can lead to severe diarrhoea with mucus or blood in the faeces. Dysentery can be caused by an amoebic parasite living in the large bowel or by bacterial invasion, commonly by *Escherichia coli* or *Salmonella* species. Crowded living conditions and poor hygiene and sanitation increase the risk of dysentery by spreading the parasite or the bacteria through contaminated water or food. Again, the picture emerges of diarrhoea and dysentery being common causes of ill health leading to death in many cases across the settlements.

Bronchitis and whooping cough were the main respiratory diseases. The conditions were more prominent in young children. Bronchitis deaths showed a typical pattern of high mortality during the first two years of life, levelling off during later childhood and early adulthood, then climbing to high frequencies after 45 years of age. Predisposing factors for acute and life-threatening symptoms for the early ages would include the unfavourable socio-economic circumstances and poor nutrition of most Aboriginal people on the settlements. A further predisposing factor would have been the dwellings, often being dusty in summer and damp during winter. Passive tobacco smoke inhalation would have been common among newborn and young Aboriginal children, further promoting the onset of bronchitis. A sharp increase in deaths from bronchitis occurred after 45 years of age. This trend was quite likely to have been a result of chronic bronchitis due to many years of smoking.

Pneumonia and the generalised 'inflammation of the lungs' caused deaths in all age ranges across the settlements but showed a pattern of increasing mortality after 15 years of age. Pneumonia as a recorded cause of death was most probably a secondary complication of other disorders, particularly influenza infections aggravated by chronic tobacco smoke inhalation and alcohol consumption, both of which were common in the settlements. The European colonists smoked a lot of tobacco, often seeing it as a necessity of the hard life in the colonies rather than as a luxury. Contact with Europeans introduced Aboriginal people to tobacco and smoking quickly became a particularly common practice among most communities. A currency of addiction was created from tobacco. The colonial governments provided Aboriginal people with regular weekly or monthly rations of tobacco, often giving extra proportions to the elderly or sick. The substance was further bartered or bought from European traders. Pastoralists often used tobacco rather than money as an enticement to Aboriginal people to work for them.

Tobacco was easily obtained in the settlements and addiction was widespread among both males and females. It took the place of indigenous narcotics such as pituri (*Duboisia hopwoodi*), which in the past had been traded through the extensive exchange networks by now largely no longer in place. In the Lake Tyers settlement in 1878, 60 people (many of them elderly women) out of just over 100 residents were addicted to tobacco. The manager of the settlement, Reverend J. Bulmer, allowed a three-monthly ration of 14kg a month for the whole settlement, which he rationed out at no more than two 'figs' per week. He could not get them to abstain from smoking tobacco, which was seen by many Aboriginal people as the only drug in the British pharmacopoeia that was of any use. Opium, when obtainable, was also smoked by some.[11]

Surprisingly, measles, which caused severe mortality when in epidemic form, particularly in 1875, was relatively low. There are two likely reasons for this. The first is that the Aboriginal people living in the settlements were to a certain extent isolated from the European population and were shielded from the measles outbreaks that occurred. The second is that many of them had contracted the disease previously, were lucky enough to survive and therefore had built up an immunity. Whatever the reason, measles would appear to be a minor cause of death after the 1875 epidemic.

Another surprise in the 'infectious disease' category was the relatively high presence of hydatids recorded as a cause of death. Hydatids disease is caused by infection from a small tapeworm (*Echinococcus granulosus*) generally passed between sheep and dogs. Human infection is caused when a sheep infected with the worm is consumed. In an attempt to be self-sufficient, to generate income and to educate the Aboriginal occupants into animal farming, sheep were kept on the settlements. Along with the ever-present settlement dogs often feeding on infected sheep carcasses, cross-infection between the natural hosts of sheep or dog and humans would have been common.

Several other recorded causes of death could not be specifically clarified to a specific infection – 'liver disorders', 'bowel disorders', 'chronic disease of stomach' and 'gastric fever'. It is difficult to make any substantial statement regarding these diseases other than to say they were often given as a cause of death. Liver disorders included 'cirrhosis of the liver',' liver enlargement', 'liver inflammation', 'tumefied liver' and 'liver complaint'. Although the liver is vulnerable to a wide range of metabolic, circulatory, toxic, microbial and neoplastic insults, the recorded cases, together with one cause of death recorded as 'hepatitis', may suggest the presence of acute hepatitis. Hepatitis (infection of the hepatic system) has been recognised by medical practitioners and observers for millennia and was usually associated with jaundice. However, the term 'jaundice' does not appear in the Aboriginal mortality records from the eight settlements examined. The reason for this may be that the condition, a yellowing tint to the skin, was less visible in darker skinned people. Acute hepatitis usually causes inflammation and necrosis of the liver, to which the above terms may apply. If so, then the disease may well have been hepatitis A. Hepatitis A is spread from person to person by the faecal–oral route, usually by oral ingestion of contaminated water or food supplies. With the poor sanitation and hygiene conditions on the Aboriginal settlements, hepatitis A would most likely be the common form of the disease and the culprit for the 'liver disorder' causes of death.

Less frequently recorded causes of death were those affecting the digestive, nervous and circulatory systems, along with perinatal conditions, neoplasms, complications of pregnancy, diseases of the genitourinary system, injuries and poisoning. No reliable epidemiological inferences can be drawn from these causes other than to note their presence among the Aboriginal people in the settlements. Disorders of the digestive system accounted for 41 deaths recorded. This grouping included abnormal conditions of the mouth, stomach, peritoneum and bowels. Hydrocephalus, meningitis and 'convulsions and fits' accounted for a further 38 causes of death, the latter most likely from any number of underlying causes.

Fifteen cases of marasmus were reported: five from the Lake Hindmarsh settlement and ten from Point McLeay. Marasmus is a form of severe malnutrition, occurring mainly in children who, for a variety of reasons, do not ingest enough protein, calories, carbohydrates and other essential nutrients in their food. All but one case, a 64-year-old female, were of children under 9 years of age. There is a causal link between chronic diarrhoea and marasmus, but it is unclear what the underlying factors on the two settlements were. However, the recording of marasmus on just two settlements is possibly due to the different diagnosis or recording practice rather than a differential occurrence with the other settlements.

Although syphilis and other sexually transmitted diseases were major causes of disease among Aboriginal people following contact, just one case was recorded in all the 714 deaths between 1876 and 1900. This was a case identified as congenital syphilis in a child. The lack of any mention of syphilis as a cause of death across the settlements is in one way no surprise. Syphilis, although present in the European, Asiatic and Aboriginal communities, was a condition embodied with revulsion, horror, guilt and often silence in general society. It was a disease that no-one wanted to admit to having. In the case of the settlement mangers, there existed a determined reluctance to admit to its presence in the official records, particularly as a cause leading to the deaths of the inmates in their charge. But I am quite sure that it was just as prevalent among the Aboriginal people of the settlements as it was in non-Aboriginal communities. Syphilis, particularly in the tertiary stage, can affect almost all the vital organs and nervous system. It is a disease of many faces and a great imitator of a wide range of other pathogenic conditions. I also have little doubt that many of the official causes of death noted in the settlement records had an underlying cause of syphilis infection.

Also of note was the absence in the mortality records of smallpox and measles, both of which were major epidemic diseases. By the beginning of the time period, in 1876, outbreaks of smallpox had largely been brought under control through quarantine restrictions by the colonial authorities, although there were several minor localised outbreaks, mainly associated with shipping arrivals, and larger outbreaks in the southern colonies in the 1880s.[12] It would appear that the Aboriginal people in the settlements were protected from these outbreaks. After the 1875 epidemic of measles, which caused excessive morbidity and mortality among Aboriginal people, the disease was no longer a problem. Outbreaks occurred among the populations of New South Wales, Victoria and South Australia in the 1880s and 1890s but had little effect on the Aboriginal settlements.[13]

Scarlet fever (scarlatina) was another disease that appears to have been largely absent on the settlements. Two deaths were reported, one in a 45-year-old (sex not recorded) and the other in a two-year-old female. The low frequency of recorded deaths from this disease reflects the general pattern in the population of south-eastern Australia for the period. In both Victoria and South Australia scarlet fever had its highest recorded death rate in 1876 and throughout the remainder of the century it was in a steady decline, with localised epidemic occurrences. While it may have entered the settlements and caused some morbidity, the disease was never a major cause of death.

Having identified the causes of death on the settlements, I wanted to get an idea of the overall health of the Aboriginal residents during the period. Was their state of health the same as the non-Aboriginal population in Victoria and South Australia or was it different? Better, worse or just the same? Examining infant mortality (deaths in the first year of life) is an accepted way of measuring the health, health services and social progress of a population. This is largely because the baby, in its first year of life, is at a critical stage of disease risk and is entirely dependent on the care of others, and their ability to provide a healthy and safe environment. It follows that the measurement of death during this period of life will be an assessment of the general health state of the community concerned. The statistics I had for Aboriginal people were from the records of births and deaths taken on the settlements and, while they were incomplete and subject to the vagaries of the recorders as to the cause of death, for the most part the age at death was recorded. So it was then a matter of extracting the number of deaths in the first year of life for the period and comparing them with the live births for the same period. This would give the infant mortality ratio (IMR) for the settlements in deaths per thousand.

$$\text{IMR} = \frac{\text{Deaths under age one for period}}{\text{Live births during period}} \text{ X } 1000$$

The next step was to do the same for the non-Aboriginal populations in the same regions and for the same period using the vital statistics kept by the colonial governments. I should say here that, while the colonial statisticians kept records of births and deaths for the European populations, they did not do so for the Aboriginal populations so the records from the Aboriginal settlements had to be relied on. Another concern with this method is that using an IMR as a measure of overall health has limitations in that it assumes that the period of greatest danger for children is only the first year of life and that it is the same for each population concerned.

This may not have been the case for the Aboriginal and European populations being compared. I suspect that the greatest danger of death for Aboriginal infants may have extended further than the first year when compared with the Europeans, so any figure coming from a comparative IMR should be viewed with this in mind.

The IMR for the Aboriginal people of the settlements was calculated at 184 deaths per thousand compared with the non-Aboriginal population (mainly of European descent) at 119 deaths per thousand. Comparing the two groups, the IMR reveals that 65 more Aboriginal infant deaths occurred for every one thousand births than for the non-Aboriginal population. Looking further afield at other communities, for example, 17th-century London (IMR 185), 19th-century Prussia (IMR 220–230), Irian Jaya before 1920 (IMR 202) and mid-20th-century Papua New Guinea islands (IMR 189), the Aboriginal IMR is not especially high, comparatively speaking.

The IMRs indicate that Aboriginal people living in the settlements were less healthy than the non-Aboriginal Victorians and South Australians but healthier than say the Irian Jaya communities then under Dutch colonial rule. The infants and children of Irian Jaya and New Guinea had to cope with similar introduced diseases but had the added risk of a high infection rate from naturally occurring malaria. Malaria was not a disease of the Aboriginal settlements.[14]

The high infant mortality among the Aboriginal children is not fully explainable without comprehensive health records of the individuals living in the settlements. These just do not exist in a form that would allow even rudimentary assessment of health. So that must be accepted. But, putting the diseases aside for the moment, among the prime contenders for the higher mortality, and by nature morbidity, into early childhood is a combination of malnutrition and diarrhoea commonly reported. Most of the diarrhoea and dysentery recorded as a cause of death in the first two years of life on the settlements possibly occurred during the weaning period of the Aboriginal children. A trend showing substantial mortality in the first year of life and extending into the early childhood years is demonstrative of the weaning process taking place in an undernourished environment. Little, however, is known about weaning practices on the settlements. There is little evidence available to indicate at what ages children were weaned, how this may have differed over time or between settlements, how much influence the European supervisors and medical practitioners had in the process and what cultural beliefs were involved. But, whatever the case, the Aboriginal children living in the settlements were subjected to an extended period of health risk that was largely, if not wholely, due to poorer nutrition, poorer living standards and less resilience to infectious disease. Whichever way it is examined, there is a substantial difference between the health status of the Aboriginal people of the settlements and the populations of colonial Victoria and South Australia during the 25-year period.

Coda: Examining the Infant Mortality Rate, Then and Now

This chapter has allowed an insight into the health of Aboriginal people living in the selected settlements in colonial Victoria and South Australia between 1876 and 1900. A health gap was assessed by infant mortality between the mainly European population of the two colonies and the Aboriginal people of the settlements. We can look at this health gap a little more closely by doing one more simple calculation. A differential rate ratio can be obtained between the infant mortality rates of the two populations by dividing the Aboriginal infant mortality by the non-Aboriginal infant mortality:

$$\frac{\text{Aboriginal infant mortality}}{\text{Non-Aboriginal infant mortality}}$$

The figure obtained represents the difference or gap in the overall health status between the two groups. The higher the figure, the larger the gap.

The Aboriginal infant mortality calculated for the period 1876 to 1900 was 184 per 1000 births and for the non-Indigenous populations 118 per 1000 births over the same period. The calculation for the differential rate ratio produces a figure of 1.5. A differential rate ratio of 1.5 means that Aboriginal infant mortality was half as much again as that of the non-Aboriginal population. Looking at the corresponding infant mortalities between the two communities today, after more than 100 years, produces an interesting comparison.

In 2018 the IMR for Aboriginal people across Australia was 6.6 for males and 5.8 for females per 1000 births. For the non-Aboriginal people, the IMR was 3.4 for males and 2.9 for females.[15] We can see immediately that there has been a significant improvement in the two figures, which relates to a far better health status for both. That is the good news. The bad news is that the corresponding differential rate ratios – the health gap between the two – produces a different picture. The differential rate ratio between the two is now 1.9 for males and 2.0 for females. That is higher today than it was more than 100 years ago. Now, I know that there are discrepancies in the data sets and the comparison of the two ratios. One set is taken over a period of 25 years, from non-official data sources in settlements in two colonies and does not separate males from females. The 2018 data set is taken nationwide from people who identify themselves as Indigenous, may live on dedicated settlements or elsewhere, separates males from females and forms a data set that is more rigorous. But looking at the two data sets is not comparing chalk and cheese or apples with oranges. It is the enumeration of infant deaths in the two data sets using very unsophisticated methods of analysis. But it is not rubbish statistics in, rubbish results out. Both sets of data and the derived ratios relate directly to two separate ethnic groups living at the same times and in the same country.

The reality is that, although the health status of each population has improved very significantly over the intervening decades, the health gap between the two has not improved. Putting just some reliability on the figures, then it seems that the gap has widened. This is despite the many attempts by state and Commonwealth governments to improve the health status of

Aboriginal people to equal that of the rest of the population of Australia. Aboriginal people were the least healthy population sector in Australia during the last 25 years of the 19th century and they still are today as we enter into the third decade of the 21st century.

Chapter 9

A PERSONAL UNDERSTANDING

On January 12th 1836, a young Charles Darwin stepped ashore in Sydney. He was on the homeward leg of that wonderful voyage aboard HMS *Beagle* that was to inspire him and ultimately change the way we consider the planet's biology and the role of humans in the great web of life he succinctly explained. Four days later, in the summer heat, he set off on an expedition to explore inland to Bathurst. On the way he was fascinated with the strangeness of the animals he saw and was able to observe, strangest of all, the platypus. On the Aboriginal people he commented:

> Wherever the European has trod, death seems to pursue the aboriginal. We may look to the wide extent of the Americas, Polynesia, the Cape of Good Hope, and Australia, and we find the same result.[1]

His next port of call was Hobart, where he made several journeys inland. It was here in Van Diemen's Land that he learned of the fate of the island's Aboriginal populations, their removal from their country, their incarceration at Wybalenna on Flinders Island and the death of many. He wrote again:

> I fear there is no doubt, that this train of evil and its consequences, originated in the infamous conduct of some of our countrymen.[2]

The focus next is on a particular individual, exampling the disease burden that dismayed Darwin and that was faced by many Indigenous people following contact with Europeans. In doing so, a deeper and more personal understanding of the disease load they suffered can be developed.

Truganini: A Biomedical History

Truganini, a Nuenonne woman, was born circa 1812, probably on Bruny Island on the south-east coast of Tasmania. She was one of the better known Tasmanian Aboriginal people of her time and was incorrectly labelled 'the last Tasmanian' in the latter part of her life. Her historical presence is still familiar in today's Tasmania, particularly with a monument to her on Bruny Island and in the capital, Hobart.

Her biographer, Cassandra Pybus, described her:

> She was a lovely young woman, diminutive girl [she stood 130cm or 4 feet 3 inches] and fine-boned, with her hair cut close to her scalp, which emphasised her lively dark eyes and a generous mouth.[3]

Documented history tells us little about her early life other than that she spent her younger years in the traditional lifestyle of her people on the south-east coast of mainland Tasmania and Bruny Island. However, she would have been well aware of the European presence on the coast, with sealers and whalers establishing bases on her lands, and of the European settlement at present-day Hobart established in 1804, before she was born.

At around the age of 16–17 years Truganini experienced the violence, trauma and distress that was to affect her people for years to come. On Bruny Island she witnessed the violent murder by European sealers of her mother and intended husband, and the abduction of her sister (who she never saw again), and was later herself abducted, to be brutally and repeatedly raped. It could have been during this event that Truganini was infected with a venereal disease, most likely syphilis or gonorrhoea. Both these diseases were prolific among the Europeans. Despite many reputed further sexual liaisons with European sealers, whalers, convicts and local timbercutters, as well as her own people throughout her lifetime, Truganini appears to have never conceived and was most likely rendered infertile in the early years of her life.[4] (However, we cannot rule out other conditions producing lifelong infertility.)

In 1829, while living with a gang of convict woodcutters across the channel from Bruny Island, Truganini met George Augustus Robinson. Robinson had come to Bruny Island in the employ of the colonial government to establish what he called 'a Friendly Mission with the Aboriginal people'[5] and to establish a government-controlled Aboriginal settlement on the island. The settlement was a failure, lasting just nine months, mainly due to an epidemic of influenza that resulted in excessive morbidity and mortality among Aboriginal people. It was likely at this time that Truganini was first exposed to influenza. She survived but saw many of her people die, largely from the secondary effects of pneumonia. While living in the settlement Truganini was again exposed to sexually transmitted disease. Robinson recorded in his diary that Truganini and two other women were sick. He recorded them as '... afflicted with a loathsome disorder' (read syphilis) that they had contracted during their cohabitation with the whalers on Bruny Island. Truganini was just 17 years of age. She was to develop a predilection for sexual relations with European convicts and whalers throughout her early life, no matter how violent these relationships may have been. One of her biographers has suggested that her repeated attraction to Europeans could have been a factor of the psychological condition known today as Stockholm syndrome,[6] a psychological response occurring when hostages or victims of abuse bond with their captors over a period of time. This bonding is considered to counteract the initial experience of terror or fear. Whether this was the case with Truganini is, of course, unclear but would go some way to explaining why she repeatedly entered into sexual liaisons with Europeans.

The 1820s had been a period of intense violence (some would say war) between the Tasmanians and the colonists and it was the government's misplaced policy to round up the Tasmanians throughout the main island and settle them in a place offshore, away from the ever-increasing European population. This became the main objective of Robinson in his role as protector and conciliator during the next decade. From 1830 to 1834 he, with Truganini by his side, together with a select group of other Tasmanians and a European escort party were to travel the coastal and inland regions of Tasmania in what were labelled by Robinson as 'Friendly Missions'.[7]

Throughout the next decade, including travelling with the Friendly Missions, Truganini spent a great deal of time far away from the colonial settlements and the constant presence of infectious diseases, alcohol, poor diet and unsanitary living conditions. But to say that she was free from further infectious diseases or the threat of death would not be quite the case. In 1831 during the first of the Friendly Missions, Truganini was exposed to what was recorded by Robinson as 'violent diarrhoea' when 50 of the west coast Tasmanians were rounded up and temporally incarcerated on Gun Carriage Island in eastern Bass Strait. Ten or more were to die and many more were ill. Truganini pleaded with Robinson to take her and the other Tasmanians off the island. The only medical assistance they had was a convict, a ticket-of-leave man, who had been appointed as the medical superintendent. He was unable to alleviate their suffering and was often drunk.[8] Such was the official government's concern for the health of the Tasmanians. It is not known how Truganini fared then, but she was to witness more sickness and death among her people in times to come.

The group, including Truganini, were then moved to Swan Island, where three more died. The medical superintendent claimed the island and the accommodation were unsuitable for the Aboriginal people and requested to find another place. Robinson blamed the ill health of the Tasmanians on the wet and windy conditions of the island. Eventually the whole group was moved to Flinders Island, where a more permanent settlement was established. Truganini's initial stay on Flinders Island was short and, while she suffered a bout of diarrhoea, she escaped falling to a severe epidemic of what was recorded as pneumonia on the settlement in 1832, when 22 deaths were recorded in one year.[9]

Resuming her travels with the Friendly Missions, Truganini twice escaped a violent death. On two occasions in the north-west the mission party came under attack by armed warriors. In one incident Truganini had to protect Robinson by assisting him across the Arthur River clutching a log (Robinson could not swim) and in a second incident she had to swim across the Henty River twice to help some of her own people to the opposite bank in order to avoid being attacked. On both occasions it was either swim across the river, risking being drowned in the cold and fast-flowing waters, or be speared to death. Truganini experienced severe hypothermia following the first rescue. Robinson recorded in his diary, 'That night she had a severe fit', presumably caused by her long immersion in the freezing waters.

> No amount of rum could mitigate the shock to Truganini's exhausted body. That night she had a severe fit. She was seriously ill and still had days to travel through thunderstorms with wind-driven hail like tiny points of glass. The wind gusts were strong.

Robinson wrote that they almost lifted him off his feet, and he was a big man, whereas Truganini was small and slight. The wonder was that the whole experience did not kill her.[10] But she appears to have recovered in the morning and there is no further reference to hypothermia.[11]

Robinson also reported that he and the group, including Truganini, were infected with 'vermin' and a skin rash of pustules covering parts of their skin. This rash appears to have been common and persistent among them. A likely cause was a form of canine scabies. The Tasmanian Aboriginal people had quickly developed a close association with dogs following their introduction to the island and would often sleep next to them.[12]

With Robinson's Friendly Missions completed by 1836, Truganini was to spend most of the next 25 years of her life as an inmate of government-controlled Aboriginal stations, again Wybalenna on Flinders Island and later at Oyster Cove on the Tasmanian mainland (ironically for Truganini her last incarceration was located immediately opposite her homeland of Bruny Island). After spending five months at Wybalenna, Truganini accompanied Robinson's son on a further expedition to the north-west of the main island to bring in a last group of Tarkina people. This expedition away from the settlement, with constant illness on the station, was highly beneficial to Truganini as she returned in particularly good health. While she had been away 19 more of its residents had died.[13]

One interlude away from Tasmania that is worth mentioning is between 1839 and 1842, when Truganini accompanied Robinson to Port Phillip (Melbourne) on the Australian mainland. Robinson by then had been appointed as the Aboriginal chief protector for that colony and had taken a small group of Aboriginal Tasmanians with him. Just prior to leaving for Victoria Truganini contracted a severe case of influenza on Flinders Island during a worldwide pandemic of the disease. She, Robinson and the rest of the group had to spend five days in isolation on their ship at Port Phillip before they were allowed ashore. Once again, leaving the Flinders Island settlement during the epidemic may well have been fortunate for Truganini, as she recovered from the disease. Eight of the Tasmanians who stayed at Wybalenna died within days of her departure from the settlement.[14]

While in Port Phillip, Robinson seems to have had no use for Truganini or the rest – Maulbyheener (Jemmy, or Bob), Peevay (Napoleon, or Jack), Plorenernoopner (Fanny) and Maytepueminer (Matilda). Feeling abandoned in a strange country the two men and three women turned to the crime of bushranging (highway robbery). They ranged though the farm settlements in the Westernport district south-east of Port Phillip. They lived off the land but repeatedly raided the small households for food, guns and ammunition. This ultimately resulted in the killing of two Europeans and led to Truganini and the four other Tasmanians being hunted down and apprehended.[15] In the early hours of the morning of November 20th 1841, while Truganini and her companions were camped, a hunting party of 25 armed men (18 mounted) made up of police, soldiers, civilians and Aboriginal trackers, all firing their weapons, swept down on the sleeping Tasmanians. Police Commissioner Powlett, who led the attack, wrote in his official report:

> On the morning of the 20th, before sunrise, we came upon the fire of the Van Diemen's land natives, so placed that there appeared to be much difficulty in surrounding it. The ground at the back was pretty open but within four yards on one side was a thick tea tree scrub. So I ordered the men, if the natives got into the scrub, to capture them if possible – if not, to shoot them. On our approaching the camping place, the two men Bob and jack [sic] and the women got into the scrub. Several

> shots were fired at jack, and one slightly grazed the woman who was making off. The three women being secured, I surrounded the scrub as well as the number would admit and finding that the natives had left their firearms at the camp, I ordered the men on no account whatever to fire another shot.[16]

One of the attackers was Samuel Rawson an ensign in the 28th Regiment, Port Phillip. During the frenzy of the attack he took deliberate aim at the head of one of the sleeping Tasmanians:

> I extended the men along the top of the hill, and then myself in the centre 6 feet apart, with orders to take them alive if possible but if they offered resistance or to escape to shoot them at once – we advanced down the hill, and were closing in upon them, I was about 6 feet from the fire, and could see them laying down, when a policeman who was on my left, catching a glimpse of a man's head, without orders, fired and missed him, he was rather behind me at the time, that I was not certain from which party the shot came – immediately out rushed dogs and men, the first at us, the latter to the shrub, everybody fired at them as they got a sight at them – I fired both barrels right and left, and I saw one drop. I had 5 pistol balls in in each barrel. I immediately ordered the men to surround the shrub and prevent their escape, and then I went to reconnoitre the camp and find out the state of their larder, as tho' I had ordered the scrub to be surrounded, in case of accidents, yet from the heavy fire opened upon them I concluded they must all be shot – while I was turning over the blankets with the end of my gun, I discovered a woman, I handed her over to a policeman to put handcuffs on her and a little further I discovered another, after they were secured, I put a pistol to their heads and told to call their companions out of the shrub if they were alive, in about a minute out came a woman covered with blood, from a wound in her head, a ball had struck the back of her head and cut the scalp open without injuring the scull, and from the size of the wound, was caused by a small ball and was the one that dropped when I fired.[17]

Despite many shots being fired at the five Tasmanians, all survived. One of the women was wounded, grazed by a shot ball to the back of the head. The wound cut into the scalp without injuring the bone of the skull.[18] Was it Truganini? The accounts are conflicting but, while the wound was minor, the violent attack was yet another potentially fatal incident in the precarious life of Truganini. The two men, Maulbyheener and Peevay, were found guilty and were hanged (the first hangings in Victoria). Truganini, Plorenernoopner and Maytepueminer escaped the gallows and were exiled back to Tasmania.[19]

Wybalenna Period

Following her return from the mainland, Truganini, now 30 years of age, was to spend the next five years on Flinders Island at the Wybalenna Aboriginal settlement. Soon after her arrival she began once again to cohabit with the European sealers based on the island. She would often abscond from the settlement for extended periods and, although 'married' to Tasmanian Alphonso, she appears to have preferred Europeans as sexual partners. The commandant of the station, Dr Henry Jeanneret, reported the presence a of 'loathsome disease' (syphilis) present among the women and it is highly likely that Truganini was among them.

There is little surviving information on the Aboriginal Tasmanians during Truganini's period at Wybalenna. Much of the official reporting from the two superintendents, Dr Jeanneret and Dr Milligan, was about their displeasures with other European staff rather than about the health and wellbeing of the Aboriginal people. When there is mention of their health, the official statements most often give the impression that they were in good health and spirit. However, a statement by an independent visitor to the station stated that 'there seemed to be an air of melancholy depression hanging around everything I saw'.[20]

But looking beyond the official reports from Wybalenna during Truganini's period and using the station's register of births and deaths, it is apparent she was exposed to local outbreaks of whooping cough, which affected all or most of the residents; a 'destructive epidemic of catarrh' (most likely equated to the influenza epidemic accompanied by pneumonia that occurred throughout Australia in 1847); and the continual presence of tuberculosis.[21] Between October 1835, when Truganini began living at Wybalenna, and February 1839, Dr James Allen, the station surgeon, performed 32 autopsies. At least 13, or 35 per cent, of all these autopsy cases involved extensive tuberculosis infection.[22]

The overall morbidity (close to 70 per cent) of the original Tasmanian inmates during the 16 years of the Flinders Island establishment was made worse by their poor diet, living conditions and excessive consumption of alcohol and tobacco. Truganini smoked a pipe for much of her life and was more than a little fond of alcohol. These habits would have made her highly susceptible to the respiratory infections affecting her fellow Tasmanians. But she survived her incarceration on the island despite being regularly exposed to the infections.

Oyster Cove Aboriginal Station

Truganini, along with 48 of the remaining Aboriginal Tasmanians, was removed from Wybalenna and spent the next 15 years at the Oyster Cove Aboriginal settlement on the main island. Ironically, Oyster Cove was within her own country, just a few kilometres from where she had been born. The settlement was established in a former convict settlement, abandoned because it was deemed unfit for health reasons. Nevertheless, it was deemed fit for Aboriginal people. They were forced to live in vermin-ridden, damp huts, cold in winter. Fresh water and traditional food were scarce and government rations, often highly salted, lacked adequate nutrition. Tea, tobacco and flour was standard and alcohol was always available off the settlement.

The mortality records at Oyster Cove are seriously defective – very messy in fact – with little attention given by managing staff to recording deaths or causes. But piecing together what reports were made during its operation there is an overall picture of exceptionally high mortality. Between 1848 and 1851 there appears to be at least 27 deaths – that is 59 per cent who died within the first four years of the settlement. In 1858 a census shows only 14 alive; in 1861 only 8 were alive (2 males and 6 females). In 1867 an outbreak of dysentery killed the remaining females, apart from Truganini, who, while ill herself, again managed to survive.

Nevertheless, despite the paucity of the official records, it was here at Oyster Cove that a more personal picture of Truganini's health emerges, from the official letters of the commandant of Oyster Cove, John Dandridge, to the colonial secretary's office in Hobart and the station visiting officers' book. Dr William Smith, a local surgeon from nearby Kingston (already mentioned in Chapter 7), made irregular records when visiting Oyster Cove regarding the health and treatment of the remaining Aboriginal people.[23] Their records for Truganini reveal the state of her health. In the winter of 1876 Truganini was ill. Dandridge wrote:

> 12 July 1867
> Lallah Rookh [a European name given to Truganini] still continues very weak, and is quite deaf; she is however in a fair way of getting well, but will require the greatest care to pull her through the winter …
>
> 15 August 1867
> Lallah Rookh, I am sorry to say is by no means well and is under medical treatment.

> 22 August 1867
> Lallah Rookh I am happy to say is somewhat better, but is still low and weak…
>
> 24 August 1867
> [Truganini] complaining of cough being troublesome, very low in spirits.

Truganini survived the 1867 winter. There are no records regarding her health for the summer months but in 1868 Dandridge again became concerned for her health. He wrote to the colonial secretary in Hobart:

> Oyster Cove
>
> 23 July 1868
>
> Sir,
>
> I have the honor to report the serious illness of Lallah Rookh an aged Aborigine, and last female of her race.
>
> Finding that she was much troubled by vermin about the body and head, I had her thoroughly washed by Mary-Ann on the 20th Inst. in a bath of warm water, then rubbed upon the worst places with a small quantity of 'blue ointment' [a mercury-based cream commonly used at this time] and dressed in a new and warm set of clothes.
>
> Though cautioned to keep indoors and out of the damp, she took her old clothing to the creek and there I presume got a chill, for on the following morning (the 21st) I found her suffering from congestion of the lungs.
>
> I had her at once put into bed in one of our rooms, applied turpentine strips, croton oil ale with the usual medicines, procured a nurse of 1/- per day, and engaged Mary-Ann's husband to supply cut up firewood at 5/- per ton.
>
> On the following morning (the 22nd) the chest symptoms were much relieved, but seeing approaching salivation [ptyalism] I went to Kingston for Dr Smith who returned with me in the afternoon and whose reports I append.
>
> The salivation reached its worst on the 27th when the glands were much swelled and the inside of her mouth and tongue one mass of ulcerations, causing great pain, inability to speak and almost to swallow.

Since that time the symptoms have gradually abated, but I cannot think she is yet out of danger, though Dr Smith considers his further attendance unnecessary.

The account of the latter I herewith forward for approval and payment, the charges are the same as heretoforth.[24]

Dr Smith had examined Truganini at Oyster Cove and recorded:

22 July 1868
I have visited the station to see Lallah Rookh who is suffering from an affection of the chest – she has had mercurial ointment rubbed into the axilla and head but has taken cold from imprudent exposure and is suffering from an attack of salivation. I recommenced her to gargle the mouth with weak brandy and water and to have brandy beaten up with eggs three or four times a day and new milk with it.

Dr Smith returned four days later:

26 July 1868
I have visited the Station today and find that Lallah has been out in the open air with apparent benefit. On examination of the mouth I find considerable ulceration going on, I strongly recommend that she should be placed upon a milk diet and that the mouth should be syringed with a solution of Carbonate of Sosa, and as she finds considerable relief from the fresh air to get out as much as possible, of course avoid undue exposure to the cold.

Carbonate of soda (sodium bicarbonate) is more commonly used today as baking soda but as a medicinal it is a natural non-toxic alkalising agent used to relieve the symptoms of acid reflux and general inflammation, and a treatment for many other ailments.

Dr Smith must have shown some concern for Truganini's health as he returned to Oyster Cove two days later:

28 July 1868
I visited the station this morning; during my visit Lallah parted with a small quantity of blood most likely from an abscess in the mouth. In some respects she appears better, but the pulse was rather hectic after parting with blood.

Six days later:

> 3 August 1868
> The swelling of the face and throat are some what abated and she takes eggs and brandy with milk well. Her nights are restless, and she does a good deal during the day. The pulse is moderate. The chest symptoms are considerable abated.[25]

The facial swelling was not previously recorded by Dr Smith but most likely reported to him by Dandridge.

Truganini again survived and appeared to be recovering something of her health. Dandridge wrote again to the colonial secretary:

> I am glad to be able to report the complete recovery of 'Lallah Rookh'. During the first 3 weeks of August she made but little progress but afterwards as the sores in her mouth and throat disappeared and she was rapidly regained her strength, and is now in a better state of health than she had been for a long period prior to her illness.[26]

The cause of Truganini's symptoms may be related to her treatment with mercury-based medicines. Mercury in its various forms was common in the medical pharmacopeia of 19th-century doctors and always carried in their medical bags.

Mercury in any of its organic or medicinal forms is toxic. The clinical effects of mercury can manifest in a variety of ways, depending on the nature of the exposure, the intensity of the exposure and the length of exposure. In its organic form mercury is primarily a neurotoxin causing tissue damage to the central nervous system, resulting in neurological and psychological disorders that are often irreversible. Chronic mercury exposure can cause severe abdominal pain and the passing of bloody stools, ashen-grey mucus membranes often described by early practitioners as 'furriness' of the mouth and excessive salivation. Other effects include mood changes, depression, muscle weakness, hypovolemic shock (an abnormal decrease in the volume of circulating fluids in the body), impairment of motor skills and cardiac arrythmia.[27]

In Truganini's case the first indication of potential mercury poisoning is the treatment by 'blue ointment' (Calomel), which was applied to her chest on July 20th. This was most likely not the first time it had been applied to Truganini, as it was also a common medicinal used by the general public and was most likely on Dandridge's shelf at Oyster Cove. After the application of blue ointment, two days later she was suffering from excessive salivation and four days later she had developed extensive ulceration of the mouth. These signs are characteristic of excessive use of the ointment. The salivation was encouraged by the medical practitioners as this was seen as another way of purging the body and resuming the balance of the humours. Mercury causes an allergic skin inflammation and reacts with the oral mucosa, causing mouth ulcers such as experienced by Truganini. By July 28th, Truganini's 'pulse was rather hectic'. Cardiac arrythmia is another sign of excessive mercury intake and by August 3rd, 13 days after the first recorded application of blue ointment, she had developed swelling to her face and was most likely suffering from insomnia. These symptoms suffered by Truganini are all consistent with excessive application of mercury-based medicines, bolstered by the recording of mercury as a treatment.[28]

While the exposure to mercury and the subsequent consequences experienced by Truganini were due to the medical treatment she received, Dr Smith, and any other well-meaning person who administered to her, should not be blamed. Smith was the product of the current state of medical understanding and practice at that time. He would have believed in the Hippocratic theory of a healthy body being in a state of equilibrium. The essence of equilibrium, as seen in Chapter 2, lay in the balance of the four perceived body fluids or the humours: blood, phlegm, black bile and yellow bile. Diseases came as a result of upsetting the equilibrium. Curing the disease meant getting rid of, or purging, any excess humours from the body. This was done by giving the patient a range of medications that largely caused vomiting, diarrhoea, excessive sweating and salivation, or by bleeding the patient (phlebotomy). These were common practices at this time, before the germ theory of infection of today became established. I am sure Dr Smith was acting within his professional paradigm and was trying to heal rather than harm.[29]

The mortality was excessively high at Oyster Cove and the colonial government decided to close the settlement in 1862. Truganini then spent her remaining years in Hobart with John Dandridge and his wife. In her last year years of life, taking short walks through the streets of Hobart with Mrs Dandridge, she became a well-known figure, albeit one of curiosity as the perceived 'last Tasmanian'. The people of Hobart would see 'a stout black woman in a dark bombazine dress with a lace collar and wearing a red turban with a pipe tucked into the fold'.[30]

On May 3rd 1876, Truganini suffered a stroke and remained in a comatose state for five days, being attended by two local medical practitioners, Dr Butler and Dr McFarlane. She was 64 years of age. Her last wish, just before she died, was for her remains to be returned to her homeland. A wish that was tragically and perfidiously not granted for one hundred years.

Immediately following her death there was strong interest from members of the Royal Society to obtain Truganini's skeleton for scientific research. She had been secretly interred in an unmarked grave at the former Female Factory cemetery in Hobart. In December 1878, two years after her death, her remains were disinterred. Her skeleton was presented on public display at the Melbourne Centennial Exhibition in 1888 as the 'last Tasmanian'. In 1904 eminent anthropologist Baldwin Spencer had casts made of her skull and skeleton. Her bones were then returned to Tasmania to become the centrepiece of an exhibition on Indigenous Tasmanians in the Hobart Museum. There they remained, articulated, on public display until 1947. After several public protests, her bones were removed from the exhibition case and stored in a box in the basement of the museum for the next 30 years. Following further protests and persistent advocacy from Indigenous Tasmanian descendants her bones were ceremoniously cremated in 1976 and with dignity scattered in the waters of D'Entrecasteaux Channel in her home country. One hundred years after her death Truganini was finally at peace.[31]

In 1971, five years before her cremation and final interment, Truganini's skeleton was examined by a student as part of an anatomical study. The examination was primarily focused on the measurements of individual bones (anthropometry) but it did reveal evidence of the trauma Truganini had experienced during her life.[32] Truganini had a healed fracture of the distal third section of her left radius (lower mid-arm); the right nasal bone displayed a healed transverse pre-mortem fracture approximately at the midpoint of the bone; and the pre-mortem loss of the left maxillary pre-molar and third molar teeth.

The arm fracture is consistent with what is termed a parrying fracture caused by the arm being held in a defensive position warding off a blow. However, such an assault was not recorded and we do not know when it occurred, if it was indeed a parrying fracture, or by whom the attack might have been made. Other skeletal collections of mainland Aboriginal people have shown these types of trauma in 10–20 per cent of adults.[33] The fracture to the nose as well as the loss of the teeth could also have been caused by trauma from an intentional blow to the face. Whether these events occurred at the same time or as separate incidents is unknown.

Disease and Trauma in the Life of Truganini

As a final glimpse into Truganini's biomedical history we can sum up the diseases she had and were exposed to and at least some of the psychological and physical trauma she experienced during her life:

Born into and grew up in an environment exposed to exotic pathogens
Witnessed violence to her close family
Suffered personal violence – broken arm, broken nose, loss of teeth
Repeatedly raped and beaten
Suffered from Stockholm syndrome?
Infected with sexually transmitted disease – syphilis and/or gonorrhoea likely on several occasions
Rendered infertile – pelvic inflammatory disease?
Influenza infection – several incidents
Violent diarrhoea – several incidents
Suffered in severe dysentery epidemic
Exposed to an epidemic of pneumonia
Escaped an attack by armed warriors on two occasions
Suffered hypothermia from swimming in cold waters while escaping
Oedema in legs
Skin rash – canine scabies?
Survived an attack by gunfire from European posse
Escaped a death sentence
Survived an epidemic of catarrh
Exposed repeatedly to tuberculosis infections – most likely infected
Consumed alcohol and tobacco
Suffered from poor diets and living conditions on settlements
Suffered vermin infections
Exposed to excessive treatments of mercury causing mercury poisoning
Cardiac arrhythmia
Deafness
Ulcerations in mouth
Suffered a fatal stroke

This list is somewhat daunting when considering that it was the experience of just one Indigenous Australian born and living during early European colonisation. The ability to construct such a biomedical profile over the greater part of a lifetime is rare, if not unique, in Australian history. It is largely because of the extant records pertaining to Truganini that it can be done. The diaries and reports of George Augustus Robinson on his journeys around Tasmania and the mainland accompanied by Truganini, and the later records, imperfect and incomplete though they are, of the Wybalenna and Oyster Cove settlements, have given this rare opportunity to glimpse into the life of Truganini. Unique as this may be in a histological sense, I do not think that uniqueness could be applied to the biomedical experiences of other Indigenous Australians of that time. By discussing the impacts of the diseases introduced into the Australian populations and the severity of the epidemics that spread across the continent, the suffering of Truganini is just one case in many thousands. The only difference is that the many went largely unrecorded.

Two main themes emerge from this personal study of Truganini. The first is the destructive effect of European colonialism on the Tasmanian Aboriginal people through the introduction of foreign infectious pathogens on populations that were immunologically naive and had little or no herd immunity to the new pathogens. The real morbidity and mortality caused by the introduced diseases will most likely never be known. But it can be construed with some confidence that they were severe and excessive to individuals and to the population as a whole, not only to Tasmanians but to the Indigenous populations Australia-wide. Along with the infectious diseases was the ever-present threat of violence from encounters with Europeans, which could often lead to death.

The second theme is the remarkable resilience of Truganini as an individual to survive for so long the foreign pathogens and violence she encountered throughout her life, when many of her fellow Tasmanians did not. Truganini encountered, and was exposed to, more infectious diseases than most other Indigenous Tasmanians of her time and she survived. Like her fellow Tasmanians she would have had little or no immunity at first to the infectious diseases that had been introduced, yet she survived to reach a reasonable age and to die quietly and in relative safety. But during that life she witnessed the constant deaths of her people. An experience that even today is hard to come to terms with.

Truganini was certainly a survivor but she was not the 'last Tasmanian', as many opinions have portrayed. There were others who lived after her, particularly on the north coast and Bass Strait islands, and produced families, predominantly of mixed ethnicity – their descendants today identify themselves as Tasmanian Aboriginal people. This biological and cultural continuity of Tasmanians, when put in context with the other Indigenous people of Australia, then speaks again to the resilience of the human species to ultimately survive periods of local and global catastrophes and life-threatening diseases.

Chapter 10

IN THE TIME OF COVID-19

There is an ominous manifestation in this discussion of epidemic diseases among the Indigenous populations of Australia. As I review the early chapters and write the final words of this book there is a fearsome new pandemic spreading throughout the world. It is essentially a respiratory disease caused by a novel virus first identified in China during the final months of 2019. By mid-2020 it had spread (or flown) its way across the world. It is caused by a recently evolved virus belonging to a family of corona viruses, some of which usually cause the mild symptoms we attribute to the common cold. But this particular variant is more serious in its pathogenic consequences in humans. The disease has been given the official name of COVID-19 (coronavirus disease identified in 2019) and the virus itself is labelled SARS-CoV-2 (severe acute respiratory syndrome caused by a second identified genetically similar coronavirus). The first SARS virus was identified during an outbreak largely limited to Asia and Canada in 2003.

At the time of writing, COVID-19 has infected millions of people across the globe, with numbers rising by the day. Deaths from the disease are also rising by the day across the world. It is indeed a world pandemic in the true sense of the phrase. It is fair to say that the pandemic has affected either biologically or socially almost everyone in the world. It is the 'next big one' (NBO) that many researchers have been predicting for some time now. And, while all humans are at some risk of infection by the virus, the First Nations people of Australia particularly are at a higher risk than the rest of the population due to an inherent inequality in health, social and economic factors.

Compared with other viral pandemics, humans across the world have experienced throughout history, such as measles, smallpox and influenza, COVID-19 has been with us just a short time. There is still a lot to learn about its aetiology, pathogenesis and epidemiology. In the coming years, as the virus will surely still be with us, a greater understanding of its nature and its consequences for the future state of human health and wellbeing will surely be gained. But here it is useful to point out a few elementary characteristics of the virus and its effects on humans.

As its name implies, the SARS-CoV-2 virus attacks the human respiratory system with similar mild to severe symptoms as influenza. The infected host experiences an initial fever and cough, which may be followed by a sore throat, headache, fatigue and myalgia, leading into respiratory distress. In many cases the host may experience mild symptoms or be asymptomatic, unaware of the infection and requiring little or no medical assistance. In more severe cases, respiratory distress increases, leading to life-threatening pneumonia-like symptoms. Autopsies have shown alveolar destruction of the lung, with severe and diffuse exudation (excessive fluid on the lungs), massive capillary congestion and pulmonary artery destruction. The heart, oesophagus, kidneys, bladder and ileum (the distal portion of the small intestine) can also be compromised. The elderly and those with underlying health problems such as high blood pressure, persistent respiratory and cardiac problems, diabetes, cancer and compromised immune systems are at a higher risk of serious illness from the virus, ultimately leading to organ failure and death.[1] COVID-19 can be a nasty piece of work. While more needs to be discovered, it seems that the virus is highly virulent and spreads easily among people in close contact via expelled respiratory droplets. When an infected person sneezes or coughs, the droplets can be inhaled by another or be deposited on nearby surfaces and transferred to another host by touch.

In Australia, the disease has been at its most severe in the main cities and urban centres due to higher densities of population. But it has spread into regional areas also by infected carriers. Worldwide, and including Australia, the disease has resulted in higher than usual morbidity and mortality, hospitalisation, extreme family and social disruption, and unimaginable economic losses. Psychological issues relating to imposed social isolation, restriction of movement, fear of the unknown and an uncertainty of what the future may hold are common side effects of the pandemic.

For this book, being concerned about the history and effects of introduced infectious epidemics that have occurred in the Indigenous communities in Australia, it is fitting to end by discussing, as far as practicable, the effects of the COVID-19 pandemic among contemporary communities. But it must be borne in mind that the pandemic is not over and the virus is still very much around. The situation regarding morbidity, mortality and accompanying social stresses is fluid and may change for the better or worse in the near future.

But first a brief background on the general health status of indigenous populations throughout the world – the lasting legacy of colonisation.

The Legacy of Colonisation

There can be no doubt that European colonisation across the world has had a severe and lasting effect on the indigenous populations who either welcomed, fought or were forced to tolerate the incursions of a strange and foreign people. Indeed, this was well known by the British colonists even before they set foot in Australia in 1788. Up until the early 20th century, successive colonial, state and federal governments considered that the Indigenous populations of Australia would slowly die out completely, and they shaped their regulating policies to such an event. Even those Europeans with a strong sense of compassion for the tragedy of the losses they saw, and who tried to help, believed that they were only easing the way of the remaining few, endeavouring to make their lives comfortable until the inevitable end. One such person, Daisy Bates, who spent most of her life in the first half of the 20th century among Aboriginal communities, administering aid and care to the ill and displaced, firmly believed that they would eventually die out – the title of her main book, *The Passing of the Aborigines*,[2] speaks to such a belief. Of course, they ultimately survived, despite the communities being ravaged by successive epidemics and chronic infections resulting in extraordinary population collapses. Truganini, the Tasmanian woman who was born into the colonial experience, suffered from introduced diseases and ultimately survived to spend her final years in a European household, typifies the human will of First Nations people to survive.

The result of global colonialism today is that there is a marked inequality in the impact and threat of infectious and non-infectious diseases among the millions of indigenous people worldwide. During an epidemic or a pandemic indigenous people suffer higher infection rates, morbidity and mortality than non-indigenous populations. The long-term effects of colonisation throughout the world have led to higher disease burdens, higher infant mortality and lower life expectations of indigenous populations.

During the 1918–19 H1N1 influenza epidemic, New Zealand Maoris died at a rate of seven times that of the European population. While this figure is startling enough, it is most likely an underestimation because many of the Maori deaths went unrecorded. Pacific Islander people and Maori were seven times more likely to be hospitalised than the Europeans during the epidemic, and three and a half times more likely to die. During the same epidemic, mortality for American Indians and Alaskan indigenous communities was four times higher than people from other ethnicities combined. The First Nations people of Canada were three times more likely to be hospitalised and six and a half times more likely to be admitted to intensive care.[3] The list goes on. In Australia during the H1N1 influenza pandemic outbreak of 1918–19 First Nations people suffered five times the diagnosis rate, eight times the hospitalisation rate and three times the intensive care admission rate than non-Indigenous people.[4]

Such an effect among the First Nations people of Australia is seen repeatedly throughout this study. The ongoing legacy of poor health is also recorded specifically in Chapter 8, where infant mortality rates among people living on the Aboriginal settlements were examined and compared with the rate in contemporary populations in 2018. The effects of colonisation in Australia have been affecting First Nations people for over 230 years now. In the Americas it has been over 500 years.

COVID-19 and Australia's First Nations People

The vulnerability of First Nations people to COVID-19 is well understood by community leaders, Indigenous medical and community organisations, non-Indigenous medical organisations and the federal, state and territory governments of Australia. In April 2020, a group of Indigenous researchers wrote in the *Medical Journal of Australia*:

> The risk for First Nations from COVID-19 taking hold are immense – the oldest continuous culture on the planet is at risk.[5]

Although this was written in the early days of the pandemic, when the number of daily cases and hospitalisations across the country were on the increase and there was high uncertainty ahead, it is a startling statement indeed. The basis of this statement, the researchers pointed out, was the stark reality of current interrelated health factors embedded in the communities, an already high burden of chronic diseases, long-standing inequity issues related to service provision, reduced access to basic health care and equally long-standing pervasive social and economic disadvantage in areas such as housing, education and employment. They were correct in being concerned for the many First Nations communities across the country, both in the cities and urban centres, and in the remote areas of Australia. To gain an understanding of this concern, it is helpful to take a brief look at some basic health-measuring statistics for Indigenous populations in Australia and elsewhere where colonial impact is still apparent, compared with a benchmark rate, presented in Tables 10.1 a and b. The countries selected are those classified by the World Bank as high income, in order to present the best literal economic comparison with Australia.[6]

Table 10.1a. Infant mortality rates of Indigenous populations in high-income countries.

Indigenous Community	Infant Mortality Rate	Benchmark Rate	Difference
Australia, Aboriginal and Torres Strait Islander	6.3	3.7	2.6
New Zealand, Maori	7.4	4.5	2.9
Canada, Inuit	10.7	5.7	5
USA, Amerindian and Alaskan	8.3	6.1	2.2

Table 10.1b. Life expectancy rates of Indigenous populations in high-income countries.

Indigenous Community	Life Expectancy Rate	Benchmark Rate	Difference
Australia, Aboriginal and Torres Strait Islander	71.4	81.4	–10
New Zealand, Maori	75.1	82.1	–7
Canada, Inuit	68.5	81.0	–12.5
USA, Amerindian and Alaskan	73.7	78.5	–4.8

Source: Extracted from Ian Anderson et al., 'Indigenous and Tribal Peoples' Health (The Lancet-Lowitja Institute Global Collaboration): A Population Study', *The Lancet*, Vol 388, 9 July 2016, pp. 131–157, https://www.thelancet.com/journals/lancet/article/PIIS0140-6736(16)00345-7/fulltext (accessed 18 January 2021).

These figures show at a glance the infant mortality rates (IMR, the number of infant deaths under one year of age per 1000 live births) for the indigenous populations are higher than the benchmark rates (rest of the population) for all. This indicates, as seen in Chapter 8, that the overall health of the indigenous populations is poorer than that of the rest of the population. More children die in their first year of life. In Australia, the IMR statistical rate difference is 2.6 (if the overall health were equal for both groups then the statistical rate would be 1). Looking at the life expectancy rates (the average number of years that a group of newborn babies would be expected to live if the current death rate of the population remained the same) shows another health inequity between the Indigenous population and the rest of the population. In Australia, the First Nations people would be expected to live 10 years less than the rest of the population, in New Zealand it is 7 years less, for Canadian Inuit 12.5

years less and for American Indians 4.8 years less. And these inequities are common with indigenous populations worldwide.[7] These inequities in health were assessed in times when there was no COVID-19 pandemic. So the concern shown by the Indigenous researchers for Australia's First Nations people when the pandemic arrived was completely justified. Little wonder then that, as the pandemic spread its way through Australia, there was concern for First Nations people. They were more vulnerable whether they lived in the high-density areas of the cities and regional areas or in the many remote settlements in central and northern Australia.

It is difficult to assess the impact of the epidemic among urban-living First Nations people in Australia as there is often no indication of ethnicity in the official daily figures of cases, intensive care hospitalisations or deaths. More research is needed and hopefully that will come. But the impact could be expected to be higher on average compared with non-Indigenous communities. Many urban First Nations people live in lower socio-economic environments. Households often comprise large groups, leading to overcrowding and inadequate personal accommodation, which in itself can pose a risk to health and wellbeing. Crowded accommodation means continual close personal contact. More so when overcrowding poses difficulties in maintaining personal hygiene, clean spaces and clothing, and respiratory problems from passive smoking. Households are more likely to be intergenerational, with babies, children and young and older adults living with grandparents and elderly relatives. This mix would potentially increase the risk of COVID-19 gaining a foothold and then spreading between households. Maintaining social distancing would be a problem within such a household, increasing the ability of the virus to spread. A low-economic situation would also reduce the ability to access appropriate healthcare and impact on healthy diets.

Then there is the psychological damage resulting from the pandemic. Living in an urban environment would reduce the ability to maintain contact with relatives elsewhere. Being distanced from traditional country and the inability to exercise cultural customs would also lead to anxiety and psychological stress. (Sound familiar?) While the impact of the COVID-19 pandemic on urban-living Indigenous people has yet to be analysed it would be expected to be more severe physically, socially and culturally than for their non-Indigenous neighbours.[8] On the upside of all this is of course those First Nations people who live in less crowded housing and have a higher economic style of living. For these it would be expected that the impact of COVID-19 would be similar to an established population mean and better than those living in crowded places.

However, the situation in remote communities across the country is reassuring. This is largely due to the responses put in place by the people themselves. In fact, the health gap between Indigenous and non-Indigenous communities that is seen in this study, and that still exists today, with diseases other than COVID-19, is reversed. The non-Indigenous communities became more susceptible and experienced more morbidity and mortality than remote Indigenous communities.

When the pandemic was realised to be a serious matter by the federal, state and territory governments of Australia, legislative measures were invoked. The federal government invoked the Biosecurity Act 2005, and the state and territory jurisdictions did similarly with their own legislative powers. The fundamental elements of the acts were to impose lockdowns within and travel restrictions in and out of Indigenous community settlements. Only necessary and approved movement was to be allowed. Those who wished to enter a community had to self-isolate for 14 days prior to entry and to be tested for the presence of the virus. Because of the isolated nature of the communities and a lack of cultural awareness by the authorities, the measures were inappropriate and frankly unworkable. Many of the Indigenous residents, as a normal part of their lives, spent time away from the settlements in the bush, sleeping out at night and participating in long-held traditional cultural practices. The self-isolation and social distancing that applied to urban populations were just not appropriate to Indigenous life in remote areas.[9]

Pre-empting by five days the World Health Organization's declaration of COVID-19 as a pandemic on 11 March 2020, the Australian Government Department of Health stepped in. A specialised taskforce was convened, together with the National Aboriginal Community Controlled Health Organisation (known by its natty acronym NACCHO). NACCHO is the national peak body representing 143 Aboriginal community-controlled health services across the country, with the objective of advising governments on health and wellbeing issues of all First Nations people. The taskforce, including the specialised Aboriginal and Torres Strait Islander Advisory Group on COVID-19, was to provide health and advisory services to remote and urban communities. The taskforce members include Aboriginal and Torres Strait Islander health sector representatives and representatives of state and territory governments. It is designed to work on a shared decision-making principle, with two-way communication with community organisations allowing self-determination and a leadership approach in decision making. The First Nations representatives have a major role in decision making.

The success of the program has been largely due to the Indigenous health experts and media services reaching out to the communities. More culturally appropriate health services of Indigenous health workers treating Indigenous patients has been a successful way of educating and informing the communities. Face-to-face contact, often in their own language, has enabled the communities to be informed about how they can minimise infection by the virus. Indigenous-tailored media messaging uses social media, radio and television platforms to expound culturally and linguistically appropriate health literature. It advises people to get tested for the virus, wash hands frequently, keep a safe distance from others where possible but at the same time stay connected to the community and, importantly, stay in touch with country and culture – keeping the 'mob' together – and look after personal health, both physical and mental, as well as others. These measures are espoused as the mainstays of success. So far this has worked within remote communities and it is hoped that it will continue to be successful while COVID-19 is with us.[10]

Borroloola and COVID-19

How have remote communities responded to the threat of further illness from COVID-19? It's a broad question that requires further investigation and research to answer, but some early research gives a glimpse into how one remote community in northern Australia has dealt with the pandemic.[11] The Yanyuwa people form a remote community at Borroloola, located in the south-west of the Gulf of Carpentaria in the Northern Territory, some 1056km from the capital, Darwin. The population of the settlement fluctuates at around 870 people with 71 per cent identifying as Indigenous. The main settlement is located on the McArthur River 45km from the coast and is serviced by road and an airstrip. The Sir Edward Pellew islands form part of Yanyuwa country.

As the pandemic began to take hold in early 2020, the Northern Territory Government quickly acted, with biosecurity restrictions controlling movement in and out of the settlement. Emergency health cases were, however, able to be transported to Darwin for care but had to go unaccompanied by a family member. The Indigenous residents of the settlement were able to move freely across their country, extending to the coast and offshore islands, and were able to visit outstations, but non-residents required specifically issued permits to enter the area.

Early on in the pandemic, anthropologists from Flinders University in Adelaide and Monash University in Melbourne conducted a series of telephone and digital conferencing interviews with Yanyuwa families living in the settlement.[12] Their aim was to investigate the long history of cultural response to illness and the threat of illness within the community and how this was translated to the present COVID-19 pandemic. What they unearthed was a culturally orientated understanding of the pandemic. As seen in earlier chapters, the belief systems surrounding unusual sickness and epidemics have often been attributed to some form of personal or group sorcery. This sorcery can come from an individual or be associated with a particular place considered to invoke illness on those who enter or transgress into it.

These beliefs have been directly associated with past epidemics that the Yanyuwa have experienced. These include the epidemic of Hong Kong influenza that struck the community in 1969 and further back to the 1918–19 influenza pandemic, both of which killed many of the elders, resulting in a loss of traditional knowledge. The cause of these epidemics has been associated with sorcery. In fact, in Yanyuwa country there is a place with a strong taboo located on Wurdaliya clan country on the coast north of Borroloola, where during the 1918–19 influenza pandemic many elders died. The place has been embedded in current culture as a site of the Flu Dreaming and to be avoided when possible. These beliefs of sorcery-induced sickness among the Yanyuwa people have been a long-standing part of their culture. Along with this origin perception, the people were also fully aware of the severity of these past diseases, the mortality they caused and how their previous generations dealt with them. Then along came COVID-19 into a world that is digitally connected.

For this new disease, COVID-19, their main source of information was through digital and media platforms available to them. They were able to tap into a range of digital sources obtaining up-to-date and day-by-day information on the course of the pandemic in Australia and the world. Using these sources, they were able to decide what preventative steps they should take to minimise exposure and infection. Much of this information was provided in digital form in language by Indigenous-controlled community organisations. With this information constantly flowing through the community, COVID-19 was viewed not as sickness caused by sorcery or association with a bad place, or as another part of the Flu Dreaming story as it was in the past, but as a worldwide pandemic, a whitefella disease.[13] With this awareness now being based on a scientific understanding of the disease but drawing on the cultural memories of past experiences, the Borroloola residents were able manage themselves effectively against the epidemic threat.

In the face of possible illness striking the community again, family ties became the guiding structure for transmission of information through the community. Key elements of their method of staying safe were education and sharing of knowledge with the young and elderly, and vice versa; going out bush with family, seeking bush foods or moving to one of the offshore islands (the Sir Edward Pellew island group); and shopping for the elderly confined to the settlement and generally looking after each other, making sure people had the right foods to eat and ensuring no-one felt lonely. They realised the benefits of washing hands frequently, practising social distancing as best they could, keeping up to date with the current information and staying away from larger urban centres. One resident, who could recall the Hong Kong influenza pandemic when it struck the community, told the researchers:

> We have been very careful this time. We follow the rules, we don't want to die, we are helping each other. Maybe if we had … known these rules when that Hong Kong flu came, people would have stayed alive.[14]

Their actions were a result of long-held cultural explanations for sickness that had previously occurred and of having the means to survive another epidemic with a new source of information available to them.

This then brings a question relating to the perceived general notion of isolation and remoteness that is given to settlements like Borroloola throughout Australia. Although over a thousand kilometres from the nearest city (Darwin) the Yanyuwa people of Borroloola, along with many other First Nations settlements across the country, may be constrained (or protected) by geography but they are still instantly in touch with the rest of the world. How this knowledge and understanding of illness and disease will be interpreted and inaugurated into the cultural Dreaming stories of the future is yet to be determined.

However, one thing is clear from the Borroloola investigation. It shows that the First Nations people of Australia can now understand the nature of such a pandemic, how it can be transmitted and how they themselves can apply their culture to integrate with modern science to protect from infection and still retain their long-held traditions in the face of it. The people who suffered the past epidemics of introduced infectious diseases did not have such advantages in the face of relentless colonial expansion in their worlds. And they suffered an immeasurable loss. Those epidemics came close to wiping them out.

NOTES

Foreword

1 Alfred W. Crosby, *Ecological Imperialism: The Biological Expansion of Europe, 900–1900* (Cambridge: Cambridge University Press, 1986).
2 Noel Butlin, *Our Original Aggression: Aboriginal Populations of Southeastern Australia 1788–1850* (Sydney: George Allen & Unwin, 1983).

Introduction: A Brief Flight over History

1 Chris Clarkson et al., 'Human Occupation of Northern Australia by 65,000 Years Ago', *Nature*, 547 (7663), July 2017, pp. 306–310; Shelia M. van Holst Pellekaan at al., 'Mitochondrial Genomics Identifies Major Haplogroups in Aboriginal Australians', *American Journal of Physical Anthropology*, 131, October 2006, p. 2.
2 Paul Memmott, *Gunyah Goondie + Wurley: The Aboriginal Architecture of Australia* (St Lucia, Qld: University of Queensland Press, 2007); Bruce Pascoe, *Dark Emu, Black Seeds: Agriculture or Accident?* (Broome: Magabala Books, 2014).
3 Charles Sturt, *Narrative of an Expedition into Central Australia* (Sydney: University of Sydney Library, 2001 (1849)), http://adc.library.usyd.edu.au/data-2/p00102.pdf (accessed May 2018).
4 George Grey, *Journals of Two Expeditions of Discovery in North-West and Western Australia*, Vol. II (London: T. and W. Boone, 1841) (Facsimile Edition, Victoria Park: Hesperion Press, 1984), pp. 12–13.
5 Richard Broome, *Aboriginal Australians: A History since 1788*, 4th edn (Sydney: Allen and Unwin, 2010) pp.195–196.
6 ibid. p. 196.
7 Samuel Furphy and Amanda Nettlebeck, *Aboriginal Protection and its Intermediaries in Britain's Antipodean Colonies*, Part 1, 'The Conception and Circulation of 'Aboriginal Protection' (New York: Routledge 2020) p. 4, http://web.a.ebscohost.com.rp.nla.gov.au/ehost/ebookviewer/ebook/bmxlYmtfXzIxNDEyNDVfX0FO0?sid=f29e93e4-7534-4691-bd36-6686fe70b8ce@sessionmgr4008&vid=0&format=EB&lpid=lp_1&rid=0 (accessed 28 October 2020).
8 S. Maddison, 'Indigenous Autonomy Matters: What's Wrong with the Australian Government's "Intervention" in Aboriginal Communities', *Australian Journal of Human Rights*, 14 (1), 2008, pp. 41–61.
9 Castan Centre, Monash University, 'What is the Northern Territory Intervention?' https://www.monash.edu/law/research/centres/castancentre/our-areas-of-work/indigenous/the-northern-territory-intervention/the-northern-territory-intervention-an-evaluation/what-is-the-northern-territory-intervention (accessed 2 November 2020).
10 Henry Reynolds, *The Other Side of the Frontier: Aboriginal Resistance to the European Invasion of Australia* (Sydney: University of New South Wales Press, 2006).
11 L. Ryan et al., 'Colonial Frontier Massacres in Central and Eastern Australia, 1788–1930', University of Newcastle, https://c21ch.newcastle.edu.au/colonialmassacres/introduction.php (accessed 15 August 2018).
12 Alfred W. Crosby, *Ecological Imperialism: The Biological Expansion of Europe, 900–1900*, 2nd edn (Cambridge: Cambridge University Press, 2015), p. 31.
13 R. S. W. Cilento and A. H. Baldwin, 'Malaria in Australia', *Medical Journal of Australia*, 1 (9), 1930, pp. 274–282; Timothy J. Gray et al., 'Imported Malaria in

the Northern Territory, Australia – 428 Consecutive Cases', *Communicable Diseases Intelligence*, 36 (1), March 2012, https://www1.health.gov.au/internet/main/publishing.nsf/Content/cda-cdi3601f.htm (accessed 1 June 2020).

14 F. Fenner, 'Sociocultural Changes and Infectious Disease', in B. Furnass (ed.), *Infectious Disease in Humans* (Canberra: Canberra Nature and Science Forum, 1998).

Chapter 1: Concepts and Consequences of Disease

1 Geoffrey Blainey, *The Tyranny of Distance* (Melbourne: Sun Books, 1982).

2 J. H. L. Cumpston, *The Health of the People* (Canberra: Roebuck Society Publication No. 19, 1978).

3 Frank M. Snowden, *Epidemics and Society: From the Black Death to the Present* (New Haven: Yale University Press, Kindle edition, 2019).

4 Cumpston, 1978, p. 3.

5 J. Reid, *Sorcerers and Healing Spirits* (Canberra: Australian National University Press, 1983); J. Reid, 'Medicine and Health: The Traditional Systems', in J. Reid (ed.), *Body, Land and Spirit: Health and Healing in Aboriginal Society* (St Lucia, Qld: University of Queensland Press, 1982); A. P. Elkin, *Aboriginal Men of High Degree: Initiation and Sorcery in the World's Oldest Tradition* (St Lucia, Qld: University of Queensland Press, 1994).

6 Quoted in Fred Cahir, Ian D. Clark and Philip A. Clarke, *Aboriginal Biocultural Knowledge in South-Eastern Australia: Perspectives of Early Colonists* (Clayton South, Vic.: CSIRO Publishing, 2018), p. 192.

7 Samuel Gason, quoted in G. Taplin, *The Folklore, Manners, Customs, and Languages of the South Australian Aborigines* (Adelaide: Government Printer, 1879) (Facsimile edition, 1989), p. 79.

8 Endeavour College of Natural Health, *Australian Indigenous Medicine*, https://source.endeavourlearninggroup.com.au/coursematerial/pdf/Documents/SOCH111_SN10_Lecture.pdf (accessed 15 January 2019).

9 Cahir, Clark and Clarke, 2018, pp. 209–277.

10 ibid., p. 213.

11 W. H. Baylie, 'On the Aborigines of the Goulburn district', in *Port Phillip Magazine*, I, 1843, pp. 86–92.

12 A. W. Crosby, 'The Virgin-soil Epidemic as a Factor in the Aboriginal Depopulation in America', *William and Mary Quarterly*, 33, 1976, pp. 289–299; W. H. McNeill, *Plagues and Peoples* (London: Penguin Books, 1976).

13 See the following for a review of the diseases and the demographic consequences: J. W. Verano and D. H. Ubelaker (eds), *Disease and Demography in the Americas* (Washington: Smithsonian Institution Press, 1992); H. F. Dobyns, *Their Numbers Become Thinned* (Knoxville: University of Tennessee Press, 1983); David S. Jones, 'Virgin Soils Revisited', in *William and Mary Quarterly*, 60 (4), October 2003, pp. 703–742; N. D. Cook, *Born to Die: Disease and New World Conquest, 1492–1650* (Cambridge: Cambridge University Press, 1998).

14 Timothy C. Winegard, *The Mosquito: A Human History of Our Deadliest Predator* (Melbourne: Text Publishing, 2019).

15 McNeill, 1976, pp. 192–195.

16 Alfred W. Crosby, *The Columbian Exchange: Biological and Cultural Consequences of 1492* (Westport, Connecticut: Greenwood Press, 1972).

17 Roy Porter, *The Greatest Benefit to Mankind: A Medical History of Humanity from Antiquity to the Present* (London: Harper Collins Publishers, 1997), p. 466.

18 Charles F. Merbs, 'A New World of Infectious Disease', *American Journal of Physical Anthropology*, 35, 1992, pp. 3–42.

19 McNeill, 1976; Winegard, 2019, pp. 166–170, 324.

20 Daniel Defoe, *A Journal of the Plague Year* (first published 1722; Alicia Editions, Kindle version, 2020).

21 Fred Cahir, *My Country All Gone, the White Men Have Stolen It: The Invasion of Wadawurrung Country, 1800–1870* (Ballarat: Australian History Matters, 2019).
22 Australian Institute of Aboriginal and Torres Strait Islander Studies, 'Indigenous Australian Languages: Celebrating 2019 International Year of Indigenous Languages', Canberra, https://aiatsis.gov.au/whats-new/news/international-year-indigenous-languages-officially-launched (accessed 3 July 2020).
23 E. Eyre, *Journals of Expeditions into Central Australia*, Vol. 2 (London: T. and W. Boone, 1845).
24 S. Webb, *Palaeopathology of Aboriginal Australians* (Cambridge, Melbourne: Cambridge University Press, 1995).
25 John Mulvaney, '"Difficult to Found an Opinion": 1788 Population Estimates', in Gordan Briscoe and Len Smith (eds), *The Aboriginal Population Revisited: 70,000 Years to the Present* (Canberra: Aboriginal History Monograph, No. 10, 2002); Bruce Pascoe, *Dark Emu, Black Seeds: Agriculture or Accident?* (Broome: Magabala Books, 2014).

Chapter 2: Smallpox

1 F. Fenner et al., *Smallpox and Its Eradication* (Geneva: World Health Organization, 1988).
2 Donald R. Hopkins, *Princes and Peasants: Smallpox in History* (Chicago: Chicago University Press, 1983), p. 3.
3 Centers for Disease Control and Prevention, 'History of Smallpox', formerly available from https://www.cdc.gov/smallpox/history/ (accessed 22 January 2018).
4 A. W. Crosby, 'Smallpox', in K. Kiple (ed.), *The Cambridge World History of Human Disease* (Cambridge: Cambridge University Press, 1993), p. 1008.
5 C. W. Dixon, *Smallpox* (London: J. and A. Churchill Ltd, 1962), pp. 193–201.
6 Fenner et al., 1988, p. 211.
7 Dixon, 1962, pp. 189–195.
8 ibid., p. 215.
9 Fenner et al., 1988, p. 24.
10 ibid., p. 214.
11 Alfred W. Crosby, *Ecological Imperialism: The Biological Expansion of Europe, 900–1900*, 2nd edn (Cambridge: Cambridge University Press, 2015), p. 196; R. G. Robertson, *Rotting Face: Smallpox and the American Indian* (Caldwell, Idaho: Caxton Press, 2001), p. 99.
12 For reviews of historical case fatality rates see: H. F. Dobyns, *Their Numbers Become Thinned* (Knoxville: University of Tennessee Press, 1983); Fenner et al., 1988.
13 Fenner et al., 1988, pp. 241–242.
14 Centers for Disease Control and Prevention, 'Poxvirus Diseases', https://www.cdc.gov/poxvirus/diseases.html (accessed January 2018).
15 ibid.
16 A. S. Benenson, *Control of Communicable Diseases in Man*, 15th edn (Washington: American Public Health Association, 1990), p. 396.
17 A. S. Benenson, 'Smallpox', in Evans A. S. (ed.), *Viral Infections of Humans* (New York: Plenum Press, 1976), p. 443.
18 Fenner et al., 1988, pp. 131–138.
19 ibid., p. 5.
20 ibid., pp. 22–38.
21 ibid., pp. 38–39.
22 Frank Fenner, 'Smallpox, "The Most Dreadful Scourge of the Human Species": Its Global Spread and Recent Eradication', *Medical Journal of Australia*, 141 (11), 1984, pp. 728–735.
23 Hopkins, 1983.

24 J. H. L. Cumpston, *The History of Small-pox in Australia, 1788–1908* (Quarantine Service Publication No. 3. Melbourne: Government Printer, 1914); P. H. Curson, *Times of Crisis: Epidemics in Sydney 1788–1900* (Sydney: Sydney University Press, 1985).

25 For example see: David Collins, *An Account of the English Colony in New South Wales*, Vol I, Reprint edited by B.H. Fletcher (Sydney: A.H. & A.W. Reed, 1985. Originally published London, 1798); John Hunter, *An Historical Journal of Events at Sydney and at Sea 1787–1779* (Facsimile Copy. Sydney: Angus & Robertson, 1968); Arthur Phillip, Letter to Lord Sydney, 13 February 1790, *Historical Records of Australia*, Series 1, Vol. 1, p. 159; Watkin Tench, *Sydney's First Four Years* (Sydney: Library of Australian History reprint, 1979, originally published as *A Complete Account of the Settlement at Port Jackson*, London: 1793).

26 For example: Boyd H. Hunter and John Carmody, 'Estimating the Aboriginal Population in Early Colonial Australia: The Role of Chickenpox Reconsidered', *Australian Economic History Review*, 55 (2), 2015, pp. 112–138; Sir J. Watt, 'The Colony's Health', in J. Hardy and A. Frost (eds), *Studies from Terra Australis to Australia* (Canberra: Australian Academy of the Humanities, 1989).

27 Noel Butlin, *Our Original Aggression: Aboriginal Populations of Southeastern Australia 1788–1850* (London: Allen and Unwin, 1983); Judy Campbell, *Invisible Invaders: Smallpox and Other Diseases in Aboriginal Australia* (Carlton South: Melbourne University Press, 2002); Cumpston, 1914; David Day, *Claiming a Continent: A History of Australia* (Pymble: Angus & Robertson, 1997); Campbell Macknight, 'The View from Marege: Australian Knowledge of Makassar and the Impact of the Trepang Industry across Two Centuries', *Aboriginal History*, 35, 2011, pp. 121–143.

28 Charles Sturt, *Two Expeditions into the Interior of Southern Australia*, Vols I and II (London: Smith, Elder and Co., 1833) (Facsimile Copy. Sydney: Doubleday, 1982).

29 Fenner, 1984, pp. 728–735, 841–846; Robert Gething, Report to the Vaccination Board, 30 January 1867, reprinted as 'The Smallpox amongst the Aborigines', *The South Australian Register*, 5 February 1867.

30 N. Irvine, *The Sirius Letters: The Complete Letters of Newton Fowell 1786–1790* (Sydney: Fairfax Press, 1988), p. 113.

31 Collins, 1798, p. 496.

32 Tench, 1793, p. 145.

33 ibid., p. 146.

34 ibid.

35 Collins, 1798, p. 496.

36 ibid., p. 146.

37 Phillip, 1790, p. 159.

38 Tench, 1793, p. 146.

39 Collins, 1798, p. 496.

40 Hunter, 1793, p. 134.

41 Tench, 1793, pp. 146–148.

42 Phillip, 1790, p. 159; Tench, 1793, p. 149.

43 Collins, 1798, p. 54; Tench, 1793, pp. 149–150.

44 Collins, 1798, p. 496.

45 These were the instructions given to Phillip by King George III, prior to leaving England, in Instructions to Governor Phillip, 25 April 1787, *Historical Records of Australia*, Series 1, Vol. 1, pp. 13–14.

46 Grace Karskens, *The Colony: A History of Early Sydney* (Crows Nest: Allen and Unwin, 2010).

47 Collins, 1798, p. 53.

48 ibid.

49 Cumpston, 1914, p. 2; Noel Butlin, *Our Original Aggression: Aboriginal Populations of Southeastern Australia 1788–1850* (London: Allen and Unwin, 1983), p. 24.

50 Collins, 1798, p. 52.

51 Hunter, 1793, pp. 138–139.
52 Phillip, 1790.
53 J. Mair, 'Observation on the Eruptive Febrile Disease which Prevailed among Several Tribes of the Aborigines in New South Wales during the Years 1830 and 31', AO NSW 4/2180, 1831.
54 J. Grant, *The Narrative of a Voyage of Discovery Performed in His Majesty's Ship the Lady Nelson* (Bell Yard, Fleet Street: C. Roworth, 1803) (Facsimile Edition. Adelaide: Libraries Board of South Australia, 1973).
55 J. Flemming, 'The Voyage of His Majesty's Schooner "Cumberland" from Sydney to King Island and Port Phillip in 1802–3. A Journal of the Explorations of Charles Grimes, Acting Surveyor-General of New South Wales', in *Port Phillip, First Survey and Settlement* (Reprinted by Legislative Assembly. Melbourne: Government Printer, 1879), p. 16.
56 Cumpston, 1914.
57 Curson, 1985, p. 51.
58 Phillip, 1790, p. 159.
59 See, for example, Fenner et al., 1988, pp. 1069–1102.
60 Arthur Phillip, Letter to Lord Sydney, 15 May 1788, *Historical Records of Australia*, Series 1, Vol. 1, p. 29.
61 J. P. White and D. J. Mulvaney, 'How Many People?', in D. J. Mulvaney and J. P. White (eds), *Australians to 1788: Australians, a Historical Library* (Sydney: Fairfax, Syme and Weldon Associates, 1987), p. 115.
62 J. L. Kohen, and R. Lampert, 'Hunters and Fishers in the Sydney Region', in D. J. Mulvaney and J. P. White (eds), 1987, p. 345.
63 P. Turbet, *The Aborigines of the Sydney District before 1788* (Sydney: Kangaroo Press, 1989), pp. 26–28.
64 C. M. Hotimsky, 'A Russian Account of New South Wales in 1822', *Melbourne Slavonic Studies*, 1 (1), 1967, pp. 82–95.
65 Collins, 1798, pp. 497.
66 Hunter, 1793, pp. 340–341.
67 ibid., pp. 165–167.
68 J. Cobley, *Sydney Cove 1789–1790* (Sydney: Angus & Robertson, 1963), p. 43.
69 Collins, 1798, p. 109.
70 Charles Sturt, *Two Expeditions into the Interior of Southern Australia*, Vol. I (London: Smith, Elder and Co., 1833) (Facsimile Copy. Sydney: Doubleday 1982).
71 J. Mair, 'Observation on the Eruptive Febrile Disease which Prevailed among Several Tribes of the Aborigines in New South Wales during the Years 1830 and 31', AO NSW 4/2180, 1831.
72 ibid.
73 ibid.
74 G. Busby, Letter to Inspector of Colonial Hospitals, 19 October 1831, Sydney, AO NSW 4/2130.
75 ibid.
76 ibid.
77 Mair, 1831.
78 J. Bowman, Letter to Colonial Secretary, 10 October 1831, AO NSW 4/2130.
79 Nancy Gray, 'Bowman, James (1784–1846)', *Australian Dictionary of Biography* (Canberra: National Centre of Biography, Australian National University), http://adb.anu.edu.au/biography/bowman-james-1812 (accessed March 2018).
80 L. D. Thompson, Minutes of the Executive Council, 29 December 1831, Minute no. 1, Part 7, AO NSW 4/1517.
81 Mair, 1831.
82 ibid.
83 ibid.

84 Thomas Mitchell, *Three Expeditions into the Interior of Eastern Australia*, Vol. I (London: T. W. Boone, 1838) (Australian Facsimile Edition No. 18. Adelaide: Libraries Board of South Australia, 1965), p. 26.
85 ibid., p. 218.
86 ibid., p. 261.
87 E. Beale, *Sturt the Chipped Idol: A Study of Charles Sturt, Explorer* (Sydney: Sydney University Press, 1979).
88 Joseph Hawdon, *The Journal of a Journey from New South Wales to Adelaide* (Melbourne: Georgian House, 1838).
89 ibid.
90 Charles Sturt, 'Overland Communication with New South Wales – Official Report of Captain Sturt', *South Australian Register*, 12 January 1839.
91 Charles Sturt, Sturt Papers, Microfiche copy (Oxford: Rhodes House, 1838), NLA G2200, Canberra.
92 J. Mair and J. Imlay, Letter to Colonial Secretary, 24 December 1831, AO NSW 4/2130.
93 P. Beveridge, Letter to Editor of *The Argus* (1877), in Cumpston, 1914, p.154.
94 Extract of anonymous article from *Adelaide Observer*, 8 July 1911.
95 E. C. Stirling, 'Preliminary Report on the Discovery of Native Remains at Swanport, River Murray: With an Inquiry into the Alleged Occurrence of a Pandemic among the Australian Aboriginals', *Transactions and Proceedings of the Royal Society of South Australia*, 35, 1911, pp. 18–19.
96 J. Hawker, 'Old Time Memories', *The Adelaide Observer*, 11 May 1901.
97 Stirling, 1911.
98 George Augustus Robinson, 'Journal of an Expedition to the Aborigines of the Eastern Interior Commencing April and Terminating October 1844', in *NSW Governors' Despatches*, Vol. 47, Jan–May 1845, ML A1236; G. Mackaness, *George Augustus Robinson's Journey into South-Eastern Australia: 1844* (Dubbo: Australian Historical Monograph Vol. XIX, Review Publications, 1941).
99 Isabel McBryde, 'Kulin Greenstone Quarries: The Social Contexts of Production and Distribution for the Mt William Site', *World Archaeology*, 16 (2), 1984, pp. 267–285.
100 J. Morgan, *The Life and Adventures of William Buckley: Thirty-two Years a Wanderer amongst the Aborigines of the Unexplored Country Round Port Phillip* (Canberra: Australian National University Press, 1980 (1852)).
101 James Dawson, *Australian Aborigines. The Languages and Customs of Several Tribes of Aborigines in the Western District of Victoria, Australia* (Melbourne: George Robertson, 1881).
102 Colin Pardoe, 'The Cemetery as Symbol: The Distribution of Prehistoric Burial Grounds in Southeastern Australia', *Archaeology in Oceania*, 23 (1), 1988, pp. 1–16.
103 E. M. Curr, *The Australian Race*, Vol. 1 (Melbourne: Government Printer, 1886).
104 Dawson, 1881.
105 ibid.
106 Judy Campbell, 'Smallpox in Aboriginal Australia, The Early 1830s', *Historical Studies*, 21 (84), 1985, pp. 336–358.
107 Stirling, 1911.
108 *The Argus*, 5 February 1877.
109 Campbell, 2002, p. 193.
110 Quoted in, Tony Austin, *Simply the Survival of the Fittest: Aboriginal Administration in South Australia's Northern Territory 1863–1910* (Darwin: Historical Society of the Northern Territory, 1992), p. 15.
111 R. J. Noye, 'Foelsche, Paul Heinrich Matthias (1831–1914)', *Australian Dictionary of Biography*, National Centre of Biography, Australian National University, http://abd.anu.edu.au/biography/foelsche-paul-heinrich-matthias-3543/text5467 (accessed 27 October 2020), first published in hardcopy 1972.

112 Paul Foelsche, 'Notes on the Aborigines of North Australia', extract in A. Breinl, 'Report on Health and Disease in the Northern Territory', *Bulletin of the Northern Territory*, 1a, July 1912, pp. 21–38.
113 Campbell, 2002, p. 86.
114 Foelsche, 1912.
115 Matthew Flinders, *A Voyage to Terra Australis*, Vol. 2 (London: G. and W. Nicol, 1814) (Facsimile Edition. Adelaide: Libraries Board of South Australia, 1966) p. 172.
116 ibid., pp. 229–233.
117 D. J. Mulvaney, *Encounters in Place: Outsiders and Aboriginal Australians 1606–1985* (St Lucia: University of Queensland Press, 1989), pp. 22–23.
118 Foelsche, 1912.
119 Robert Gething, Report to the Vaccination Board, 30 January 1867, reprinted as 'The Smallpox amongst the Aborigines', *The South Australian Register*, 5 February 1867.
120 ibid.
121 *South Australian Register*, Letter to the Editor, 2 April 1867.
122 J. P. Buttfield, Letter to Acting Protector of Aborigines, 1 April 1867, PRO SA, GRG 52/1/1867/138.
123 Fenner, 1984, pp. 728–735, 841–846.
124 J. B. Cleland, 'Some Diseases Peculiar to, Or of Interest in, Australia', in J. H. L. Cumpston, 1914.
125 H. Goodall, 'Colonialism and Catastrophe: Contested Memories of Nuclear Testing and Measles Epidemics at Ernabella', in K. Darian-Smith and P. Hamilton (eds), *Memory and History in Twentieth-Century Australia* (Oxford: Oxford University Press, 1994).
126 Fenner, 1984, p. 732.
127 Cumpston, 1914.
128 Charles Sturt, *Narrative of an Expedition into Central Australia* (Sydney: University of Sydney Library, 2001 (1849)), http://adc.library.usyd.edu.au/data-2/p00102.pdf (accessed May 2018).
129 ibid., p. 290.
130 Mike Smith, *The Archaeology of Australia's Deserts* (Cambridge: Cambridge University Press, 2013), pp. 266–270.
131 D. J. Mulvaney, *The Prehistory of Australia* (Ringwood: Penguin Australia, 1975), p. 111; John Mulvaney and Johan Kamminga, *Prehistory of Australia* (Sydney: Allen and Unwin, 1999), p. 97.
132 Rupert Gerritsen, *Beyond the Frontier: Explorations in Ethnohistory* (Canberra: Batavia Online Publishing, 2011), p. 25.
133 Cited in E. Couper Black, 'Population and Tribal Distribution', in B. C. Cotton (ed.), *Aboriginal Man in South and Central Australia*, Part 1 (Adelaide: Government Printer, 1966), pp. 98–99.
134 Elizabeth Williams, 'The Archaeology of Lake Systems in the Middle Cooper Basin, North-Eastern South Australia', *Records of the South Australian Museum*, 30, 1997–1998, pp. 69–91.
135 Mike Smith, *The Archaeology of Australia's Deserts* (Cambridge: Cambridge University Press, 2013).
136 Williams, 1997–1998.
137 Harry Lourandos, *Continent of Hunter-Gatherers: New Perspectives in Australian Prehistory* (Cambridge: Cambridge University Press, 1997), pp. 183–194.
138 Gething, 1867.
139 Quoted in Campbell, 2002, p. 196.
140 Daisy Bates Papers, National Library of Australia, MS 365, folio 33/1-30.
141 ibid., folio 33/72-80.
142 F. Fenner, 'Smallpox in Australia', Letter to the Editor, *Medical Journal of Australia* 142, 1985, p. 278.

143 *Adelaide Observer*, Report on the Meeting of the Royal Society of South Australia, 17 June 1882.
144 Fenner, 1984, p. 731.
145 Stephen Gapps, *The Sydney Wars: Conflict in the Early Colony 1788–1817* (Sydney: New South Publishing, 2018).
146 Governor Phillip, Letter to Lord Sydney, 30 October 1788, *Historical Records of Australia*, Series 1, Vol. 1, p. 96.
147 Phillip to Lord Sydney, 1788.
148 Gipps, 2018.

Chapter 3: Measles

1 Robert Dawson, *The Present State of Australia* (London: Smith, Elder and Co., 1830), p. 323.
2 Maritime Museum of Tasmania, 'The Journey – by Sailing Ship', http://www.maritimetas.org/collection-displays/displays/over-seas-stories-tasmanian-migrants/journey-sailing-ship (accessed 1 February 2017).
3 A. Cliff, P. Haggett and M. Smallman-Raynor, *Measles: An Historical Geography of a Major Human Viral Disease, from Global Expansion to Local Retreat, 1840–1990* (Oxford: Blackwell Publishers, 1993).
4 W. H. McNeill, *Plagues and Peoples* (London: Penguin Books, 1976).
5 N. D. Cook, *Born to Die: Disease and New World Conquest, 1492–1650* (Cambridge: Cambridge University Press, 1998), pp. 85–94.
6 N. McArthur, *Island Populations of the Pacific* (Canberra: Australian National University Press, 1967); A. D. Cliff and P. Haggett, *The Spread of Measles in Fiji and the Pacific* (Canberra: Australian National University, 1985).
7 Robert C. Schmitt and Eleanor C. Nordyke, 'Death in Hawai'i: The Epidemics of 1848–1849', in *The Hawaiian Journal of History*, 35, 2001, pp. 1–13.
8 Robert, J. Wolfe, 'Alaska's Great Sickness, 1900: An Epidemic of Measles and Influenza in a Virgin Soil Population', *Proceedings of the American Philosophical Society*, 126 (2), 1982, pp. 91–121.
9 L. E. (Rev.) Threlkeld, 'Annual Report of the Mission to the Aborigines, Lake Macquarie,' 1835, Threlkeld Papers, ML A382.
10 ibid.
11 Charles Darwin, *A Naturalist's Voyage. Journal of Researches into the Natural History and Geology of the Countries Visited during the Voyage of H. M. S. 'Beagle' Round the World* (London: John Murray, 1889), p. 520.
12 Threlkeld, 1835.
13 William Clindening, Letter, July 6, in *South Australian Register*, 4 August 1854, p. 3.
14 Samuel Schumack, 'Canberra Blacks', *Sydney Morning Herald*, 11 June 1927, p. 9.
15 J. Flood, *The Moth Hunters: Aboriginal Prehistory of the Australian Alps* (Canberra: Australian Institute of Aboriginal Studies, 1980).
16 ibid., pp. 68–69.
17 William Smith, Entries in the Oyster Cove Aboriginal Station Visiting Officers Book (1858–1869) AO Tas., CSO/89/A171/3.
18 P. Dowling, '"A Great Deal of Sickness": Introduced Diseases among the Aboriginal People of Colonial Southeast Australia 1788–1900' (Canberra: PhD thesis, Australian National University, 1997), https://digitalcollections.anu.edu.au/handle/1885/7529 (accessed July 2016).
19 J. Burton Cleland, *A Contribution to the History of Disease in Australia*, Paper, Australian Medical Congress, Sydney, September 1911.
20 M. Morgan, *Nosological Index 1863 and Staff and Registrars of the Registrar-General's Department Victoria 1862* (Blackburn: Marjorie Morgan Publications, 1987).

21 James Gibson, Reports, in 'Annual Report of the Board for the Protection of the Aborigines', Papers Presented to Parliament, Legislative Assembly, *Victorian Parliamentary Papers*, Vol. 4, 1869; Vol. 3, 1871; Vol. 3, Part 2, 1872; Vol. 3, Part 1, 873; Vol. 3, Part 1, 1874; Vol. 3, 1875–76.

22 J. H. L. Cumpstson, *The History of Diphtheria, Scarlet Fever, Measles and Whooping Cough in Australia* (Canberra: Government Printer, 1927), p. 223.

23 Gibson, 1873.

24 ibid.

25 W. McCrea, Enclosure in 'Aborigines. Report and Correspondence Relative to the Mortality amongst the Residents of the Aboriginal Stations of Victoria', in Papers Presented to Parliament, Legislative Assembly, *Victorian Parliamentary Papers*, Vol. 3, 1879.

26 A. Massola, *Coranderrk. A History of the Aboriginal Station* (Kilmore: Lowden Publishing, 1975).

27 H. E. Brewer, Reports, 2 Jan and 29 April 1874, in 'Eleventh Report of the Board for the Protection of the Aborigines', Papers Presented to Parliament, Legislative Assembly, *Victorian Parliamentary Papers*, Vol. 3, 1875.

28 ibid.

29 J. Jamieson, Letter, 3 May 1876, in 'Eleventh Annual Report of the Board for the Protection of the Aborigines', Papers Presented to Parliament, Legislative Assembly, *Victorian Parliamentary Papers*, Vol. 3, 1875–76.

30 Reverend F. A. Hagenauer, Prepared Statement, 23 May 1877, in 'Royal Commission on the Aborigines', Papers Presented to Parliament, Legislative Assembly', *Victorian Parliamentary Papers*, Vol. 3, 1877–78.

31 P. H. Curson, *Times of Crisis: Epidemics in Sydney 1788–1900* (Sydney: Sydney University Press, 1985).

32 A. D. Cliff and P. Haggett, *The Spread of Measles in Fiji and the Pacific* (Canberra: Australian National University, 1985).

33 E. L. Hamilton, 'Yearly Report for the Year Ending 31 December 1875', in *South Australian Government Gazette*, 6 April 1876.

34 E. L. Hamilton, 'Half-year Report, for Period Ending 31 December 1874', in *South Australian Government Gazette*, 18 March 1875.

35 Hamilton, 1876.

36 Melba Turner, 'A First-Hand Account of the 1948 Measles Epidemic by Sister Melba Turner Sister-in-Charge at the Time', in W. Hilliard, *The People in Between. The Pitjantjatjara People of Ernabella* (London: Hodder and Stoughton, 1968), Appendix II, pp. 230–236); Rani Kerin, '"Natives Allowed to Remain Naked": An Unorthodox Approach to Medical Work at Ernabella Mission', *Health and History*, 8 (1), 2006, pp. 80–99.

37 Isabel McBryde, 'Goods from Another Country: Exchange Networks and the People of the Lake Eyre Basin', in D. J. Mulvaney and J. P. White (eds), *Australians to 1788: Australians, a Historical Library* (Sydney, Fairfax, Syme and Weldon Associates, 1987), pp. 252–273.

38 Hamilton, 1876.

39 ibid.

40 ibid.

41 *South Australian Government Gazette* 18 March 1875, 6 April 1876.

42 G. Taplin, Letter to Sub-Protector of Aborigines, 17 January 1876, PRO SA. GRG 52/1/1876/35.

43 Hamilton, 1876.

44 Taplin, 1876.

45 Peggy Brock and Dawn Kartinyeri, *Poonindie: The Rise and Destruction of an Aboriginal Agricultural Community* (Adelaide: Aboriginal Heritage Branch, Department of Environment and Planning, 1989).

46 Hamilton, 1876.

47 Legislative Council, Western Australia, 'Report of a Commission to Inquire into the Treatment of Aboriginal Native Prisoners of the Crown in this Colony', *Votes and Proceedings of the Legislative Council* (Perth: Government Printer, 1884).
48 Reverend F. A Hagenauer, Report, 18 July 1887, in 'Twenty-third Annual Report of the Board for the Protection of the Aborigines', Papers Presented to Parliament, Legislative Assembly, *Victorian Parliamentary Papers*, Vol. 3, 1887.
49 Edward Frosby, 'Protection of the Aborigines, Report of the Board', in *NSW Votes and Proceedings of the Legislative Assembly*, Part I, 1894.
50 ibid.
51 Report of the Annual Meeting of the Aborigines Friends' Association, Adelaide, *South Australian Register*, 1 September 1894.
52 Francis Gillen, 'Report to Minister Controlling the Northern Territory', *Adelaide Observer*, 11 March 1898.
53 Daisy Bates, *The Passing of the Aborigines: A Lifetime Spent among the Natives of Australia*, 2nd Australian edn (London: Murray, 1947), pp. 84–88.
54 B. R. Adels and D. C. Gajdusek, 'Survey of Measles Patterns in New Guinea, Micronesia and Australia', *American Journal of Hygiene*, 77 (3), 1963, pp. 317–343.
55 Cliff and Haggett, 1985; McNeill, 1976; J. V. Neel, et al., 'Notes on the Effect of Measles and Measles Vaccine in a Virgin-soil Population of South American Indians', *American Journal of Epidemiology*, 91 (4), 1970, pp. 418–429.
56 Cliff and Haggett, 1985.
57 Cliff and Haggett, 1985.
58 N. McArthur, *Island Populations of the Pacific* (Canberra: Australian National University Press, 1967).
59 ibid.
60 Neel et al., 1970; Adels and Gajdusek, 1963; F. L. Black, 'Measles Endemicity in Insular Populations: Critical Community Size and Its Evolutionary Implication', *Journal of Theoretical Biology*, 11 (2), 1966, pp. 207–211.
61 Robert Kim-Farley, 'Measles', in K. Kiple (ed.), *The Cambridge Historical Dictionary of Disease* (Cambridge: Cambridge University Press, 2003), pp. 211–214; Mark Cohen, *Health and the Rise of Civilization* (New Haven: Yale University Press, 1989).
62 Neel et al., 1970.
63 Dowling, 1997.
64 Australian Medical Association, 'Australia Declared Measles-free' (29 April 2014), https://ama.com.au/ausmed/australia-declared-measles-free (accessed October 2018).
65 Centers for Disease Control and Prevention, 'Global Measles Outbreaks', in Global Immunization, https://www.cdc.gov/globalhealth/measles/globalmeaslesoutbreaks.htm (accessed 28 October 20).
66 National Centre for Immunisation Research and Surveillance of Vaccine Preventable Diseases, 'Vaccine Preventable Diseases and Vaccination Coverage in Aboriginal and Torres Strait Islander People, Australia 2006–2010', *Communicable Diseases Intelligence*, 37, Supp., December 2013, http://www.health.gov.au/internet/publications/publishing.nsf/Content/cda-cdi37suppl.htm/$FILE/cdi37suppl.pdf (accessed October 2018).

Chapter 4: Syphilis beyond the Colonial Boundaries

1 H. J. Gibney, 'Sturt, Charles (1795–1869)', in *Australian Dictionary of Biography* (Canberra: National Centre of Biography, Australian National University), http://adb.anu.edu.au/biography/sturt-charles-2712 (accessed Februry2016).
2 Charles Sturt, *Two Expeditions into the Interior of Southern Australia,* Vol. 2 (London: Smith, Elder and Co., 1830) (Facsimile Copy. Sydney: Doubleday, 1982).
3 ibid.
4 ibid, p. 83.
5 ibid., p. 96.

6 ibid., p. 125.
7 ibid., p. 131.
8 ibid., p. 135.
9 ibid., p. 148.
10 Ann G. Carmichael, 'Leprosy (Hansen's Disease)', in K. Kiple (ed.), *The Cambridge World History of Human Disease* (Cambridge: Cambridge University Press, 1993), pp. 192–195; Diana N. J. Lockwood, in David A. Warrell et al. (eds), *Oxford Textbook of Medicine*, Vol. 1, 4th edn (Oxford: Oxford University Press 2003), pp. 575–583.
11 H. Basedow, 'Diseases of the Australian Aborigines', *Journal of Tropical Medicine and Hygiene,* 15 June to 15 September (1932), p. 13; J. B. Cleland, 'Disease among the Australian Aborigines', *Journal of Tropical Medicine and Hygiene,* (5), 1928, pp. 53–59; J. H. L. Cumpston, in M. J. Lewis (ed.), *Health and Disease in Australia: A History* (Canberra: Australian Government Printing Service, 1989); J. J. Elphinstone, 'The Health of Australian Aborigines with No Previous Association with Europeans, *Medical Journal of Australia*, 2 (6), 1971, p. 130.
12 Carmichael, 1993, p. 203; R. T. Steinbock, *Paleopathological Diagnosis and Interpretation: Bone Disease in Ancient Populations* (Springfield: Charles C. Thomas, 1976).
13 Judy Campbell, *Invisible Invaders: Smallpox and Other Diseases in Aboriginal Australia 1780–1880* (Melbourne: Melbourne University Press, 2002), pp. 119–124.
14 Frank Fenner et al., *Smallpox and Its Eradication* (Geneva, World Health Organization, 1988).
15 P. Dowling, '"A Great Deal of Sickness": Introduced Diseases among the Aboriginal People of Colonial Southeast Australia 1788–1900' (Canberra: PhD thesis, Australian National University, 1997), https://digitalcollections.anu.edu.au/handle/1885/7529 (accessed July 2016).
16 ibid., pp. 77–79.
17 E. Beale, *Sturt, the Chipped Idol: A Study of Charles Sturt, Explorer* (Sydney: University Press, 1979).
18 W. H. McNeill, *Plagues and Peoples* (London: Penguin Books, 1976).
19 A. King and C. Nicol, *Venereal Diseases* (London: Baillière, Tindall and Cassell, 1975), p. 197.
20 Cecil J. Hackett, *Diagnostic Criteria of Syphilis, Yaws and Treponarid (Treponematoses) and of Some Other Diseases in Dry Bones* (New York: Springer-Verlag (1976); S. Webb, *Palaeopathology of Aboriginal Australians: Health and Disease across a Hunter-Gatherer Continent* (Cambridge: Cambridge University Press, 1995).
21 Denise Donlon, 'Aboriginal Skeletal Collections and Research in Physical Anthropology: An Historical Perspective', *Australian Archaeology* (39), 1994, pp. 73–82.
22 ibid., p. 78.
23 ibid.
24 K. M. Domett et al., 'Late Holocene Human Remains from Northwest Queensland Australia: Archaeology and Paleopathology', *Archaeology in Oceania*, 41 (1), 2006, pp. 25–36.
25 Flinders University, *Roonka Bioarchaelogy Research Project,* Adelaide, Flinders University, https://www.flinders.edu.au/ehl/archaeology/research-profile/current-projects/roonka-bioarchaeology-redearch-project.cfm (accessed July 2016); C. Smith and J. Littleton, 'Experiencing Childhood at Roonka: An Analysis of Enamel Hypoplasia on the Permanent Dentition of Australian Aboriginal Hunter-Gatherers', *American Journal of Physical Anthropology*, 159, 2016, pp. 294–295.
26 Judith Littleton and Harry Allen, 'Hunter-Gatherer Burials and the Creation of Persistent Places in Southeastern Australia', *Journal of Anthropological Archaeology*, 26 (2), 2007, pp. 283–298.
27 Webb, 1995.
28 Dowling, 1997, pp. 76–78.

29 Hackett, 1976.
30 Kristin N. Harper et al., 'The Origin and Antiquity of Syphilis Revisited: An Appraisal of Old World Pre-Columbian Evidence for Treponemal Infection', *American Journal of Physical Anthropology*, 146 (Suppl. 53), 2011, pp. 99–133, doi:10.1002/ajpa.2163; D. Ortner, *Identification of Pathological Conditions in Human Skeletal Remains*, 2nd edn (San Diego: Academic Press, 2003).
31 Lorenzo Glacabi and Shelia A. Lukehart, 'The Endemic Treponematoses', *Clinical Microbiological Reviews*, 27 (1), 2014, pp. 89–115; Arthur C. Aufderheide and Conrado Rodriguez-Martin, *The Cambridge Encyclopedia of Human Paleopathology* (Cambridge: Cambridge University Press, 1998; reprinted 2003); Ortner 2003.
32 Aufderheide and Rodriguez-Martin, 1998.
33 Webb, 1995, p. 98.
34 J. J. Elphinstone, 'The Health of Australian Aborigines with No Previous Association with Europeans,'*Medical Journal of Australia*, 2, 1971, pp. 293–301.
35 Cleland, 1928, p. 144.
36 Hackett, 1936.
37 Basedow, 1932.
38 Cleland, 1928, p. 141.
39 P. Pirie, 'The Effects of Treponematosis and Gonorrhoea on the Populations of the Pacific Islands', *Human Biology in Oceania*, 1, 1972, p. 189.
40 World Health Organization, 'Yaws' (Fact Sheet), http://www.who.int/mediacentre/factsheets/fs316/en/ (accessed 18 February 2016).
41 Steinbock, 1976, p. 142.
42 Ortner, 2003.
43 ibid.
44 Dowling, 1997, pp. 128–130.
45 Pirie, 1972, p. 192.
46 G. Taplin, *Folklore, Manners and Customs of the South Australian Aborigines* (Adelaide: Government Printer, 1879).
47 Cleland, 1928, p. 142.
48 Dowling, 1997, p. 106.
49 David Collins, *An Account of the English Colony in New South Wales*, Vol I, Reprint edited by B.H. Fletcher (Sydney: A.H. & A.W. Reed, 1985. Originally published London, 1798).
50 Dowling, 1997, pp. 109–111.
51 J. Critchett, *A Distant Field of Murder* (Melbourne: Melbourne University Press, 1990); Dowling, 1997, p. 110.
52 Critchett, 1990.
53 H. D. Moore, 'Notes on the Early Settlers in South Australia prior to 1836', *Proceedings of the Royal Geographical Society of Australasia, South Australian Branch*, 25, 1923, pp. 81–135.
54 J. Summers, 'Colonial Race Relations', in E. Richards (ed.), *Flinders History of South Australia: Social History* (Adelaide: Wakefield Press, 1986), p. 285.
55 ibid., p. 121.
56 Letter from J. M. Mcfarlane to E. Stephens, 1837, Public Records Office, GRG 24/90/366, Adelaide.
57 Cleland, 1928, p. 121.
58 McNeill, 1976, p. 63.
59 A. W. Crosby, 'The Virgin-soil Epidemic as a Factor in the Aboriginal Depopulation in America', *William and Mary Quarterly*, 33, 1976, pp. 289–299.
60 L. B. Marshall, 'Disease Ecologies of Australia and Oceania', in K. Kipple (ed.), *The Cambridge World History of Human Disease* (Cambridge: Cambridge University Press, 1993), p. 490.

Chapter 5: Sexually Transmitted Disease after Colonial Expansion

1 Sir J. Watt, 'The Colony's Health', in J. Hardy and A. Frost (eds), *Studies from Terra Australis to Australia* (Canberra: Australian Academy of the Humanities, 1989).
2 J. White, 'State of Sick Convicts and Marines', 1787, *Historical Records of Australia*, Series 1, Vol. 1, p. 16.
3 David Collins, *An Account of the English Colony in New South Wales*, Vol I, Reprint edited by B.H. Fletcher (Sydney: A.H. & A.W. Reed, 1985. Originally published London, 1798); M. J. Lewis, *Thorns on the Rose: The History of Sexually Transmitted Diseases in Australia in International Perspective* (Canberra: Australian Government Publishing Service, 1998), pp. 20–28.
4 P. H. Curson, *Times of Crisis: Epidemics in Sydney 1788–1900* (Sydney: Sydney University Press, 1985).
5 Collins, 1798, p. 496.
6 ibid.
7 Arthur Phillip, Letter, to Secretary Stevens, 10 July 1788, *Historical Records of Australia*, Series 1, Vol. 1, p. 63.
8 Collins, 1798, p. 29.
9 Peter Cunningham, *Two Years in New South Wales*, Vol. II (London: Henry Colburn, 1827).
10 P. Cussen, Letter to G. A. Robinson, 6 May 1839, Robinson Papers, Vol. 54, ML, A7075-1.
11 P. Cussen, Letter to C. J. La Trobe, 18 November 1839, in M. Cannon (ed.), *Historical Records of Victoria*, Vol. 2B (Melbourne: Victorian Government Printing Office, 1983).
12 C. W. Sievwright, Letter to G. A. Robinson, 5 May 1839, in M. Cannon (ed.), *Historical Records of Victoria*, Vol. 2B (Melbourne: Victorian Government Printing Office, 1983), p. 460.
13 Foster Fyans, Undated letter (c. 1853) in T. F. Bride (ed.), *Letters From Victorian Pioneers* (Melbourne: Heineman, 1969).
14 Edward Parker, Letter to Robinson, 31 December 1840, PRO Vic., VPRS 11 unit 4/156.
15 J. Dredge, Report of the Operations of the Assistant Protector of Aborigines in the Goulburn District from the 1st of July 1839 to the 29th February 1840 Inclusive, PRO Vic., VPRS 4410 Unit 2/47.
16 George Augustus Robinson, 'Journal of an Expedition to the Aborigines of the Eastern Interior Commencing April and Terminating October 1844', in *NSW Governors' Despatches*, Vol. 47, Jan–May 1845, ML A1236.
17 C. Huon et al., Letter to G. A. Robinson, October 3, 1844, in *NSW Governors' Despatches*, Vol. 47, Jan–May 1845, ML A1236.
18 T. H. Goodwin, Letter, 26 November 1860, in 'First Annual Report of the Board for the Protection of the Aborigines', Papers Presented to Parliament, Legislative Assembly, *Victorian Parliamentary Papers*, Vol. 3, Part 1, 1861–62.
19 N. Campbell, Letter to G. A. Robinson, 1 March 1867, Robinson Papers, ML A7078-2 Vol. 57.
20 W. B. Wilmot, Letter to Protector Robinson, 17 August 1842, 'Robinson Papers', Vol. 55, p. 257, ML A7076.
21 A. S. Benenson, *Control of Communicable Diseases in Man*, 15th edn (Washington: American Public Health Association, 1990) pp. 81–82.
22 William Wyatt, in 'Report of the Select Committee of the Legislative Council upon The Aborigines', SAPP No. 165, 1860.
23 M. Moorhouse, Letter to Governor, 19 July 1844, PRO SA GRG 24/6/1844/772.
24 J. Summers, 'Colonial Race Relations', in E. Richards (ed.), *Flinders History of South Australia: Social History* (Adelaide: Wakefield Press, 1986).

25 M. Moorhouse, Protector of Aborigines Quarterly Report, 15 March 1853, *South Australian Government Gazette*, 24 March 1853.

26 J. P. Buttfield, Letter to Acting Protector of Aborigines, 1 April 1867, PRO SA, GRG 52/1/1867/138; Letter to Acting Protector of Aborigines, 18 May 1867, PRO SA, GRG 52/1/1867/246.

27 J. P. Buttfield, Letter to Commissioner for Crown Lands, 11 May 1874, PRO SA, GRG 52/1/1874/163.

28 B. C. Beasley, Annual Report, 11 April 1888, PRO SA 52/1/1888/112.

29 C. A. Meyer, Letter to Sub-Protector of Aborigines, Adelaide, 1880, PRO SA, GRG 52/1/1880/125.

30 C. Stevens, *White Man's Dreaming: Killalpaninna Mission 1866–1915* (Melbourne: Oxford University Press, 1994).

31 C. A. Meyer, Letter to Sub-Protector of Aborigines, Adelaide, 15 January 1885, PRO SA GRG 52/1/1885/125.

32 G. Taplin, Letter to Protector of Aborigines, 20 July 1868, PRO SA GRG 52/1/1868/286.

33 Jade Louise Stingemore, 'Surviving the "Cure": Life on Bernier and Dorre Islands under the Lock Hospital Regime' (Perth: PhD thesis, University of Western Australia, 2010).

34 Mary Anne Jebb, 'The Lock Hospital Experiment: Europeans, Aborigines and Venereal Disease', in Bob Reece and Tom Savage (eds), *European-Aboriginal Relations in Western Australian History* (Nedlands: University of Western Australia, 1984), pp. 68–87.

35 D. J. Mulvaney, *Encounters in Place: Outsiders and Aboriginal Australians 1606–1985* (St Lucia, Qld: University of Queensland Press, 1989).

36 Richard Henry Wace, Submission to Western Australian Government, *Royal Commission on the Condition of the Natives, Report, Appendix C, Minutes of Evidence* (Perth: Government Printer, 1904).

37 Jebb, 1984; Mulvaney, 1989.

38 Cited in Mulvaney, 1989, p. 186.

39 Jebb, 1984; Mulvaney, 1989.

40 Jebb, 1984; Frederick Lovegrove in *Report of the Chief Protector of Aborigines for the Year Ending 30th June 1909* (Perth: Government Printer, 1909).

41 Bates cited in Jebb, 1984.

42 Watson cited in Jebb, 1984.

43 Mulvaney, 1989.

44 P. Dowling, 'Mercury Poisoning at Oyster Cove? Suspected Cases of Unintentional Poisoning of Tasmanian Aboriginal Internees', *Tasmanian Historical Studies*, 11, 2006, pp. 59–68.

45 Lovegrove, 1909; Jebb, 1984.

46 J. R. Hickenbotham and J. Burton Cleland, 'Ulcerative Granuloma of the Pudenda in the Gascoyne District of Western Australia', *Australasian Medical Congress, Transactions of the Eighth Session* (Melbourne: Australian Government Printer, 1909), p. 265.

47 ibid., p. 266.

48 Jacki J. Mein, Nick M. Anstey and Frank J. Bowden, 'Missing the Diagnosis of Donovanosis in Northern Australia', *Medical Journal of Australia*, 170 (1), January 1999, p. 48.

49 Jebb, 1984.

50 Amy Bright and Johanna Dups, 'Infectious and Congenital Syphilis Notifications Associated with an Ongoing Outbreak in Northern Australia', *CDI*, 40 (1), 2016, pp. e7–e10, https://www.health.gov.au/internet/main/publishing.nsf/content/cda-cdi4001-pdf-cnt.htm/$FILE/cdi4001b.pdf (accessed 22 August 2018); Australian Department of Health, 'Multijurisdictional Syphilis Outbreak Surveillance Report: June 2018',

formerly available from http://www.health.gov.au/internet/main/publishing.nsf/Content/71E8A32E7518E532CA25801A0009A217/$File/3rd-Surveil-Report-June-18.pdf (accessed 22 August 2018).

51 Bright and Dups, 2016 (accessed 30 October 2020).

52 Australian Indigenous HealthInfoNet, *Overview of Australian Indigenous and Torres Strait Islander Health Status, 2015* (Perth, WA: Australian Indigenous HealthInfoNet, 2016), http://www.healthinfonet.ecu.edu.au/uploads/resources/31110_31110.pdf (accessed 21 December 2016).

53 Australian Health Protection Principal Committee (AHPPC) Governance Group, *Action Plan: Enhanced Response to Addressing Sexually Transmissible Infections (and Blood Borne Viruses) in Indigenous Populations*, http://www.health.gov.au/internet/main/publishing.nsf/Content/71E8A32E7518E532CA25801A0009A217/$File/Action-Plan-May18.pdf (accessed August 2018).

Chapter 6: Tuberculosis among Aboriginal Populations 1788–1901

1 J. Beaglehole, *The Journals of Captain James Cook on his Voyages of Discovery. The Voyage of the Endeavour 1768–1771* (Cambridge: Hakluyt Society, 1955), p. 307 and footnote 2, http://www.gutenberg.org/files/8106/8106-h/8106-h.htm#ch7 (accessed 3 December 2016).

2 C. A. Roberts and J. E. Buikstra, *The Bioarchaeology of Tuberculosis: A Global View on a Reemerging Disease* (Gainesville: University Press of Florida, 2003).

3 Arthur C. Aufderheide and Conrado Rodriguez-Martin, *The Cambridge Encyclopedia of Human Paleopathology* (Cambridge: Cambridge University Press, 1998; reprinted 2003).

4 M. C. Gutierrez et al., 'Ancient Origin and Gene Mosaicism of the Progenitor of *Mycobacterium tuberculosis*', *PloS Pathogens*, 1 (1) e5, 2005, pp. 55–61; W. T. Johnston, 'Tuberculosis', in K. Kiple (ed.), *The Cambridge Historical Dictionary of Disease* (Cambridge: Cambridge University Press, 2003).

5 Roberts and Buikstra, 2003, p. 6.

6 Roberts and Buikstra, 2003, p. 4.

7 A. McMichael (with A. Woodward and C. Muir), *Climate Change and the Health of Nations* (New York: Cambridge University Press, 2017).

8 W. Farr, 'Statistical Nosology with Explanations', in *Statistical Register of Victoria* (Melbourne: Government Printer, 1854); S. Waksman, *The Conquest of Tuberculosis* (London: Robert Hale Ltd, 1964).

9 World Health Organization, 'Tuberculosis' (Fact Sheet), http://www.who.int/mediacentre/factsheets/fs104/en/ (accessed 11 December 2016).

10 P. Dowling, '"A Great Deal of Sickness": Introduced Diseases among the Aboriginal People of Colonial Southeast Australia 1788–1900' (Canberra: PhD thesis, Australian National University, 1997), https://digitalcollections.anu.edu.au/handle/1885/7529 (accessed July 2016); S. Webb, *Palaeopathology of Aboriginal Australians: Health and Disease across a Hunter-Gatherer Continent* (Cambridge: Cambridge University Press, 1995); Charles MacKay, 'Some Pathological Changes in Australian Aboriginal Bones', Reprint from *Medical Journal of Australia*, 14, 1938, p. 537.

11 Judith Littleton, et al., 'The End of a Plague? Tuberculosis in New Zealand', in D. A. Herring and A. C. Swedlund (eds), *Plagues and Epidemics: Infected Spaces Past and Present* (Oxford: Berg, 2010); L. Bryder, 'Tuberculosis in New Zealand', in A. J. Proust (ed.), *History of Tuberculosis in Australia, New Zealand and Papua New Guinea* (Canberra: Brolga Press, 1991), pp. 79–102.

12 Dowling, 1997; Webb, 1995; Mackay, 1938.

13 Roberts and Buikstra, 2003, p. 92.

14 H. D. Donoghue et al., 'Ancient DNA Analysis – An Established Technique in Charting the Evolution of Tuberculosis and Leprosy', *Tuberculosis*, 95 (Supp. 1), June 2015, pp. S140–S144, http://www.sciencedirect.com/science/article/pii/S1472979215000219 (accessed 9 December 2016).

15 Denise Donlon, 'Aboriginal Skeletal Collections and Research in Physical Anthropology: An Historical Perspective', *Australian Archaeology*, (39), 1994, pp. 73–82.
16 B. Gandevia and J. Cobley, 'Mortality at Sydney Cove, 1788–1792', in *Australian and New Zealand Journal of Medicine*, 4 (2), 1974, pp. 111–125.
17 C. Bateson, *The Convict Ships, 1787–1868* (Glasgow: Brown, Son and Ferguson Ltd, 1959); (Sir) J. Watt, 'The Colony's Health', in J. hardy and A. Frost (eds), *Studies from Terra Australis to Australia* (Canberra, Australian Acadamy of the Humanities, 1989).
18 S. Waksman, 'The Conquest of Tuberculosis' (London: Robert Hale, 1965), pp. 106–108.
19 T. Jamieson, Letter, 3 May 1876, in Eleventh Annual Report of the Board for the Protection of the Aborigines', Papers Presented to Parliament, Legislative Assembly, *Victorian Parliamentary Papers*, Vol. 3, 1875–76.
20 P. G. King, Letter to Nepean 7 August 1803, *Historical Records of Australia*, Series 1, Vol. 4, p. 370.
21 ibid.
22 Gandevia and Cobley, 1974, p. 122.
23 J. H. L. Cumpston, in M. J. Lewis (ed.), *Health and Disease in Australia: A History* (Canberra: Australian Government Printing Service, 1989) p. 276; A. J. Proust, 'Tuberculosis in Australia: Part 1', in A. J. Proust (ed.), *History of Tuberculosis in Australia, New Zealand and Papua New Guinea* (Canberra: Brolga, 1991) p. 5.
24 C. M. H. Clarke, *A History of Australia*, Vol. I (Melbourne: Melbourne University, 1981) p. 123.
25 Cumpston, 1989, p. 276.
26 H. G. Royle, 'The State of Health in New South Wales in the 1820's', in *Medical Journal of Australia* 1 (19), 1973, pp. 950–953.
27 N. J. B. Plomley, *Weep in Silence: A History of the Flinders Island Aboriginal Settlement* (Hobart: Blubber Head Press, 1987), pp. 917–947.
28 ibid., p. 172; L. Ryan, *The Aboriginal Tasmanians*, 2nd edn (Sydney: Allen and Unwin, 1996), p. 203.
29 A. Austin, Autopsy Report, 1837, Robinson Papers, ML A7067; M. Walsh, Autopsy Reports, 1838, Robinson Papers, ML A7070; Plomley, 1987, Appendix II.
30 Dowling, 1997, Appendix A.
31 J. Allen, Letter to G. A. Robinson, 10 September 1837, pp. 201-21, Robinson Papers, ML A7067.
32 Plomley, 1987, Appendix II.
33 C. W. Sievwright, Letter to G. A. Robinson, 5 May, in M. Cannon (ed.), *Historical Records of Victoria*, Vol. 2B (Melbourne: Victorian Government Printing Office, 1983), p. 460.
34 P. Cussen, Letter to G. A. Robinson, 6 May 1839, Robinson Papers Vol. 54, ML A7075-1.
35 J. Watton, Report of Medical and Surgical Cases treated at the Aboriginal Establishment, Mount Rouse, 1 January to 30 November 1840, Public Records Office Vic VPRS 12.
36 J. Watton, 'Quarterly Report of Medical Cases Treated', 1843, Robinson Papers, ML A7077.
37 K. Baylie, Letter to G. A. Robinson, 23 November 1841, Robinson Papers, Vol. 54, ML A 7075.
38 E. M. Curr, *The Australian Race*, Vol. 1 (Melbourne: Government Printer, 1886), p. 227.
39 E. Eyre, 'Manners and Customs of the Aborigines', in *Journals of Expeditions of Discovery*, Vol. 2 (London: T. and W. Boone, 1856), p. 379.
40 W. Thomas, Appendix to 'First Report of the Central Board Appointed to Watch over the Interests of the Aborigines in the Colony of Victoria', in Papers Presented to Both Houses Parliament, *Victorian Parliamentary Papers*, Vol. 3 No. 39, 1861–62, pp. 27–28.
41 Thomas, 1861–62.

42 J. Ann Horne, 'Beveridge, Peter (1829–1885)', *Australian Dictionary of Biography* (Canberra: National Centre of Biography, Australian National University, 1969), http://adb.anu.edu.au/biography/beveridge-peter-2992 (accessed 13 December 2016).
43 P. Beveridge, *The Aborigines of Victoria and Riverina* (Melbourne: M. L. Hutchinson, 1889).
44 A. Lourie, 'From the Paddock to the Page: Squatter Peter Beveridge's Ethnological Writing about the Wadi Wadi in Colonial Victoria', in *Oceania*, 86 (3), 2016, pp. 244–261.
45 A. Noymer, 'Epidemics and Time: Influenza and Tuberculosis during and after the 1918–1919 Pandemic', in D. A Herring and A. C. Swedlund (eds), *Plagues and Epidemics: Infected Spaces Past and Present* (Oxford: Berg, 2010).
46 H. D. Moore, 'Notes on the Early Settlers in South Australia prior to 1836', in *Proceedings of the Royal Geographical Society of Australasia, South Australian Branch*, 25, 1923, pp. 81–135; J. Summers, 'Colonial Race Relations', in E. Richards (ed.), *Flinders History of South Australia: Social History* (Adelaide: Wakefield Press, 1986).
47 Dowling, 1997.
48 G. Taplin, Letter, 'The Diseases of the Aborigines of South Australia', 20 January 1876, PRO SA, GRG 52/1/1876/36; G. Taplin, *The Folklore, Manners, Customs, and Languages of the South Australian Aborigines* (Adelaide: Government Printer, 1879) (Facsimile Edition, 1989), p. 44.
49 Dowling, 1997, pp. 141–175.
50 G. Taplin, Letter to Sub-Protector of Aborigines, 17 January 1876, PRO SA, GRG 52/1/1876/35.
51 P. Webb and C. Bain, *Essential Epidemiology: An Introduction for Students and Health Professionals* (Cambridge: Cambridge University Press, 2011), p. 239.
52 E. M. Curr and A. C. Le Souef, Letter, 21 May 1879, in 'Fifteenth Annual Report of the Board for the Protection of the Aborigines', Papers Presented to Parliament, Legislative Assembly, *Victorian Parliamentary Papers*, Vol. 3, 1879.
53 Australian Government, 'The Australian Gold Rush', formerly available from www.australia.gov.au/about-australia/australian-story/austn-gold-rush (accessed 10 January 2017).
54 Registrar General, 'Births, Deaths and Marriages of the Colony of Victoria', 'Third Annual Report of the Board for the Protection of the Aborigines', Papers Presented to Parliament, Legislative Assembly, *Victorian Parliamentary Papers*, Vol. 4, Part 1, 1856–57.
55 W. L. Richardson, 'Notes on Some of the Diseases Prevalent in Victoria, Australia', *Edinburgh Medical Journal*, 14, 1869, pp. 802–812.
56 Dowling, 1997.
57 E. H. Ruddock, *On Consumption and Tuberculosis of the Lungs*, 2nd edn (London: Homeopathic Publishing Company, 1873).
58 W. T. Johnston, 'Tuberculosis', in K. Kiple (ed.), *The Cambridge World History of Human Disease* (Cambridge: Cambridge University Press, 1993), pp. 1061–1062.
59 Proust, 'Tuberculosis in Australia: Part 1',1991.
60 J. B. Cleland, 'Some Early References to Tuberculosis in Australia', *Medical Journal of Australia*, 1, 1938, pp. 256–258.
61 A. J. Proust, 'Migration of Consumptives to Australia', in A. J. Proust (ed.), *History of Tuberculosis in Australia, New Zealand and Papua New Guinea* (Canberra: Brolga Press, 1991).
62 Cumpston, 1989, pp. 276–299; M. J. Lewis, 'Medicine in Colonial Australia, 1788–1900', *Medical Journal of Australia*, 201 (1), Supplement, 'History of Australian Medicine', 2014, pp. S5-S10.
63 P. Dowling, 'Mercury Poisoning at Oyster Cove? Suspected Cases of Unintentional Poisoning of Tasmanian Aboriginal Internees', *Tasmanian Historical Studies*, 11, 2006, pp. 59–68.

64 Australian Indigenous HealthInfoNet, *Overview of Australian Indigenous and Torres Strait Islander Health Status, 2015* (Perth, WA: Australian Indigenous HealthInfoNet, 2016), http://www.healthinfonet.ecu.edu.au/uploads/resources/31110_31110.pdf (accessed 21 December 2016).

Chapter 7: Influenza

1 C. W. Potter, 'A History of Influenza', *Journal of Applied Microbiology*, 91 (4), 2001, pp. 572–579.

2 Richard Sisley, *Epidemic Influenza: Notes on the Origin and Method of Spread* (New York: Longman Green and Co., 1891).

3 W. Ramsay Smith, *The Control of Communicable Diseases in South Australia* (Adelaide: Government Printer, 1919).

4 Centers for Disease Control and Prevention, 'Types of Influenza Viruses', formerly available from www.cdc.gov/flu/about/viruses/type.htm (accessed 24 May 2017).

5 Scott Krauss and Robert G. Webster, 'Avian Influenza Virus Surveillance and Wild Birds: Past and Present', *Avian Diseases*, 54 (Supp. 1), March 2010, pp. 394–398.

6 Richard Falcon and H. Bradford Hawley, 'Influenza', in *Magill's Medical Guide*, 4th edn (Pasadena: Salem Press, 2008).

7 For reviews of influenza introduction in the New World populations see: H. F. Dobyns, *Their Numbers Become Thinned* (Knoxville: University of Tennessee Press, 1983); F. Guerra, 'The Earliest American Epidemic: The Influenza of 1493', *Social Science and History*, 12 (3), 1988, pp. 305–25; J. W. Verano and D. H. Ubelaker (eds), *Disease and Demography in the Americas* (Washington: Smithsonian Institution Press, 1992).

8 For reviews of influenza introduction in the Pacific see: R. Lange, 'Plagues and Pestilence in Polynesia: The Nineteenth-century Cook Islands Experience', *Bulletin of the History of Medicine*, 58, 1984, pp. 325–46; R. Macleod and M. Lewis (eds), *Disease, Medicine and Empire: Perspectives on Western Medicine and the Experience of European Expansion* (London: Routledge, 1988); L. B. Marshall, 'Disease Ecologies of Australia and Oceania', in K. Kipple (ed.), *The Cambridge World History of Human Disease* (Cambridge: Cambridge University Press, 1993).

9 J. H. L. Cumpston, *Influenza and Maritime Quarantine in Australia* (Quarantine Service Publication No. 18. Melbourne: Government Printer, 1919).

10 Simon Chapple, 'Death and Disease at the Dawn of New Zealand's History', The Turnbull Library Record No. 50, 2018, https:/www.researchgate.net/publication/327427166 (accessed September 2018).

11 D. McLeod, 'Questions Proposed by the Royal College of Physicians', in *NSW Governors' Despatches to the Sec of State for the Colonies*, Vol. 17, Jan–April 1830, ML A1206.

12 Epidemic dates sourced from: W. I. B. Beveridge, *Influenza: The Last Great Plague. An Unfinished Story of Discovery* (London: Heinemann, 1977); A. W. Crosby, 'Influenza', in Kiple, 1993; J. H. L. Cumpston, *Influenza and Maritime Quarantine in Australia*, Commonwealth of Australia Quarantine Service Publication No. 18 (Melbourne: Government Printer, 1919); M. J. Lewis (ed.), *Health and Disease in Australia: A History* (Canberra: Australian Government Printing Service, 1989); H. O. Lancaster, 'The Mortality in Australia from Influenza and from Diseases of the Respiratory System', *Medical Journal of Australia*, 2, 1953, pp. 672–676; M. F. Warburton, 'Epidemiology of Influenza in Australia and Papua New Guinea', *Medical Journal of Australia*, 1 (Special Supp.), 1973, pp. 14–18.

13 *Australian Almanac of Sydney*, 'A Chronologic Table of Remarkable Events from the Foundation of the Colony to the Close of the Year 1832', *Australian Almanac of Sydney: Directory for the Year of Our Lord 1834*, p. 245.

14 P. Cunningham, *Two Years in New South Wales*, Vol. II (London: Henry Colburn, 1827).
15 Cited in H. G. Royle, 'The State of Health in New South Wales in the 1820's', *Medical Journal of Australia*, 1 (19), 1973, pp. 950–953.
16 J. H. L. Cumpston, in M. J. Lewis (ed.), *Health and Disease in Australia: A History* (Canberra: Australian Government Printing Service, 1989), pp. 313–314.
17 P. H. Curson, *Times of Crisis: Epidemics in Sydney 1788–1900* (Sydney: Sydney University Press, 1985, p. 125).
18 'Medical Gentleman' Letter to Editor, *Sydney Gazette*, 16 December 1820.
19 Cumpston, 1989, p. 313.
20 L. E. (Rev.) Threlkeld, 'Annual Report of the Mission to the Aborigines, Lake Macquarie,' 1835, Threlkeld Papers, ML A382.
21 N. J. B. Plomley, *Weep in Silence: A History of the Flinders Island Aboriginal Settlement* (Hobart: Blubber Head Press, 1987.
22 ibid., p. 328.
23 ibid., p. 35.
24 Cumpston, 1989, p. 313.
25 L. Ryan, *The Aboriginal Tasmanians*, 2nd edn (Sydney: Allen and Unwin, 1996), pp. 66–67; L. Ryan, *Tasmanian Aborigines: A History since 1803* (Sydney: Allen and Unwin, 2012), pp. 186–187.
26 Plomley, 1987, p. 938.
27 ibid.; Ryan, 1996, p. 186.
28 Ryan, 1996, p. 186; Ryan, 2012, p. 228.
29 Plomley, 1987, pp. 92–94.
30 Plomley, 2008, p. 932; Plomley, 1987, pp. 91–92; Ryan, 1996, p. 196.
31 Plomley 1987, pp. 937–946.
32 ibid., p. 916.
33 J. Allen, Letter to G. A. Robinson, 10 September 1837, Robinson Papers, ML A7067 pp. 201–21; Plomley, 1987, pp. 923–924.
34 ibid.
35 Plomley, 1987, pp. 940–941.
36 ibid.
37 M. Walsh, Autopsy Report to G. A. Robinson, 25 October 1837, Robinson Papers, ML A7068 pp. 53–4; ML A7069.
38 Plomley, 1987, p. 785.
39 ibid.
40 Ryan, 1996, p. 193; Ryan, 2012, p. 237.
41 George Robinson, Jnr., Journal, 24 February to 22 March 1839, ML A7071 pp. 217–235.
42 Plomley, 1987, p. 942.
43 ibid., p. 787.
44 Plomley, 1987, p. 162.
45 Ryan, 1996, pp. 205–212; Ryan, 2012, p. 257.
46 J. Bonwick, *The Last of the Tasmanians: Or the Black War of Van Diemen's Land* (London: Sampson, Low, Son and Marston, 1870), pp. 276–285.
47 Ryan, 1996, pp. 205–214; Ryan, 2012.
48 Plomley, 1987, pp. 186–187.
49 William Smith, Entries in the Oyster Cove Aboriginal Station Visiting Officers Book (1858–1869), AO Tas., CSO/89/A171/3.
50 Smith, 1858–69; Plomley, 1987, p. 945.
51 Plomley, 1987, p. 798; Ryan 1996, pp. 124, 131.
52 Plomley, 1987, p. 833; Ryan 1996, p. 214.
53 Plomley, 1987, p. 945.

54 Journal of William Thomas, 17 and 18 January 1839, 12 February 1839, in M. Cannon (ed.), *Historical Records of Victoria*, vol. 2B (Melbourne: Victorian Government Printing Office, 1983).
55 George Augustus Robinson, Journal entry, 20 February 1839, in N. J. B. Plomley (ed.), *Weep in Silence: A History of the Flinders Island Aboriginal Settlement* (Hobart: Blubber Head Press, 1987).
56 George Augustus Robinson, Letter, 30 March 1839, Col. Sec. Papers, AO NSW 4/2471.
57 ibid.
58 Thomas, Journal, January 1839, in Canon, 1983.
59 P. Cussen, Letter to G. A. Robinson, 6 May 1839, Robinson Papers, Vol. 54, ML A7075-1.
60 *Port Phillip Gazette*, 8 May 1839.
61 E. A. Addis, Letter to Governor Gipps, 28 December 1839, Gipps Despatches, Vol. 38, ML A1227.
62 J. Clerk, Letter to Sub-Protector Sievwright, 9 August 1839, in Cannon, M. (ed.), *Historical Records of Victoria*, Vol. 2B (Melbourne: Victorian Government Printing Office, 1983).
63 Thomas, 1839, in Canon, 1983.
64 Cumpston, 1989, p. 313.
65 George Augustus Robinson, Chief Protector's Report for 1845, PRO Vic VPRS 4399 Unit 1/1.
66 ibid.
67 Cumpston, 1989, p. 313.
68 W. Thomas, Letter, July 1852, in Despatches from the Lieutenant Governor of Victoria to the Secretary of State for the Colonies, No. 34, ML A2342.
69 W. Thomas, Appendix to 'First Annual Report of the Board for the Protection of the Aborigines', Papers Presented to Parliament, Legislative Assembly, *Victorian Parliamentary Papers*, Vol. 3, 1861–62.
70 J. Gibson, reports, in 'Annual Report of the Board for the Protection of the Aborigines', Papers Presented to Parliament, Legislative Assembly, *Victorian Parliamentary Papers*, Vol. 4, 1869; Vol. 3, 1871; Vol. 3, Part 2, 1872; Vol. 3, Part 1, 1873; Vol. 3, Part 1, 1874; Vol. 3, 1875–76.
71 W. Farr, 'Statistical Nosology with Explanations', *Statistical Register of Victoria* (Melbourne: Government Printer, 1854).
72 H. Basedow, 'Diseases of the Australian Aborigines', *Journal of Tropical Medicine and Hygiene*, Reprint, 15 June to 15 September (1932); Cumpston, 1989, p. 330.
73 Cumpston, 1989, p. 331.
74 J. H. Stahle, Report, 8 August 1889, in 'Twenty-sixth Annual Report of the Board for the Protection of the Aborigines', Papers Presented to Parliament, Legislative Assembly, *Victorian Parliamentary Papers*, Vol. 4, 1890.
75 M. Moorhouse, Letter to Governor, 19 July 1844, PRO SA GRG 24/6/1844/772.
76 M. Moorhouse, Protector of Aborigines Quarterly Report, 15 October 1850, *South Australian Government Gazette*, 31 October 1850, p. 611.
77 ibid., 8 July 1843, in Papers Relating to Australia, *British Parliamentary Papers*, Vol. 8.
78 ibid., 7 October 1843, PRO SA GRG 24/4/1843/132; ibid., 15 October, *South Australian Government Gazette*, 31 October 1850.
79 *South Australian Register*, 25 July 1855.
80 M. Moorhouse, Protector of Aborigines Quarterly Report, 15 March, *South Australian Government Gazette,* 24 March 1853.
81 ibid., 8 July, *South Australian Government Gazette*, 15 July 1852.
82 ibid., 15 March, *South Australian Government Gazette,* 24 March 1853.
83 Archdeacon Hale, Extract of Quarterly Report on Poonindie Mission, 24 December 1853, *Adelaide Observer.*

84 O. Hammond, 'State of Health at Poonindie Mission', Report, 19 September, *South Australian Parliamentary Papers*, Vol. 2, 1857–58.
85 G. Taplin, Letter to Protector of Aborigines, 20 July 1868, PRO SA GRG 52/1/1868/286.
86 J. P. Buttfield, Letter to Acting Protector of Aborigines, 5 July 1866, PRO SA, GRG 52/1/1866/115.
87 G. Taplin, Letter to Protector of Aborigines, 20 July 1868, PRO SA GRG 52/1/1868/286.
88 E. L Hamilton, 'Yearly Report for the Year Ending 31 December 1878', in *South Australian Government Gazette,* 20 March 1879.
89 *South Australian Government Gazette*, 20 August 1874, pp. 1673–1674; 18 March 1875, p. 516; 6 April 1876, pp. 643–4, Table II Showing the Number of Aborigines, Males and Females, in each County and Pastoral District of South Australia, at the Date of the Census of 1871 and 1876, p. 798; 'Summary Showing the Number of Aborigines in Each County and Pastoral District of the Province of South Australia, at Date of Census', 20 March 1879.
90 E. L. Hamilton, Report, 15 March 1874, *South Australian Government Gazette*, 18 March 1874; J. P. Buttfield, Letter to Commissioner for Crown Lands, 11 May 1874, PRO SA, GRG 52/1/1874/163.
91 M. Williams, 'The Spread of Settlement in South Australia', in F. Gale and G. H. Lawton (eds), *Settlement and Encounter* (London: Oxford University Press, 1969), p. 26.
92 J. P. Buttfield, Letter to Commissioner for Crown Lands, 6 June 1870, PRO SA, GRG 52/1/1870/124.
93 J. P. Buttfield, Letter to Commissioner for Crown Lands, 6 August 1870, PRO SA, GRG 52/1/1870/248.
94 ibid., 23 May 1871 and 6 June 1871, PRO SA, GRG 52/1/1871/109.
95 C. Stevens, *White Man's Dreaming: Killalpaninna Mission 1866–1915* (Melbourne: Oxford University Press, 1994), p. 112.
96 Cumpston, 1989, p. 331.
97 Beasley, 1888, cited in *The Advertiser*, 29 March 1893.
98 Alfred R. Waylen, M.D., 'Report by the Colonial Surgeon on the Condition of the Sick Native Prisoners at Rottnest Prison', *Legislative Council of Western Australia* (Perth: Government Printer, 1883).
99 ibid.
100 P. Curson and K. McCracken, 'An Australian Perspective of the 1918–1919 Influenza Pandemic', *NSW Public Health Bulletin*, 17 (7–8), 2006, p. 106.
101 G. Briscoe, *Queensland Aborigines and the Spanish Influenza Pandemic of 1918–1919*, Occasional Paper No. 3/1996 (Canberra: Australian Institute of Aboriginal and Torres Strait Islander Studies, 1996).
102 ibid., p. 13.
103 *Morning Bulletin* (Rockhampton), 9 June 1919, p. 8.
104 J. Atherton Young (ed.), *Jane Bardsley's Outback Letterbook, Across the Years 1896–1936* (Sydney: Angus and Robertson, 1987), p. 206.
105 J. H. L. Cumpston, *Influenza and Maritime Quarantine in Australia* (Quarantine Service Publication No. 18. Melbourne: Government Printer, 1919).
106 P. H. Curson, *Times of Crisis: Epidemics in Sydney 1788–1900* (Sydney: Sydney University Press, 1985), p. 9.
107 Ryan, 1996, pp. 66–72; M. Johnson and I. McFarlane, *Van Diemen's Land: An Aboriginal History* (Sydney: University of New South Wales Press, 2015), pp. 116–124.
108 R. A. Fitzgerald, *A History of Queensland from the Dreaming to 1915* (St Lucia: University of Queensland Press, 1982), p. 135; N. Loos, *Invasion and Resistance: Aboriginal–European Relations on the North Queensland Frontier 1861–1897* (Canberra: Australian National University Press, 1982), p. 31.

109 A. Breinl and M. J. Holmes, 'Medical Report on the Data Collected During a Journey Through Some Districts of the Northern Territory', *Bulletin of the Northern Territory*, 15, December 1915.
110 Daisy Bates, *The Passing of the Aborigines: A Lifetime Spent among the Natives of Australia*, 2nd Australian edn (London: Murray, 1947), p. 169.
111 *South Australian Weekly Chronicle*, 2 March 1861.

Chapter 8: Disease in Aboriginal Settlements, Victoria and South Australia

1 P. Dowling, '"A Great Deal of Sickness": Introduced Diseases among the Aboriginal People of Colonial Southeast Australia 1788–1900' (Canberra: PhD thesis, Australian National University, 1997), https://digitalcollections.anu.edu.au/handle/1885/7529 (accessed July 2016).
2 'Royal Commission on the Aborigines', Census of the Aboriginal Natives in the Colony of Victoria, *Victorian Parliamentary Papers*, Vol. 3, 1877–78; G. Taplin, Letter, 'The Diseases of the Aborigines of South Australia', 20 January 1876, PRO SA, GRG 52/1/1876/36; South Australian Government, 'Summary Showing the Number of Aborigines in Each County and Pastoral District of the Province of South Australia, at Date of Census' (Adelaide: South Australian Government Printer, 1879).
3 J. P. M. Long, *Aboriginal Settlements: A Survey of Institutional Communities in Eastern Australia* (Canberra: Australian National University Press, 1970), p. 15; Richard Broome, *Aboriginal Australians: A History Since 1788*, 4th edn (Sydney: Allen and Unwin, 2010), pp. 149–171.
4 Diane Barwick, 'Coranderrk and Cumeroogunga: Pioneers and Policy', in T. Scarlett Epstein and D. H. Penny (eds), *Opportunity and Response: Case Studies in Economic Development* (London: C. Hurst and Co., 1972).
5 W. McCrea, Enclosure in 'Aborigines. Report and Correspondence Relative to the Mortality amongst the Residents of the Aboriginal Stations of Victoria', in *Papers Presented to Parliament, Legislative Assembly, Victorian Parliamentary Papers*, Vol. 3, 1879.
6 ibid.
7 Phillip Pepper and Tess De Arago, *What Did Happen to the Aborigines of Victoria: The Kurnai of Gippsland*, Vol. 1 (Melbourne: Hyland House, 1985).
8 ibid.
9 For more detailed information about the living conditions on the Aboriginal settlements see: P. Brock, *Outback Ghettos: Aborigines, Institutionalisation and Survival* (Cambridge: Cambridge University Press, 1993); R. Broome, *Aboriginal Australians: Black Response to White Dominance 1788–1980* (Sydney: Allen and Unwin, 1993); G. Jenkin, *Conquest of the Ngarrindjeri: The Story of the Lower Murray Lakes Tribes* (Adelaide: Rigby, 1979); A. Massola, *Aboriginal Mission Stations in Victoria* (Melbourne: The Hawthorn Press, 1970).
10 M. Morgan, *Nosological Index 1863 and Staff and Registrars of the Registrar-General's Department Victoria 1862* (Blackburn: Marjorie Morgan Publications, 1987).
11 J. Bulmer, 'Fifteenth Report of the Board for the Protection of the Aborigines', Papers Presented to Parliament, Legislative Assembly, *Victorian Parliamentary Papers*, Vol. III, 1879.
12 J. H. L. Cumpston, 'Smallpox', in M. J. Lewis (ed.), *Health and Disease in Australia: A History* (Canberra: Australian Government Printing Service, 1989).
13 Cumpston, 'Measles', ibid.
14 Dowling, 1997, pp. 304–305.
15 Australian Indigenous HealthInfoNet, *Overview of Aboriginal and Torres Strait Islander Health Status, 2017* (Perth, WA: Australian Indigenous HealthInfoNet, 2018), p. 9.

Chapter 9: A Personal Understanding

1 Charles Darwin, *The Voyage of the Beagle*, Harvard Classics, Vol. 29 (New York: P. F. Collier and Son, 1909), p. 424, http://www.homeworknow.com/uploads/59b6087ad3def86fd94edef9c0ec5ce4.pdf (accessed 14 August 2020).
2 ibid., p. 435.
3 Cassandra Pybus, *Truganini: Journey through the Apocalypse* (Sydney: Allen and Unwin, 2020), p. 12.
4 Rae-Ellis, 1976, p. 35.
5 Pybus, 2020, p. 24.
6 ibid.
7 N. J. B. Plomley (ed.), *Friendly Mission: The Tasmanian Journals and Papers of George Augustus Robinson 1829–1834* 2nd edition (Hobart: Queen Victoria Museum and Art Gallery, Hobart: Quintus, 2008).
8 Pybus, 2020, p. 84.
9 Plomley, 2008, Appendix II.
10 Pybus, 2020, p. 149.
11 Rae-Ellis, 1976, p. 67.
12 Vivienne Rae-Ellis, 'Truganini', *Tasmanian Historical Research Association. Papers and Proceedings*, 23 (2), 1976, pp. 26–43; Peter J. Roberts-Thompson, 'Impact of Introduced Disease into Tasmanian Aboriginal Populations and Its Role in Depopulation', *Tasmanian Historical Research Association, Papers and Proceedings*, 61 (2–3), December 2014, pp. 119–135.
13 Pybus, 2020, p. 175.
14 N. J. B. Plomley, *Weep in Silence: A History of the Flinders Island Aboriginal Settlement* (Hobart: Blubber Head Press, 1987), Appendix II.
15 Pybus, 2020, pp. 206–220.
16 Powlett to Superintendent C. J. Latrobe, in Ian MacFarlane, *1842: The Public Executions at Melbourne* (Melbourne: Public Records Office, 1984).
17 Samuel Rawson, *Journal of an Expedition after Some Van Diemen's Land Blacks Who Were Committing Depredations at Western Port on the Southern Coast of New Holland, October–November 1841*, National Library of Australia, MS 204/1.
18 Kate Auty and Lynette Russell, *Hunt Them, Hang Them: The Tasmanians in Port Phillip, 1841–42* (Melbourne: Justice Press, 2016); Rawson, National Library of Australia, MS 204/1; Marguerita Stephens, *The Journal of William Thomas: Assistant Protector of the Aborigines of Port Phillip and Guardian of the Aborigines of Victoria 1839–1867*, Vol. One: 1839 to 1843 (Melbourne: Victorian Aboriginal Corporation for Languages, 2004), p. 410; MacFarlane, 1984.
19 Cassandra Pybus, 'Journey through the Apocalypse: Ria Warrawah, Wooredy and Truganini', *Griffith Review*, 58, October 2017, https://griffithreview.com/articles/journey-through-the-apocalypse-ria-warrah-wooredy-truganini/ (accessed 10 September 2019).
20 J. Broadfoot, quoted in Plomley, 1987, p. 145.
21 Plomley, 1987, pp. 915–937.
22 ibid., Appendix II.
23 Letters from J. S. Dandridge Commandant Oyster Cove to Colonial Secretary Hobart, AO Tas., CSD4/77/231; William Smith, Entries in the Oyster Cove Aboriginal Station Visiting Officers Book (1858–1869), AO Tas., CSO/89/A171/3.
24 J. S. Dandridge to Colonial Secretary, Hobart, AO Tas., CSD4/77/231.
25 W. Smith, CSO/89/A171/3.
26 J. S. Dandridge to Colonial Secretary, Hobart, AO Tas., CSD4/77/231.
27 P. Dowling, 'Mercury Poisoning at Oyster Cove? Suspected Cases of Unintentional Poisoning of Tasmanian Aboriginal Internees', *Tasmanian Historical Studies*, 11, 2006, pp. 59–68.
28 ibid., pp. 66–68.
29 ibid., p. 68.

30 Pybus, 2020, pp. 262–263.
31 ibid., pp. 265–267.
32 Frank Olaf Meumann, 'An Anthroposcopic and Anthropometric Study of the Skeleton of a Full-blood Female Tasmanian Aborigine (Truganini)' (Tasmania: B. Med Sc. Thesis, University of Tasmania, 1971).
33 S. Webb, *Palaeopathology of Aboriginal Australians: Health and Disease across a Hunter-Gatherer Continent* (Cambridge: Cambridge University Press, 1995).

Chapter 10: In the Time of COVID-19

1 'Corona Virus Disease 2019 (COVID-19)', *British Medical Journal, Best Practice*, https://bestpractice.bmj.com/topics/en-us/3000168/aetiology (accessed 29 September 2020).
2 Daisy Bates, *The Passing of the Aborigines: A Lifetime Spent among the Natives of Australia*, 2nd Australian edn (London: Murray, 1947).
3 Mark Mousseau, 'H1N1 in Retrospect: A Review of Risk Factors and Policy Recommendations', *International Indigenous Policy Journal* 4 (2), April, 2013, https://search.proquest.com/openview/1ec2ee701aa7c0306abbc825b240ed9a/1?pq-origsite=gscholar&cbl=1996357 (accessed 22 September 2020); Tamara Power et al., 'COVID-19 and Indigenous Peoples: An Imperative for Action', *Journal of Clinical Nursing* 29, pp. 2737-2741), https://onlinelibrary.wiley.com/doi/full/10.1111/jocn.15320 (accessed 22 September 2020).
4 Kristy Crooks, Dawn Casey and James S. Ward, 'First Nations People Leading the Way in the COVID-19 Pandemic: Planning, Response and Management', *Medical Journal of Australia*, Preprint, 29 April 2020.
5 ibid.
6 World Bank List of Economies 2020, https://datahelpdesk.worldbank.org/knowledgebase/articles/906519 (accessed 28 September 2020).
7 Ian Anderson et al., 'Indigenous and Tribal Peoples' Health (The Lancet-Lowitja Institute Global Collaboration): A Population Study', *The Lancet*, Vol 388, 9 July 2016, pp. 131–157, https://www.thelancet.com/journals/lancet/article/PIIS0140-6736(16)00345-7/fulltext (accessed 18 January 2021).
8 Extracted from the transcript by Adrian Carson et al., 'Urban Aboriginal People Face Unique Challenges in the Fight against Coronavirus', *The Conversation*, 24 April 2020, https://theconversation.com/urban-aboriginal-people-face-unique-challenges-in-the-fight-against-coronavirus-136050 (accessed 23 September 2020).
9 Dianne Smith, 'Governing the Pandemic: Implications for Indigenous Self-Determination and self-Government, in F. Markham, D. Smith and F. Morphy (eds), *Indigenous Australians and the COVID-19 Crisis: Perspectives on Public Policy*, https://openresearch-repository.anu.edu.au/bitstream/1885/202733/1/CAEPR_TI_no1_2020_Markham_Smith_Morphy.pdf (accessed 21 September 2020).
10 Aboriginal and Torres Strait Islander Advisory Group on COVID-19, Communique 17 August 2020, https://www.health.gov.au/sites/default/files/documents/2020/08/aboriginal-and-torres-strait-islander-advisory-group-on-covid-19-communiques-17-august-2020-communique_1.pdf (accessed 21 September 2020); Crooks, Casey and Ward, 2020.
11 Yanyuwa Families, Amanda Kearney and John Bradley, 'From Sorcery to Laboratory: Pandemics and Yanyuwa Experiences of Viral Vulnerability', *Oceania*, Special Issue, 'Oceanic Societies in COVID-19', 2020.
12 ibid.
13 ibid.
14 'Lessons from Previous Pandemics Help Indigenous Community Keep Out COVID-19', Lens, Monash University, 7 August 2020, https://lens.monash.edu/@politics-society/2020/08/07/1381018/lessons-from-previous-pandemics-help-indigenous-community-keep-covid-19-out (accessed 29 September 2020.

BIBLIOGRAPHY

Archival Sources

Archives Office of New South Wales

Bowman, J., Letter to Colonial Secretary, 10 October 1831, AO NSW 4/2130.

Busby, G., Letter to Inspector of Colonial Hospitals, 19 October 1831, AO NSW 4/2130.

Mair, J., 'Observation on the Eruptive Febrile Disease which Prevailed among Several Tribes of the Aborigines in New South Wales during the Years 1830 and 31', AO NSW 4/2180, 1831.

Mair, J., and J. Imlay, Letter to Colonial Secretary, 24 December 1831, AO NSW 4/2130.

Robinson, George Augustus, Letter, 30 March 1839, Col. Sec. Papers, AO NSW 4/2471.

Thompson, L. D., Minutes of the Executive Council, 29 December 1831, AO NSW 4/1517.

Archives Office of Tasmania

Dandridge, J. S., Commandant Oyster Cove, Letters to Colonial Secretary Hobart, AO Tas., CSD4/77/231.

Smith, William, Entries in the Oyster Cove Aboriginal Station Visiting Officers Book (1858–1869), AO Tas., CSO/89/A171/3.

Historical Records of Australia

King George III, Instructions to Governor Phillip, 25 April 1787, *Historical Records of Australia*, Series 1, Vol. 1.

King, P. G., Letter to Nepean, 7 August 1803, *Historical Records of Australia*, Series 1, Vol. 4.

Phillip, Arthur, Letter to Lord Sydney, 15 May 1788, *Historical Records of Australia*, Series 1, Vol. 1.

Phillip, Arthur, Letter to Secretary Stevens, 10 July 1788, *Historical Records of Australia*, Series 1, Vol. 1.

Phillip, Arthur, Letter to Lord Sydney, 30 October 1788, *Historical Records of Australia*, Series 1, Vol. 1.

Phillip, Arthur, Letter to Lord Sydney, 13 February 1790, *Historical Records of Australia*, Series 1, Vol. 1.

White, J., 'State of Sick Convicts and Marines', 1787, *Historical Records of Australia*, 1 (1), p. 16.

Mitchell Library

Addis, E. A., Letter to Governor Gipps, 28 December 1839, Gipps Despatches Vol. 38, ML A1227.

Allen, J., Letter to G. A. Robinson, 10 September 1837, Robinson Papers, ML A7067.

Austin, A., Autopsy Report, 1837, Robinson Papers, ML A7067.

Baylie, K., Letter to G. A. Robinson, 23 November 1841, Robinson Papers, Vol. 54, ML A7075.

Campbell, N., Letter to G. A. Robinson, 1 March 1867, Robinson Papers, ML A7078-2 Vol. 57.

Cussen, P., Letter to G. A. Robinson, 6 May 1839, Robinson Papers, Vol. 54, ML A7075-1.

Huon, C., R. Rae, A. Huon, W. Huon and R. Brown, Letter to G. A. Robinson, 3 October 1844, in *NSW Governors' Despatches* Vol. 47, Jan–May 1845, ML A1236.

McLeod, D., 'Questions Proposed by the Royal College of Physicians', in *NSW Governors' Despatches to the Sec of State for the Colonies*, Vol. 17, Jan–April 1830, ML A1206.

Robinson, George Jnr, Journal, 24 February to 22 March 1839, ML A7071.

Robinson, George Augustus, 'Journal of an Expedition to the Aborigines of the Eastern Interior Commencing April and Terminating October 1844', in *NSW Governors' Despatches*, Vol. 47, Jan–May 1845, ML A1236.

Thomas, W., Letter from the Lieutenant Governor of Victoria to the Secretary of State for the Colonies, July 1852, in Despatches, No. 34, ML A2342.

Threlkeld, L. E. (Rev.), 'Annual Report of the Mission to the Aborigines, Lake Macquarie,' 1835, Threlkeld Papers, ML A382.

Walsh, M., Autopsy Report to G. A. Robinson, 25 October 1837, Robinson Papers, ML A7068 pp. 53–4; ML A7069.

Walsh, M., Autopsy Reports, 1838, Robinson Papers, ML A7070.

Watton, J., 'Quarterly Report of Medical Cases Treated', 1843, Robinson Papers, ML A7077.

Wilmot, W. B., Letter to Protector Robinson, 17 August 1842, Robinson Papers, Vol. 55, p. 257, ML A7076.

National Library of Australia

Bates, Daisy, Papers, National Library of Australia, MS 365, folio 33/1-30.

Bates, Daisy, Papers, National Library of Australia, MS 365, folio 33/72-80.

Rawson, Samuel, *Journal of an Expedition after Some Van Diemen's Land Blacks Who Were Committing Depredations at Western Port on the Southern Coast of New Holland, October–November 1841,* National Library of Australia, MS 204/1.

Sturt, Charles, Sturt Papers, Microfiche copy (Oxford: Rhodes House, 1838) NLA G2200.

New South Wales Parliamentary Papers

Frosby, Edward, 'Protection of the Aborigines, Report of the Board', in *NSW Votes and Proceedings of the Legislative Assembly*, Part I, 1894.

Public Record Office South Australia

Beasley, B. C., Annual Report, 11 April 1888, PRO SA 52/1/1888/112.

Buttfield, J. P., Letter to Acting Protector of Aborigines, 5 July 1866, PRO SA, GRG 52/1/1866/115.

Buttfield, J. P., Letter to Acting Protector of Aborigines, 1 April 1867, PRO SA, GRG 52/1/1867/138.

Buttfield, J. P., Letter to Acting Protector of Aborigines, 18 May 1867, PRO SA, GRG 52/1/1867/246.

Buttfield, J. P., Letter to Commissioner for Crown Lands, 6 June 1870, PRO SA, GRG 52/1/1870/124.

Buttfield, J. P., Letter to Commissioner for Crown Lands, 6 August 1870, PRO SA, GRG 52/1/1870/248.

Buttfield, J. P., Letters to Commissioner for Crown Lands, 23 May 1871, PRO SA, GRG 52/1/1871/109.

Buttfield, J. P., Letters to Commissioner for Crown Lands, 6 June 1871, PRO SA, GRG 52/1/1871/109.

Buttfield, J. P., Letter to Commissioner for Crown Lands, 11 May 1874, PRO SA, GRG 52/1/1874/163.

Mcfarlane, J. M., Letter to E. Stephens, 1837, PRO SA, GRG 24/90/366.

Meyer, C. A., Letter to Sub-Protector of Aborigines, Adelaide, 1880, PRO SA, GRG 52/1/1880/125.

Meyer, C. A., Letter to Sub-Protector of Aborigines, Adelaide, 15 January 1885, PRO SA GRG 52/1/1885/125.

Moorhouse, M., Protector of Aborigines Quarterly Report, 7 October 1843, PRO SA GRG 24/4/1843/132.

Moorhouse, M., Letter to Governor, 19 July 1844, PRO SA GRG 24/6/1844/772.

Taplin, G., Letter to Protector of Aborigines, 20 July 1868, PRO SA GRG 52/1/1868/286.

Taplin, G., Letter to Sub-Protector of Aborigines, 17 January 1876, PRO SA, GRG 52/1/1876/35.

Taplin, G., Letter, 'The Diseases of the Aborigines of South Australia', 20 January 1876, PRO SA, GRG 52/1/1876/36.

Public Record Office Victoria

Campbell, N., Medical Report, Goulburn River District, PRO Vic., VPRS 4410, Unit 12 (1842).

Dredge, J., Report of the Operations of the Assistant Protector of Aborigines in the Goulburn District from the 1st of July, 1839 to the 29th February 1840 Inclusive, PRO Vic., VPRS 4410 Unit 2/47.

Letter 21 June, PRO Vic., VPRS 11 Unit 1/21 (1843).

Letter 1 October, PRO Vic., VPRS 11, Unit 1/24 (1845).

Medical Reports, PRO Vic., VPRS 4410, Unit 1/1-11 (1841–1842).

Parker, Edward, Letter to Robinson, 31 December 1840, PRO Vic., VPRS 11 unit 4/156.

Robinson, George Augustus, Chief Protector's Report for 1845, PRO Vic., VPRS 4399 Unit 1/1.

Watton, J., Report of Medical and Surgical Cases treated at the Aboriginal Establishment, Mount Rouse, 1 January to 30 November 1840, PROV Vic., VPRS 12.

South Australian Parliamentary Papers

Hammond, O., 'State of Health at Poonindie Mission', Report, 19 September, SAPP 1857–58, Vol. 2.

Wyatt, William, in, 'Report of the Select Committee of the Legislative Council upon The Aborigines', SAPP No. 165, 1860.

Victorian Parliamentary Papers

Brewer, H. E., Reports. 2 January and 29 April 1874, in 'Eleventh Report of the Board for the Protection of the Aborigines', Papers Presented to Parliament, Legislative Assembly, *Victorian Parliamentary Papers*, Vol. 3, 1875.

Bulmer, J., 'Fifteenth Report of the Board for the Protection of the Aborigines', Papers Presented to Parliament, Legislative Assembly, *Victorian Parliamentary Papers*, Vol. 3, 1879.

Curr, E. M., and A. C. Le Souef, Letter, 21 May 1879, in 'Fifteenth Annual Report of the Board for the Protection of the Aborigines', Papers Presented to Parliament, Legislative Assembly, *Victorian Parliamentary Papers*, Vol. 3, 1879.

Gibson, J., Reports, in 'Annual Report of the Board for the Protection of the Aborigines', Papers Presented to Parliament, Legislative Assembly, *Victorian Parliamentary Papers*, Vol. 4, 1869.

Gibson, J., Reports, in 'Annual Report of the Board for the Protection of the Aborigines', Papers Presented to Parliament, Legislative Assembly, *Victorian Parliamentary Papers*, Vol. 3, 1871.

Gibson, J., Reports, in 'Annual Report of the Board for the Protection of the Aborigines', Papers Presented to Parliament, Legislative Assembly, *Victorian Parliamentary Papers*, Vol. 3, Part 2, 1872.

Gibson, J., Reports, in 'Annual Report of the Board for the Protection of the Aborigines', Papers Presented to Parliament, Legislative Assembly, *Victorian Parliamentary Papers*, Vol. 3, Part 1, 1873.

Gibson, J., Reports, in 'Annual Report of the Board for the Protection of the Aborigines', Papers Presented to Parliament, Legislative Assembly, *Victorian Parliamentary Papers*, Vol. 3, Part 1, 1874.

Gibson, J., Reports, in 'Annual Report of the Board for the Protection of the Aborigines', Papers Presented to Parliament, Legislative Assembly, *Victorian Parliamentary Papers*, Vol. 3, 1875–76.

Goodwin, T. H., Letter, 26 November 1860, in 'First Annual Report of the Board for the Protection of the Aborigines', Papers Presented to Parliament, Legislative Assembly, *Victorian Parliamentary Papers*, Vol. 3, Part 1, 1861–62.

Hagenauer, Fredrick, Report, 18 July 1887, in 'Twenty-third Annual Report of the Board for the Protection of the Aborigines', Papers Presented to Parliament, Legislative Assembly, *Victorian Parliamentary Papers*, Vol 3, 1887.

Hagenauer, F. A. (Rev.), Prepared Statement, 23 May 1877, in 'Royal Commission on the Aborigines', Papers Presented to Parliament, Legislative Assembly', *Victorian Parliamentary Papers*, Vol. 3, 1877–78.

Jamieson, J., Letter, 3 May 1876, in 'Eleventh Annual Report of the Board for the Protection of the Aborigines', Papers Presented to Parliament, Legislative Assembly, *Victorian Parliamentary Papers*, Vol. 3, 1875–76.

McCrea, W., Enclosure in 'Aborigines. Report and Correspondence Relative to the Mortality amongst the Residents of the Aboriginal Stations of Victoria', in Papers Presented to Parliament, Legislative Assembly, *Victorian Parliamentary Papers*, Vol. 3, 1879.

Moorhouse, M., Protector of Aborigines Quarterly Report, 8 July 1843, in Papers Relating to Australia, *British Parliamentary Papers*, Vol. 8.

Registrar General, 'Births, Deaths and Marriages of the Colony of Victoria', 'Third Annual Report of the Board for the Protection of the Aborigines', Papers Presented to Parliament, Legislative Assembly, *Victorian Parliamentary Papers*, Vol. 4, Part 1, 1856–57.

'Royal Commission on the Aborigines', Census of the Aboriginal Natives in the Colony of Victoria, *Victorian Parliamentary Papers*, Vol. 3, 1877–78.

Stahle, J. H., Report, 8 August 1889, in 'Twenty-sixth Annual Report of the Board for the Protection of the Aborigines', Papers Presented to Parliament, Legislative Assembly, *Victorian Parliamentary Papers*, Vol. 4, 1890.

Thomas, W., Appendix to 'First Annual Report of the Board for the Protection of the Aborigines', Papers Presented to Parliament, Legislative Assembly, *Victorian Parliamentary Papers*, Vol. 3, 1861–62.

Thomas, W., Appendix to 'First Report of the Central Board Appointed to Watch over the Interests of the Aborigines in the Colony of Victoria', in Papers Presented to Both Houses Parliament, *Victorian Parliamentary Papers*, Vol. 3, No. 39, 1861–62.

Western Australian Parliamentary Papers

Legislative Council, Western Australia, 'Report of a Commission to Inquire into the Treatment of Aboriginal Native Prisoners of the Crown in this Colony', *Votes and Proceedings of the Legislative Council* (Perth: Government Printer, 1884).

Waylen, Alfred R., 'Report by the Colonial Surgeon on the Condition of the Sick Native Prisoners at Rottnest Prison', *Legislative Council of Western Australia* (Perth: Government Printer, 1883).

Newspapers

Adelaide Observer, 24 December 1853.

Adelaide Observer, 17 June 1882.

Adelaide Observer, 11 March 1898.

Adelaide Observer, 11 May 1901.

Adelaide Observer, 8 July 1911.

The Advertiser, 29 March 1893.

The Argus, 5 February 1877.
Bulletin of the Northern Territory, July 1912.
Morning Bulletin (Rockhampton), 9 June 1919.
Port Phillip Gazette, 8 May 1839.
South Australian Government Gazette, 31 October 1850.
South Australian Government Gazette, 15 July 1852.
South Australian Government Gazette, 24 March 1853.
South Australian Government Gazette, 18 March 1874.
South Australian Government Gazette, 20 August 1874.
South Australian Government Gazette, 18 March 1875.
South Australian Government Gazette, 6 April 1876.
South Australian Government Gazette, 20 March 1879.
South Australian Register, 12 January 1839.
South Australian Register, August 4 1854.
South Australian Register, 25 July 1855.
South Australian Register, 5 February 1867.
South Australian Register, 2 April 1867.
South Australian Register, 1 September 1894.
South Australian Weekly Chronicle, 2 March 1861.
Sydney Gazette, 16 December 1820.
Sydney Morning Herald, 11 June 1927.

Other Published Sources

Aboriginal and Torres Strait Islander Advisory Group on COVID-19, Communique 17 August 2020, https://www.health.gov.au/sites/default/files/documents/2020/08/aboriginal-and-torres-strait-islander-advisory-group-on-covid-19-communiques-17-august-2020-communique_1.pdf (accessed 21 September 2020)

Adels, B. R., and D. C. Gajdusek, 'Survey of Measles Patterns in New Guinea, Micronesia and Australia', *American Journal of Hygiene*, 77 (3), 1963, pp. 317–343.

Anderson, Ian, Bridget Robson, Michele Connolly, Fadwa Al-Yaman, Prof Espen Bjertness, Alexandra King, et al., 'Indigenous and Tribal Peoples' Health (The Lancet-Lowitja Institute Global Collaboration): A Population Study', *The Lancet*, Vol 388, 9 July 2016, pp. 131–157, https://www.thelancet.com/journals/lancet/article/PIIS0140-6736(16)00345-7/fulltext (accessed 18 January 2021).

Atherton Young, J. (ed.), *Jane Bardsley's Outback Letterbook, Across the Years 1896–1936* (Sydney: Angus & Robertson, 1987).

Aufderheide, Arthur C., and Conrado Rodriguez-Martin, *The Cambridge Encyclopedia of Human Paleopathology* (Cambridge: Cambridge University Press, 1998; reprinted 2003).

Austin, Tony, *Simply the Survival of the Fittest: Aboriginal Administration in South Australia's Northern Territory 1863–1910* (Darwin: Historical Society of the Northern Territory, 1992).

Australian Almanac of Sydney, 'A Chronologic Table of Remarkable Events from the Foundation of the Colony to the Close of the Year 1832', Australian Almanac of Sydney Directory for the Year of Our Lord 1834.

Australian Department of Health, *Multijurisdictional Syphilis Outbreak Surveillance Report: June 2018*, formerly available from http://www.health.gov.au/internet/main/publishing.nsf/Content/71E8A32E7518E532CA25801A0009A217/$File/3rd-Surveil-Report-June-18.pdf (accessed 22 August 2018).

Australian Government, 'The Australian Gold Rush', formerly available from www.australia.gov.au/about-australia/australian-story/austn-gold-rush (accessed 10 January 2017).

Australian Health Protection Principal Committee (AHPPC) Governance Group, *Action Plan: Enhanced Response to Addressing Sexually Transmissible Infections (and Blood Borne*

Viruses) in Indigenous Populations, http://www.health.gov.au/internet/main/publishing.nsf/Content/71E8A32E7518E532CA25801A0009A217/$File/Action-Plan-May18.pdf (accessed August 2018).
Australian Indigenous HealthInfoNet, *Overview of Australian Indigenous and Torres Strait Islander Health Status, 2015* (Perth, WA: Australian Indigenous HealthInfoNet, 2016), http://www.healthinfonet.ecu.edu.au/uploads/resources/31110_31110.pdf (accessed 21 December 2016).
Australian Indigenous HealthInfoNet, *Overview of Aboriginal and Torres Strait Islander Health Status, 2017* (Perth, WA: Australian Indigenous HealthInfoNet, 2018).
Australian Institute of Aboriginal and Torres Strait Islander Studies, 'Indigenous Australian Languages: Celebrating 2019 International Year of Indigenous Languages', Canberra, https://aiatsis.gov.au/whats-new/news/international-year-indigenous-languages-officially-launched (accessed 3 July 2020).
Australian Medical Association, 'Australia Declared Measles-free', 29 April 2014, https://ama.com.au/ausmed/australia-declared-measles-free (accessed October 2018).
Auty, Kate, and Lynette Russell, *Hunt Them, Hang Them: The Tasmanians in Port Phillip, 1841–42* (Melbourne: Justice Press, 2016).
Barwick, Diane, 'Coranderrk and Cumeroogunga: Pioneers and Policy', in T. Scarlett Epstein and D. H. Penny (eds), *Opportunity and Response: Case Studies in Economic Development* (London: C. Hurst and Co., 1972).
Basedow, H., 'Diseases of the Australian Aborigines', *Journal of Tropical Medicine and Hygiene*, Reprint, 15 June to 15 September 1932.
Bates, Daisy, *The Passing of the Aborigines: A Lifetime Spent among the Natives of Australia*, 2nd Australian edn (London: Murray, 1947).
Bateson, C., *The Convict Ships, 1787–1868* (Glasgow: Brown, Son and Ferguson Ltd, 1959).
Baylie, W. H., 'On the Aborigines of the Goulburn District', *Port Phillip Magazine* I, 1843, pp. 86–92.
Beaglehole, J., *The Journals of Captain James Cook on his Voyages of Discovery. The Voyage of the Endeavour 1768–1771* (Cambridge: Hakluyt Society, 1955), http://www.gutenberg.org/files/8106/8106-h/8106-h.htm#ch7 (accessed 3 December 2016).
Beale, E., *Sturt the Chipped Idol: A Study of Charles Sturt, Explorer* (Sydney: Sydney University Press, 1979).
Benenson, A. S., 'Smallpox', in A. S. Evans (ed.), *Viral Infections of Humans* (New York: Plenum Press, 1976).
Benenson, A. S., *Control of Communicable Diseases in Man*, 15th edn (Washington: American Public Health Association, 1990).
Beveridge, P., *The Aborigines of Victoria and Riverina* (Melbourne: M. L. Hutchinson, 1889).
Beveridge, W. I. B., *Influenza: The Last Great Plague. An Unfinished Story of Discovery* (London: Heinemann, 1977).
Black, E. Couper, 'Population and Tribal Distribution', in B. C. Cotton (ed.), *Aboriginal Man in South and Central Australia*, Part 1 (Adelaide: Government Printer, 1966).
Black, F. L., 'Measles Endemicity in Insular Populations: Critical Community Size and Its Evolutionary Implication', *Journal of Theoretical Biology*, 11 (2), 1966, pp. 207–211.
Blainey, Geoffrey, *The Tyranny of Distance* (Melbourne: Sun Books, 1982).
Bonwick, J. *The Last of the Tasmanians: Or the Black War of Van Diemen's Land* (London: Sampson, Low, Son and Marston, 1870).
Breinl, A., 'Report on Health and Disease in the Northern Territory', *Bulletin of the Northern Territory,* 1a, July 1912.
Breinl, A., and M. J. Holmes, 'Medical Report on the Data Collected during a Journey through Some Districts of the Northern Territory', *Bulletin of the Northern Territory*, 15, December 1915.
Bride, T. F. (ed.), *Letters From Victorian Pioneers* (Melbourne: Heineman, 1969).

Bright, Amy and Johanna Dups, 'Infectious and Congenital Syphilis Notifications Associated with an Ongoing Outbreak in Northern Australia', *CDI*, 40 (1), 2016, pp. e7–e10, https://www1.health.gov.au/internet/main/publishing.nsf/content/cda-cdi4001b.htm (accessed 30 October 2020).

Briscoe, G., *Queensland Aborigines and the Spanish Influenza Pandemic of 1918–1919*, Occasional Paper No. 3/1996 (Canberra: Australian Institute of Aboriginal and Torres Strait Islander Studies, 1996).

Briscoe, Gordan, and Len Smith (eds), *The Aboriginal Population Revisited: 70,000 Years to the Present* (Canberra: Aboriginal History Monograph, No. 10, 2002).

Brock, P., *Outback Ghettos: Aborigines, Institutionalisation and Survival* (Cambridge: Cambridge University Press, 1993).

Brock, Peggy, and Dawn Kartinyeri, *Poonindie: The Rise and Destruction of an Aboriginal Agricultural Community* (Adelaide: Aboriginal Heritage Branch, Department of Environment and Planning, 1989).

Broome, R., *Aboriginal Australians: Black Response To White Dominance 1788–1980* (Sydney: Allen and Unwin, 1993).

Broome, Richard, *Aboriginal Australians: A History Since 1788*, 4th edn (Sydney: Allen and Unwin, 2010).

Bryder, L., 'Tuberculosis in New Zealand', in A. J. Proust (ed.), *History of Tuberculosis in Australia, New Zealand and Papua New Guinea* (Canberra: Brolga Press, 1991).

Burton, Cleland J., *A Contribution to the History of Disease in Australia*, Paper, Australian Medical Congress, Sydney, September 1911.

Butlin, Noel, *Our Original Aggression: Aboriginal Populations of Southeastern Australia 1788–1850* (London: Allen and Unwin, 1983).

Cahir, Fred, *My Country All Gone, the White Men Have Stolen It: The Invasion of Wadawurrung Country, 1800–1870* (Ballarat: Australian History Matters, 2019).

Cahir, Fred, Ian D. Clark and Philip A. Clarke, *Aboriginal Biocultural Knowledge in South-Eastern Australia: Perspectives of Early Colonists* (Clayton South, Vic.: CSIRO Publishing, 2018).

Campbell, Judy, 'Smallpox in Aboriginal Australia, the Early 1830s', *Historical Studies*, 21 (84), 1985, pp. 336–358.

Campbell, Judy, *Invisible Invaders: Smallpox and Other Diseases in Aboriginal Australia 1780–1880* (Melbourne: Melbourne University Press, 2002).

Cannon, M. (ed.), *Historical Records of Victoria*, Vol. 2B (Melbourne: Victorian Government Printing Office, 1983).

Carmichael, Ann G., 'Leprosy (Hansen's Disease)', in K. Kiple (ed.), *The Cambridge World History of Human Disease* (Cambridge: Cambridge University Press, 1993).

Carson, Adrian, Donisha Duff, Francine Eades and Lesley Nelson, 'Urban Aboriginal People Face Unique Challenges in the Fight against Coronavirus', *The Conversation*, 24 April 2020, https://theconversation.com/urban-aboriginal-people-face-unique-challenges-in-the-fight-against-coronavirus-136050 (accessed 23 September 2020).

Castan Centre, Monash University, 'What is the Northern Territory Intervention?' https://www.monash.edu/law/research/centres/castancentre/our-areas-of-work/indigenous/the-northern-territory-intervention/the-northern-territory-intervention-an-evaluation/what-is-the-northern-territory-intervention (accessed 2 November 2020).

Centers for Disease Control and Prevention, 'Global Measles Outbreaks', in Global Immunization, https://www.cdc.gov/globalhealth/measles/globalmeaslesoutbreaks.htm (accessed 28 October 20).

Centers for Disease Control and Prevention, 'History of Smallpox', formerly available from https://www.cdc.gov/smallpox/history/ (accessed 22 January 2018).

Centers for Disease Control and Prevention, 'Poxvirus Diseases', https://www.cdc.gov/poxvirus/diseases.html (accessed January 2018).

Centers for Disease Control and Prevention, 'Types of Influenza Viruses', formerly available from www.cdc.gov/flu/about/viruses/type.htm (accessed 24 May 2017).
Chapple, Simon, 'Death and Disease at the Dawn of New Zealand's History', The Turnbull Library Record No. 50, 2018, https:/www.researchgate.net/publication/327427166 (accessed September 2018).
Cilento, R. S. W., and A. H. Baldwin, 'Malaria in Australia', *Medical Journal of Australia*, 1 (9), 1930, pp. 274–282.
Clarke, C. M. H., *A History of Australia*, Vol. I (Melbourne: Melbourne University, 1981).
Clarkson, Chris, Zenobia Jacobs, Ben Marwick and Richard Fullagar, 'Human Occupation of Northern Australia by 65,000 Years Ago', *Nature*, 547 (7663), July 2017, pp. 306–310.
Cleland, J. B., 'Disease among the Australian Aborigines', *Journal of Tropical Medicine and Hygiene*, (5), 1928, pp. 53–59.
Cleland, J. B., 'Some Diseases Peculiar to, or of Interest in, Australia', in J. H. L. Cumpston(ed.), *The History of Small-pox in Australia, 1788–1908* (Quarantine Service Publication No. 3. Melbourne: Government Printer, 1914).
Cleland, J. B., 'Some Early References to Tuberculosis in Australia', *Medical Journal of Australia*, 1938, 1, pp. 256–258.
Cliff, A., P. Haggett and M. Smallman-Raynor, *Measles: An Historical Geography of a Major Human Viral Disease, from Global Expansion to Local Retreat, 1840–1990* (Oxford: Blackwell Publishers, 1993).
Cliff, A. D., and P. Haggett, *The Spread of Measles in Fiji and the Pacific* (Canberra: Australian National University, 1985).
Cobley, J., *Sydney Cove 1789–1790* (Sydney: Angus & Robertson, 1963).
Cohen, Mark, *Health and the Rise of Civilization* (New Haven: Yale University Press, 1989).
Collins, David, *An Account of the English Colony in New South Wales*, Vol I, Reprint edited by B. H. Fletcher (Sydney: A.H. & A.W. Reed, 1985. Originally published London, 1798).
Cook, N. D., *Born to Die: Disease and New World Conquest, 1492–1650* (Cambridge: Cambridge University Press, 1998).
'Corona Virus Disease 2019 (COVID-19)', *British Medical Journal, Best Practice*, https://bestpractice.bmj.com/topics/en-us/3000168/aetiology (accessed 29 September 2020).
Critchett, Jan, *A Distant Field of Murder: Western District Frontiers 1834–1848* (Melbourne: Melbourne University Press, 1990).
Crooks, Kristy, Dawn Casey and James S. Ward, 'First Nations People Leading the Way in the COVID-19 Pandemic: Planning, Response and Management', *Medical Journal of Australia*, Preprint, 29 April 2020.
Crosby, A. W., 'The Virgin-soil Epidemic as a Factor in the Aboriginal Depopulation in America', *William and Mary Quarterly*, 33, 1976, pp. 289–299.
Crosby, A. W., 'Influenza', in K. Kiple (ed.), *The Cambridge World History of Human Disease*, Cambridge: Cambridge University Press, 1993).
Crosby, A. W., 'Smallpox', in K. Kiple (ed.), *The Cambridge World History of Human Disease* (Cambridge: Cambridge University Press, 1993).
Crosby, Alfred W., *Ecological Imperialism: The Biological Expansion of Europe, 900–1900*, 2nd edn (Cambridge: Cambridge University Press, 2015).
Crosby, Alfred W., *The Columbian Exchange: Biological and Cultural Consequences of 1492* (Westport, Connecticut: Greenwood Press, 1972).
Cumpston, J. H. L., *The History of Small-pox in Australia, 1788–1908* (Quarantine Service Publication No. 3. Melbourne: Government Printer, 1914).
Cumpston, J. H. L., *Influenza and Maritime Quarantine in Australia* (Quarantine Service Publication No. 18. Melbourne: Government Printer, 1919).
Cumpston, J. H. L., *The History of Diphtheria, Scarlet Fever, Measles and Whooping Cough in Australia* (Canberra: Government Printer, 1927).

Cumpston, J. H. L., *The Health of the People* (Canberra: Roebuck Society Publication No. 19, 1978).

Cumpston, J. H. L., *Health and Disease in Australia: A History*, M. J. Lewis (ed.), (Canberra: Australian Government Printing Service, 1989).

Cunningham, Peter, *Two Years in New South Wales*, Vol. II (London: Henry Colburn, 1827).

Curr, E. M., *The Australian Race*, Vol. 1 (Melbourne: Government Printer, 1886).

Curson, P. H., *Times of Crisis: Epidemics in Sydney 1788–1900* (Sydney: Sydney University Press, 1985).

Curson, P., and K. McCracken, 'An Australian Perspective of the 1918–1919 Influenza Pandemic', *NSW Public Health Bulletin*, 17 (7–8), 2006, p. 106.

Cussen, P., Letter to C. J. La Trobe, 18 November 1839, in M. Cannon. (ed.), *Historical Records of Victoria*, Vol. 2B (Melbourne: Victorian Government Printing Office, 1983).

Darwin, Charles, *A Naturalist's Voyage. Journal of Researches into the Natural History and Geology of the Countries Visited during the Voyage of H. M. S. 'Beagle' Round the World* (London: John Murray, 1889).

Darwin, Charles, *The Voyage of the Beagle*, Harvard Classics, Vol. 29 (New York: P. F. Collier and Son, 1909), http://www.homeworknow.com/uploads/59b6087ad3def86fd94edef9c0ec5ce4.pdf (accessed 14 August 2020).

Dawson, James, *Australian Aborigines. The Languages and Customs of Several Tribes of Aborigines in the Western District of Victoria, Australia* (Melbourne: George Robertson, 1881).

Dawson, Robert, *The Present State of Australia* (London: Smith, Elder and Co., 1830).

Day, David, *Claiming a Continent: A History of Australia* (Pymble: Angus & Robertson, 1997).

Defoe, Daniel, *A Journal of the Plague Year* (first published 1722; Alicia Editions, Kindle version, 2020).

Dixon, C. W., *Smallpox* (London: J. and A. Churchill Ltd, 1962).

Dobyns, H. F., *Their Numbers Become Thinned* (Knoxville: University of Tennessee Press, 1983).

Domett, K. M., L. A. Wallis, D. Kynuna, A. Kynina and H. Smith, 'Late Holocene Human Remains from Northwest Queensland Australia: Archaeology and Paleopathology', *Archaeology in Oceania*, 41 (1), 2006, pp. 25–36.

Donlon, Denise, 'Aboriginal Skeletal Collections and Research in Physical Anthropology: An Historical Perspective', *Australian Archaeology* (39), 1994, pp. 73–82.

Donoghue, H. D., Mark Spigelman, Justin O'Grady, Ildiko Szikossy, IIdiko Pap, Oona Y-C Lee, Houdini H. iko T Wu, Gurdyal S. Besra and David E. Minnikin, 'Ancient DNA Analysis – An Established Technique in Charting the Evolution of Tuberculosis and Leprosy', *Tuberculosis*, 95 (Supp. 1), June 2015, pp. S140–S144, http://www.sciencedirect.com/science/article/pii/S1472979215000219 (accessed 9 December 2016).

Dowling, P., '"A Great Deal of Sickness": Introduced Diseases among the Aboriginal People of Colonial Southeast Australia 1788–1900' (Canberra: PhD thesis, Australian National University, 1997), https://digitalcollections.anu.edu.au/handle/1885/7529 (accessed July 2016).

Dowling, P., 'Mercury Poisoning at Oyster Cove? Suspected Cases of Unintentional Poisoning of Tasmanian Aboriginal Internees', *Tasmanian Historical Studies*, 11, 2006, pp. 59–68.

Elkin, A. P., *Aboriginal Men of High Degree: Initiation and Sorcery in the World's Oldest Tradition* (St Lucia, Qld: University of Queensland Press, 1994).

Elphinstone, J. J., 'The Health of Australian Aborigines with No Previous Association with Europeans', *Medical Journal of Australia*, 2 (6), 1971, pp. 293–301.

Endeavour College of Natural Health, *Australian Indigenous Medicine*, https://source.endeavourlearninggroup.com.au/coursematerial/pdf/Documents/SOCH111_SN10_Lecture.pdf (accessed 15 January 2019).

Eyre, E., *Journals of Expeditions into Central Australia*, Vol. 2 (London: T. and W. Boone, 1845).
Eyre, E., 'Manners and Customs of the Aborigines', in *Journals of Expeditions of Discovery*, Vol. 2 (London: T. and W. Boone, 1856).
Falcon, Richard, and H. Bradford Hawley, 'Influenza', in *Magill's Medical Guide*, 4th edn (Pasadena: Salem Press, 2008).
Farr, W., 'Statistical Nosology with Explanations', in *Statistical Register of Victoria'* (Melbourne: Government Printer, 1854).
Fenner, F., 'Smallpox, "The Most Dreadful Scourge of the Human Species": Its Global Spread and Recent Eradication', *Medical Journal of Australia*, 141 (11 and 12–13), 1984, pp. 728–735, 841–846.
Fenner, F., 'Smallpox in Australia', Letter to the Editor, *Medical Journal of Australia*, 142, 1985, p. 278.
Fenner, F., 'Sociocultural Changes and Infectious Disease', in B. Furnass (ed.), *Infectious Disease in Humans* (Canberra: Canberra Nature and Science Forum, 1998).
Fenner, F., D. A. Henderson, I. Arita, Z. Jezek and I. D. Ladnyi, *Smallpox and Its Eradication* (Geneva: World Health Organization, 1988).
Fitzgerald, R. A., *A History of Queensland from the Dreaming to 1915* (St Lucia, Qld: University of Queensland Press, 1982).
Flemming, J., 'The Voyage of His Majesty's Schooner "Cumberland" from Sydney to King Island and Port Phillip in 1802–3. A Journal of the Explorations of Charles Grimes, Acting Surveyor-General of New South Wales', in *Port Phillip, First Survey and Settlement* (Reprinted by Legislative Assembly. Melbourne: Government Printer, 1879).
Flood, J., *The Moth Hunters: Aboriginal Prehistory of the Australian Alps* (Canberra: Australian Institute of Aboriginal Studies, 1980).
Flinders, Matthew, *A Voyage to Terra Australis*, Vol. 2 (London: G. and W. Nicol, 1814) (Facsimile Edition. Adelaide: Libraries Board of South Australia, 1966).
Flinders University, *Roonka Bioarchaelogy Research Project*, Adelaide, Flinders University, formerly available from https://www.flinders.edu.au/ehl/archaeology/research-profile/current-projects/roonka-bioarchaeology-redearch-project.cfm (accessed July 2016).
Foelsche, Paul, 'Notes on the Aborigines of North Australia', extract in A. Breinl, 'Report on Health and Disease in the Northern Territory', *Bulletin of the Northern Territory*, 1a, July 1912, pp. 21–38.
Furphy, Samuel, and Amanda Nettlebeck, *Aboriginal Protection and its Intermediaries in Britain's Antipodean Colonies*, Part 1, 'The Conception and Circulation of 'Aboriginal Protection' (New York: Routledge 2020), http://web.a.ebscohost.com.rp.nla.gov.au/ehost/ebookviewer/ebook/bmxlYmtfXzIxNDEyNDVfX0FO0?sid=f29e93e4-7534-4691-bd36-6686fe70b8ce@sessionmgr4008&vid=0&format=EB&lpid=lp_1&rid=0 (accessed 28 October 2020).
Gandevia, B., and J. Cobley, 'Mortality at Sydney Cove, 1788–1792', *Australian and New Zealand Journal of Medicine*, 4 (2), 1974, pp. 111–125.
Gapps, Stephen, *The Sydney Wars: Conflict in the Early Colony 1788–1817* (Sydney: New South Publishing, 2018).
Gerritsen, Rupert, *Beyond the Frontier: Explorations in Ethnohistory* (Canberra: Batavia Online Publishing, 2011).
Gibney, H. J., 'Sturt, Charles (1795–1869)', in *Australian Dictionary of Biography* (Canberra: National Centre of Biography, Australian National University), http://adb.anu.edu.au/biography/sturt-charles-2712 (accessed Februry 2016).
Glacabi, Lorenzo, and Shelia A. Lukehart, 'The Endemic Treponematoses', *Clinical Microbiological Reviews*, 27 (1) 2014, pp. 89–115.
Goodall, H., 'Colonialism and Catastrophe: Contested Memories of Nuclear Testing and Measles Epidemics at Ernabella', in K. Darian-Smith and P. Hamilton (eds), *Memory and History in Twentieth-Century Australia* (Oxford: Oxford University Press, 1994).

Grant, J., *The Narrative of a Voyage of Discovery Performed in His Majesty's Ship the Lady Nelson* (Bell Yard, Fleet Street: C. Roworth, 1803) (Facsimile Edition. Adelaide: Libraries Board of South Australia, 1973).

Gray, Nancy, 'Bowman, James (1784–1846)', in *Australian Dictionary of Biography* (Canberra: National Centre of Biography, Australian National University), http://adb.anu.edu.au/biography/bowman-james-1812 (accessed March 2018).

Gray, Timothy J., James M. Trauer, Merv Fairley, Vicki L. Krause and Peter G. Markey, 'Imported Malaria in the Northern Territory, Australia – 428 Consecutive Cases', *Communicable Diseases Intelligence*, 36 (1), March 2012, https://www1.health.gov.au/internet/main/publishing.nsf/Content/cda-cdi3601f.htm (accessed 1 June 2020).

Grey, George, *Journals of Two Expeditions of Discovery in North-West and Western Australia*, Vol. II (London: T. and W. Boone, 1841) (Facsimile Edition. Victoria Park: Hesperion Press, 1984).

Guerra, F., 'The Earliest American Epidemic: The Influenza of 1493', *Social Science and History*, 12 (3), 1988, pp. 305–25.

Gutierrez, M. Cristina, Sylvain Brisse, Roland Brosch, Michel Fabre, Bahia Omaïs, Magali Marmiesse, Philip Supply and Veronique Vincent, 'Ancient Origin and Gene Mosaicism of the Progenitor of *Mycobacterium tuberculosis*', *PloS Pathogens*, 1 (1) e5, 2005, pp. 55–61.

Hackett, Cecil J., *Diagnostic Criteria of Syphilis, Yaws and Treponarid (Treponematoses) and of Some Other Diseases in Dry Bones* (New York: Springer-Verlag, 1976).

Harper, Kristin N., Molly K. Zuckerman, Megan L. Harper, John D. Kingston and George J. Armelagos, 'The Origin and Antiquity of Syphilis Revisited: An Appraisal of Old World Pre-Columbian Evidence for Treponemal Infection', *American Journal of Physical Anthropology*, 146 (Suppl. 53), 2011, pp. 99–133, doi:10.1002/ajpa.2163.

Hawdon, Joseph, *The Journal of a Journey from New South Wales to Adelaide* (Melbourne: Georgian House, 1838).

Hickenbotham, J. R., and J. Burton Cleland, 'Ulcerative Granuloma of the Pudenda in the Gascoyne District of Western Australia', in *Australasian Medical Congress, Transactions of the Eighth Session* (Melbourne: Australian Government Printer, 1909).

Hilliard, W., *The People in Between. The Pitjantjatjara People of Ernabella* (London: Hodder and Stoughton, 1968).

Hopkins, Donald R., *Princes and Peasants: Smallpox in History* (Chicago: Chicago University Press, 1983).

Horne, J. Ann, 'Beveridge, Peter (1829–1885)', in *Australian Dictionary of Biography* (Canberra: National Centre of Biography, Australian National University, 1969), http://adb.anu.edu.au/biography/beveridge-peter-2992 (accessed 13 December 2016).

Hotimsky, C. M., 'A Russian Account of New South Wales in 1822', *Melbourne Slavonic Studies*, 1 (1), 1967, pp. 82–95.

Hunter, Boyd H., and John Carmody, 'Estimating the Aboriginal Population in Early Colonial Australia: The Role of Chickenpox Reconsidered', *Australian Economic History Review*, 55 (2), 2015, pp. 112–138.

Hunter, John, *An Historical Journal of Events at Sydney and at Sea 1787–1779* (Facsimile Copy. Sydney: Angus & Robertson, 1968).

Irvine, N., *The Sirius Letters: The Complete Letters of Newton Fowell 1786–1790* (Sydney: Fairfax Press, 1988).

Jebb, Mary Anne, 'The Lock Hospital Experiment: Europeans, Aborigines and Venereal Disease', in Bob Reece and Tom Savage (eds), *European-Aboriginal Relations in Western Australian History* (Nedlands: University of Western Australia, 1984).

Jenkin, G., *Conquest of the Ngarrindjeri: The Story of the Lower Murray Lakes Tribes* (Adelaide: Rigby, 1979).

Johnson, M., and I. McFarlane, *Van Diemen's Land: An Aboriginal History* (Sydney: University of New South Wales Press, 2015).

Johnston, W. T., 'Tuberculosis', in K. Kiple (ed.), *The Cambridge World History of Human Disease* (Cambridge: Cambridge University Press, 1993).
Johnston, W. T., 'Tuberculosis', in K. Kiple (ed.), *The Cambridge Historical Dictionary of Disease* (Cambridge: Cambridge University Press, 2003).
Jones, David S., 'Virgin Soils Revisited', *William and Mary Quarterly*, 60 (4), October 2003, pp. 703–742.
Karskens, Grace, *The Colony: A History of Early Sydney* (Sydney: Allen and Unwin, 2010).
Kerin, Rani, '"Natives Allowed to Remain Naked": An Unorthodox Approach to Medical Work at Ernabella Mission', *Health and History*, 8 (1), 2006, pp. 80–99.
Kim-Farley, Robert, 'Measles', in K. Kiple (ed.), *The Cambridge Historical Dictionary of Disease* (Cambridge: Cambridge University Press, 2003).
King, A., and C. Nicol, *Venereal Diseases* (London: Baillière, Tindall and Cassell, 1975).
Kiple, K. (ed.), *The Cambridge World History of Human Disease* (Cambridge: Cambridge University Press, 1993).
Kiple, K. (ed.), *The Cambridge Historical Dictionary of Disease* (Cambridge: Cambridge University Press, 2003).
Kohen, J. L., and R. Lampert, 'Hunters and Fishers in the Sydney Region', in D. J. Mulvaney and J. P. White (eds), *Australians to 1788: Australians, a Historical Library* (Sydney: Fairfax, Syme and Weldon Associates, 1987).
Krauss, Scott, and Robert G. Webster, 'Avian Influenza Virus Surveillance and Wild Birds: Past and Present', *Avian Diseases*, 54 (Supp. 1), March 2010, pp. 394–398.
Lancaster, H. O., 'The Mortality in Australia from Influenza and from Diseases of the Respiratory System', *Medical Journal of Australia*, 2, 1953, pp. 672–676.
Lange, R., 'Plagues and Pestilence in Polynesia: The Nineteenth-century Cook Islands Experience', *Bulletin of the History of Medicine*, 58, 1984, pp. 325–46.
'Lessons from Previous Pandemics Help Indigenous Community Keep Out COVID-19, Lens, Monash University, 7 August 2020, https://lens.monash.edu/@politics-society/2020/08/07/1381018/lessons-from-previous-pandemics-help-indigenous-community-keep-covid-19-out (accessed 29 September 2020.
Lewis, M. J. (ed.), *Health and Disease in Australia: A History* (Canberra: Australian Government Printing Service, 1989).
Lewis, M. J., *Thorns on the Rose: The History of Sexually Transmitted Diseases in Australia in International Perspective* (Canberra: Australian Government Publishing Service, 1998).
Lewis, M. J., 'Medicine in Colonial Australia, 1788–1900, *Medical Journal of Australia*, 201 (1), Supplement, 'History of Australian Medicine', 2014, pp. S5–S10.
Littleton, Judith, and Harry Allen, 'Hunter-Gatherer Burials and the Creation of Persistent Places in Southeastern Australia', *Journal of Anthropological Archaeology*, 26 (2), 2007, pp. 283–298.
Littleton, Judith, Julie Park and Linda Bryder, 'The End of a Plague? Tuberculosis in New Zealand', in D. A. Herring and A. C. Swedlund (eds), *Plagues and Epidemics: Infected Spaces Past and Present* (Oxford: Berg, 2010).
Lockwood, Diana N. J., in David A. Warrell, Timothy M. Cox and John D. Firth (eds), *Oxford Textbook of Medicine*, Vol. 1, 4th edn (Oxford: Oxford University Press, 2003).
Long, J. P. M., *Aboriginal Settlements: A Survey of Institutional Communities in Eastern Australia* (Canberra: Australian National University Press, 1970.)
Loos, N., *Invasion and Resistance: Aboriginal–European Relations on the North Queensland Frontier 1861–1897* (Canberra: Australian National University Press, 1982).
Lourandos, Harry, *Continent of Hunter-Gatherers: New Perspectives in Australian Prehistory* (Cambridge: Cambridge University Press, 1997).
Lourie, A., 'From the Paddock to the Page: Squatter Peter Beveridge's Ethnological Writing about the Wadi Wadi in Colonial Victoria', *Oceania*, 86 (3), 2016, pp. 244–261.
MacFarlane, Ian, *1842, The Public Executions at Melbourne* (Melbourne: Public Record Office, 1984).

Mackaness, G., *George Augustus Robinson's Journey into South-Eastern Australia – 1844* (Dubbo: Australian Historical Monograph Vol. XIX, Review Publications, 1941).

MacKay, Charles, 'Some Pathological Changes in Australian Aboriginal Bones', Reprint from *Medical Journal of Australia*, 1, 1938, pp. 537–55.

Macknight, Campbell, 'The View from Marege: Australian Knowledge of Makassar and the Impact of the Trepang Industry across Two Centuries', *Aboriginal History*, 35, 2011, pp. 121–143.

Macleod, R., and M. Lewis (eds), *Disease, Medicine and Empire: Perspectives on Western Medicine and the Experience of European Expansion* (London: Routledge, 1988).

Maddison, S., 'Indigenous Autonomy Matters: What's Wrong with the Australian Government's "Intervention" in Aboriginal Communities', *Australian Journal of Human Rights*, 14 (1), 2008, pp. 41–61.

Maritime Museum of Tasmania, 'The Journey – by Sailing Ship', http://www.maritimetas.org/collection-displays/displays/over-seas-stories-tasmanian-migrants/journey-sailing-ship (accessed 1 February 2017).

Marshall, L. B., 'Disease Ecologies of Australia and Oceania', in K. Kipple (ed.), *The Cambridge World History of Human Disease* (Cambridge: Cambridge University Press, 1993).

Massola, A., *Aboriginal Mission Stations in Victoria* (Melbourne: The Hawthorn Press, 1970).

Massola, A., *Coranderrk. A History of the Aboriginal Station* (Kilmore: Lowden Publishing, 1975).

McArthur, N., *Island Populations of the Pacific* (Canberra: Australian National University Press, 1967).

McBryde, Isabel, 'Kulin Greenstone Quarries: The Social Contexts of Production and Distribution for the Mt William Site', *World Archaeology*, 16 (2), 1984, pp. 267–285.

McBryde, Isabel, 'Goods from Another Country: Exchange Networks and the People of the Lake Eyre Basin', in D. J. Mulvaney and J. P. White (eds), *Australians to 1788: Australians, a Historical Library* (Sydney: Fairfax, Syme and Weldon Associates, 1987).

McMichael, A. (with A. Woodward and C. Muir), *Climate Change and the Health of Nations* (New York: Cambridge University Press, 2017).

McNeill, W. H., *Plagues and Peoples* (London: Penguin Books, 1976).

Mein, Jacki J., Nick M. Anstey and Frank J. Bowden, 'Missing the Diagnosis of Donovanosis in Northern Australia', *Medical Journal of Australia*, 170 (1), January 1999, p. 48.

Memmott, Paul, *Gunyah Goondie + Wurley: The Aboriginal Architecture of Australia* (St Lucia, Qld: University of Queensland Press, 2007).

Merbs, Charles F., 'A New World of Infectious Disease', *American Journal of Physical Anthropology*, 35, 1992, pp. 3–42.

Meumann, Frank Olaf, 'An Anthroposcopic and Anthropometric Study of the Skeleton of a Full-blood Female Tasmanian Aborigine (Truganini)' (Tasmania: B. Med Sc. thesis, University of Tasmania, 1971).

Mitchell, Thomas, *Three Expeditions into the Interior of Eastern Australia*, Vol. I (London: T. W. Boone, 1838) (Australian Facsimile Editions No. 18. Adelaide: Libraries Board of South Australia, 1965).

Moore, H. D., 'Notes on the Early Settlers in South Australia prior to 1836', *Proceedings of the Royal Geographical Society of Australasia, South Australian Branch*, 25, 1923, pp. 81–135.

Morgan, J., *The Life and Adventures of William Buckley: Thirty-two Years a Wanderer amongst the Aborigines of the Unexplored Country Round Port Phillip* (Canberra: Australian National University Press, 1980 (1852)).

Morgan, M., *Nosological Index 1863 and Staff and Registrars of the Registrar-General's Department Victoria 1862* (Blackburn: Marjorie Morgan Publications, 1987).

Mousseau, Mark, 'H1N1 in Retrospect: A Review of Risk Factors and Policy Recommendations', *International Indigenous Policy Journal* 4 (2), April 2013, https://search.proquest.com/openview/1ec2ee701aa7c0306abbc825b240ed9a/1?pq-origsite=gscholar&cbl=1996357 (accessed 22 September 2020).

Mulvaney, D. J., *The Prehistory of Australia* (Ringwood: Penguin Australia, 1975).

Mulvaney, D. J., *Encounters in Place: Outsiders and Aboriginal Australians 1606–1985* (St Lucia, Qld: University of Queensland Press, 1989).

Mulvaney, John, '"Difficult to Found an Opinion": 1788 Population Estimates', in Gordan Briscoe and Len Smith (eds), *The Aboriginal Population Revisited: 70,000 Years to the Present* (Canberra: Aboriginal History Monograph, No. 10, 2002).

Mulvaney, John, and Johan Kamminga, *Prehistory of Australia* (Sydney: Allen and Unwin, 1999).

National Centre for Immunisation Research and Surveillance of Vaccine Preventable Diseases, 'Vaccine Preventable Diseases and Vaccination Coverage in Aboriginal and Torres Strait Islander People, Australia 2006–2010', *Communicable Diseases Intelligence*, 37, Supp., December 2013, http://www.health.gov.au/internet/publications/publishing.nsf/Content/cda-cdi37suppl.htm/$FILE/cdi37suppl.pdf (accessed October 2018).

Neel, J. V., W. R. Centrewall, N. A. Chagnon and H. L. Casey, 'Notes on the Effect of Measles and Measles Vaccine in a Virgin-soil Population of South American Indians', *American Journal of Epidemiology*, 91 (4), 1970, pp. 418–429.

Noye, R. J., 'Foelsche, Paul Heinrich Matthias (1831–1914), *Australian Dictionary of Biography*, National Centre of Biography, Australian National University, http://abd.anu.edu.au/biography/foelsche-paul-heinrich-matthias-3543/text5467 (accessed 27 October 2020), first published in hardcopy 1972.

Noymer, A., 'Epidemics and Time: Influenza and Tuberculosis during and after the 1918–1919 Pandemic', in D. A Herring and A. C. Swedlund (eds), *Plagues and Epidemics: Infected Spaces Past and Present* (Oxford: Berg, 2010).

Ortner, D., *Identification of Pathological Conditions in Human Skeletal Remains*, 2nd edn (San Diego: Academic Press, 2003).

Pardoe, Colin, 'The Cemetery as Symbol: The Distribution of Prehistoric Burial Grounds in Southeastern Australia', *Archaeology in Oceania*, 23 (1), 1988, pp. 1–16.

Pascoe, Bruce, *Dark Emu, Black Seeds: Agriculture or Accident?* (Broome: Magabala Books, 2014).

Pepper, Phillip, and Tess De Arago, *What Did Happen to the Aborigines of Victoria: The Kurnai of Gippsland*, Vol. 1 (Melbourne: Hyland House, 1985).

Pirie, P., 'The Effects of Treponematosis and Gonorrhoea on the Populations of the Pacific Islands', *Human Biology in Oceania*, 1, 1972, pp. 187–206.

Plomley, N. J. B., *Weep in Silence: A History of the Flinders Island Aboriginal Settlement* (Hobart: Blubber Head Press, 1987).

Plomley, N. J. B. (ed.), *Friendly Mission: The Tasmanian Journals and Papers of George Augustus Robinson 1829–1834* 2nd edition (Hobart: Queen Victoria Museum and Art Gallery, Hobart: Quintus, 2008).

Porter, Roy, *The Greatest Benefit to Mankind: A Medical History of Humanity from Antiquity to the Present* (London: Harper Collins Publishers, 1997).

Potter, C. W., 'A History of Influenza', *Journal of Applied Microbiology*, 91 (4), 2001, pp. 572–579.

Power, Tamara, Denise Wilson, Odette Best, Teresa Brockie, Lisa Bourque Bearskin, Eugenia Millender and John Lowe, 'COVID-19 and Indigenous Peoples: An Imperative for Action', *Journal of Clinical Nursing* 29, pp. 2737–2741, https://onlinelibrary.wiley.com/doi/full/10.1111/jocn.15320 (accessed 22 September 2020).

Proust, A. J. (ed.), *History of Tuberculosis in Australia, New Zealand and Papua New Guinea* (Canberra: Brolga, 1991).

Proust, A. J., 'Migration of Consumptives to Australia', in A. J. Proust (ed.), *History of Tuberculosis in Australia, New Zealand and Papua New Guinea* (Canberra: Brolga Press, 1991).

Proust, A. J., 'Tuberculosis in Australia: Part 1', in A. J. Proust (ed.), *History of Tuberculosis in Australia, New Zealand and Papua New Guinea* (Canberra: Brolga, 1991).

Pybus, Cassandra, 'Journey through the Apocalypse: Ria Warrawah, Wooredy and Truganini', *Griffith Review*, 58, October 2017, https://griffithreview.com/articles/journey-through-the-apocalypse-ria-warrah-wooredy-truganini/ (accessed 10 September 2019).

Pybus, Cassandra, *Truganini: Journey through the Apocalypse* (Sydney: Allen and Unwin, 2020).

Rae-Ellis, Vivienne, *Truganini: Queen or Traitor* (Hobart: O.B.M. Publishing Company, 1976a).

Rae-Ellis, Vivienne, 'Truganini', *Tasmanian Historical Research Association. Papers and Proceedings*, 23 (2), 1976b, pp. 26–43.

Reid, J., 'Medicine and Health: The Traditional Systems', in J. Reid (ed.), *Body Land and Spirit: Health and Healing in Aboriginal Society* (St Lucia, Qld: University of Queensland Press, 1982).

Reid, J., *Sorcerers and Healing Spirits* (Canberra: Australian National University Press, 1983).

Report of the Chief Protector of Aborigines for the Year Ending 30th June 1909 (Perth: Government Printer, 1909).

Reynolds, Henry, *The Other Side of the Frontier: Aboriginal Resistance to the European Invasion of Australia* (Sydney: University of New South Wales Press, 2006).

Richardson, W. L., 'Notes on Some of the Diseases Prevalent in Victoria, Australia', *Edinburgh Medical Journal*, 14, 1869, pp. 802–812.

Roberts, C. A., and J. E. Buikstra, *The Bioarchaeology of Tuberculosis: A Global View on a Reemerging Disease* (Gainesville: University Press of Florida, 2003).

Roberts-Thompson, Peter J., 'Impact of Introduced Disease into Tasmanian Aboriginal Populations and Its Role in Depopulation', *Tasmanian Historical Research Association, Papers and Proceedings*, 61 (2–3), December 2014, pp. 119–135.

Robertson, R. G., *Rotting Face: Smallpox and the American Indian* (Caldwell, Idaho: Caxton Press, 2001).

Royal Commission on the Condition of the Natives, Report, Appendix C, Minutes of Evidence (Perth: Government Printer, 1904).

Royle, H. G., 'The State of Health in New South Wales in the 1820's', *Medical Journal of Australia*, 1 (19), 1973, pp. 950–953.

Ruddock, E. H., *On Consumption and Tuberculosis of the Lungs*, 2nd edn (London: Homeopathic Publishing Company, 1873).

Ryan, L., *The Aboriginal Tasmanians*, 2nd edn (Sydney: Allen and Unwin, 1996).

Ryan, L., *Tasmanian Aborigines: A History since 1803* (Sydney: Allen and Unwin, 2012).

Ryan, Lyndall, William Pascoe, Jennifer Debenham, Stephanie Gilbert, Jonathan Richards, Robyn Smith et al., 'Colonial Frontier Massacres in Central and Eastern Australia, 1788–1930', University of Newcastle, https://c21ch.newcastle.edu.au/colonialmassacres/introduction.php (accessed 15 August 2018).

Schmitt, Robert C., and Eleanor C. Nordyke, 'Death in Hawai'i: The Epidemics of 1848–1849', *The Hawaiian Journal of History*, 35, 2001, pp. 1–13.

Sievwright, C. W., Letter to G. A. Robinson, 5 May 1839, in M. Cannon (ed.), *Historical Records of Victoria*, Vol. 2B (Melbourne: Victorian Government Printing Office, 1983).

Sisley, Richard, *Epidemic Influenza. Notes on the Origin and Method of Spread* (New York: Longman Green and Co., 1891).

Smith, C., and J. Littleton, 'Experiencing Childhood at Roonka: An Analysis of Enamel Hypoplasia on the Permanent Dentition of Australian Aboriginal Hunter-Gatherers', *American Journal of Physical Anthropology*, 159, 2016, pp. 294–295.

Smith, Dianne, 'Governing the Pandemic: Implications for Indigenous Self-Determination and self-Government, in F. Markham, D. Smith and F. Morphy (eds), *Indigenous Australians and the COVID-19 Crisis: Perspectives on Public Policy*, https://openresearch-repository.anu.edu.au/bitstream/1885/202733/1/CAEPR_TI_no1_2020_Markham_Smith_Morphy.pdf (accessed 21 September 2020).

Smith, Mike, *The Archaeology of Australia's Deserts* (Cambridge: Cambridge University Press, 2013).

Smith, W. Ramsay, *The Control of Communicable Diseases in South Australia* (Adelaide: Government Printer, 1919).

Snowden, Frank M., *Epidemics and Society: From the Black Death to the Present* (New Haven: Yale University Press, Kindle edition, 2019).

South Australian Government, 'Summary Showing the Number of Aborigines in Each County and Pastoral District of the Province of South Australia, at Date of Census' (Adelaide: South Australian Government Printer, 1879).

Steinbock, R. T., *Paleopathological Diagnosis and Interpretation: Bone Disease in Ancient Populations* (Springfield: Charles C. Thomas, 1976).

Stephens, Marguerita, *The Journal of William Thomas: Assistant Protector of the Aborigines of Port Phillip and Guardian of the Aborigines of Victoria 1839–1867*, Vol. One: 1839 to 1843 (Melbourne: Victorian Aboriginal Corporation for Languages, 2004).

Stevens, C., *White Man's Dreaming: Killalpaninna Mission 1866–1915* (Melbourne: Oxford University Press, 1994).

Stingemore, Jade Louise, 'Surviving the "Cure": Life on Bernier and Dorre Islands under the Lock Hospital Regime' (Perth: PhD thesis, University of Western Australia, 2010).

Stirling, E. C., 'Preliminary Report on the Discovery of Native Remains at Swanport, River Murray: With an Inquiry into the Alleged Occurrence of a Pandemic among the Australian Aboriginals', *Transactions and Proceedings of the Royal Society of South Australia*, 35, 1911, pp. 18–19.

Sturt, Charles, *Two Expeditions into the Interior of Southern Australia*, Vols I and II (London: Smith, Elder and Co., 1833) (Facsimile Copy. Sydney: Doubleday, 1982).

Sturt, Charles, *Narrative of an Expedition into Central Australia* (Sydney: University of Sydney Library, 2001 (1849)), http://adc.library.usyd.edu.au/data-2/p00102.pdf (accessed May 2018).

Summers, J., 'Colonial Race Relations', in E. Richards (ed.), *Flinders History of South Australia: Social History* (Adelaide: Wakefield Press, 1986).

Taplin, G., *The Folklore, Manners, Customs, and Languages of the South Australian Aborigines* (Adelaide: Government Printer, 1879) (Facsimile edition. 1989).

Tench, Watkin, *Sydney's First Four Years* (Sydney: Library of Australian History reprint, 1979, originally published as *A Complete Account of the Settlement at Port Jackson*, London, 1793).

Turbet, P., *The Aborigines of the Sydney District before 1788* (Sydney: Kangaroo Press, 1989).

Turner, Melba, 'A First-Hand Account of the 1948 Measles Epidemic by Sister Melba Turner Sister-in-Charge at the Time', Appendix II in W. Hilliard, *The People in Between: The Pitjantjatjara People of Ernabella* (London: Hodder and Stoughton, 1968.)

van Holst Pellekaan, Shelia M., Max Ingman, June Roberts-Thomson and Rosalind M. Harding, 'Mitochondrial Genomics Identifies Major Haplogroups in Aboriginal Australians', *American Journal of Physical Anthropology*, 131, October 2006, p. 2.

Verano, J. W., and D. H. Ubelaker (eds), *Disease and Demography in the Americas* (Washington: Smithsonian Institution Press, 1992).

Wace, Richard Henry, Submission to Western Australian Government, *Royal Commission on the Condition of the Natives, Report, Appendix C, Minutes of Evidence* (Perth: Government Printer, 1904).

Waksman, S., *The Conquest of Tuberculosis* (London: Robert Hale Ltd, 1964).

Warburton, M. F., 'Epidemiology of Influenza in Australia and Papua New Guinea', *Medical Journal of Australia*, 1 (Special Supp.), 1973, pp. 14–18.

Watt, Sir J., 'The Colony's Health', in J. Hardy and A. Frost (eds), *Studies from Terra Australis to Australia* (Canberra: Australian Academy of the Humanities, 1989).

Webb, P., and C. Bain, *Essential Epidemiology: An Introduction for Students and Health Professionals* (Cambridge: Cambridge University Press, 2011).

Webb, S., *Palaeopathology of Aboriginal Australians: Health and Disease across a Hunter-Gatherer Continent* (Cambridge: Cambridge University Press, 1995).

White, J. P., and D. J. Mulvaney, 'How Many People', in D. J. Mulvaney and J. P. White (eds), *Australians to 1788: Australians, a Historical Library* (Sydney: Fairfax, Syme and Weldon Associates, 1987).

Williams, Elizabeth, 'The Archaeology of Lake Systems in the Middle Cooper Basin, North-Eastern South Australia', *Records of the South Australian Museum*, 30, 1997–1998, pp. 69–91.

Williams, M., 'The Spread of Settlement in South Australia', in F. Gale and G. H. Lawton (eds), *Settlement and Encounter* (London: Oxford University Press, 1969).

Winegard, Timothy C., *The Mosquito: A Human History of Our Deadliest Predator* (Melbourne: Text Publishing, 2019).

Wolfe, Robert, J., 'Alaska's Great Sickness, 1900: An Epidemic of Measles and Influenza in a Virgin Soil Population', *Proceedings of the American Philosophical Society*, 126 (2), 1982, pp. 91–121.

World Bank List of Economies 2020, https://datahelpdesk.worldbank.org/knowledgebase/articles/906519 (accessed 28 September 2020).

World Health Organization, 'Yaws' (Fact Sheet), http://www.who.int/mediacentre/factsheets/fs316/en/ (accessed 18 February 2016).

World Health Organization, 'Tuberculosis' (Fact Sheet) http://www.who.int/mediacentre/factsheets/fs104/en/ (accessed 11 December 2016).

Yanyuwa Families, Amanda Kearney and John Bradley, 'From Sorcery to Laboratory: Pandemics and Yanyuwa Experiences of Viral Vulnerability', *Oceania*, Special Issue, 'Oceanic Societies in COVID-19', 2020.

INDEX

ABOUT THE AUTHOR

Peter Dowling holds a PhD in archaeology and biological anthropology from the Australian National University. He has written and lectured on Australian history, archaeology, Indigenous and European biological contact history and Australian cultural heritage assessment. He dabbles in military history and has organised and led local, national and overseas tours in history, archaeology and heritage. In a previous life Dr Dowling spent twenty years in signals intelligence with the Royal Australian Navy. He now lives quietly but busily in retirement with his wife and visiting bird families in the Tuggeranong Valley of Canberra.

CPSIA information can be obtained
at www.ICGtesting.com
Printed in the USA
DWIIW041102?9001021
620260BV00002B/107

9 781922 464460